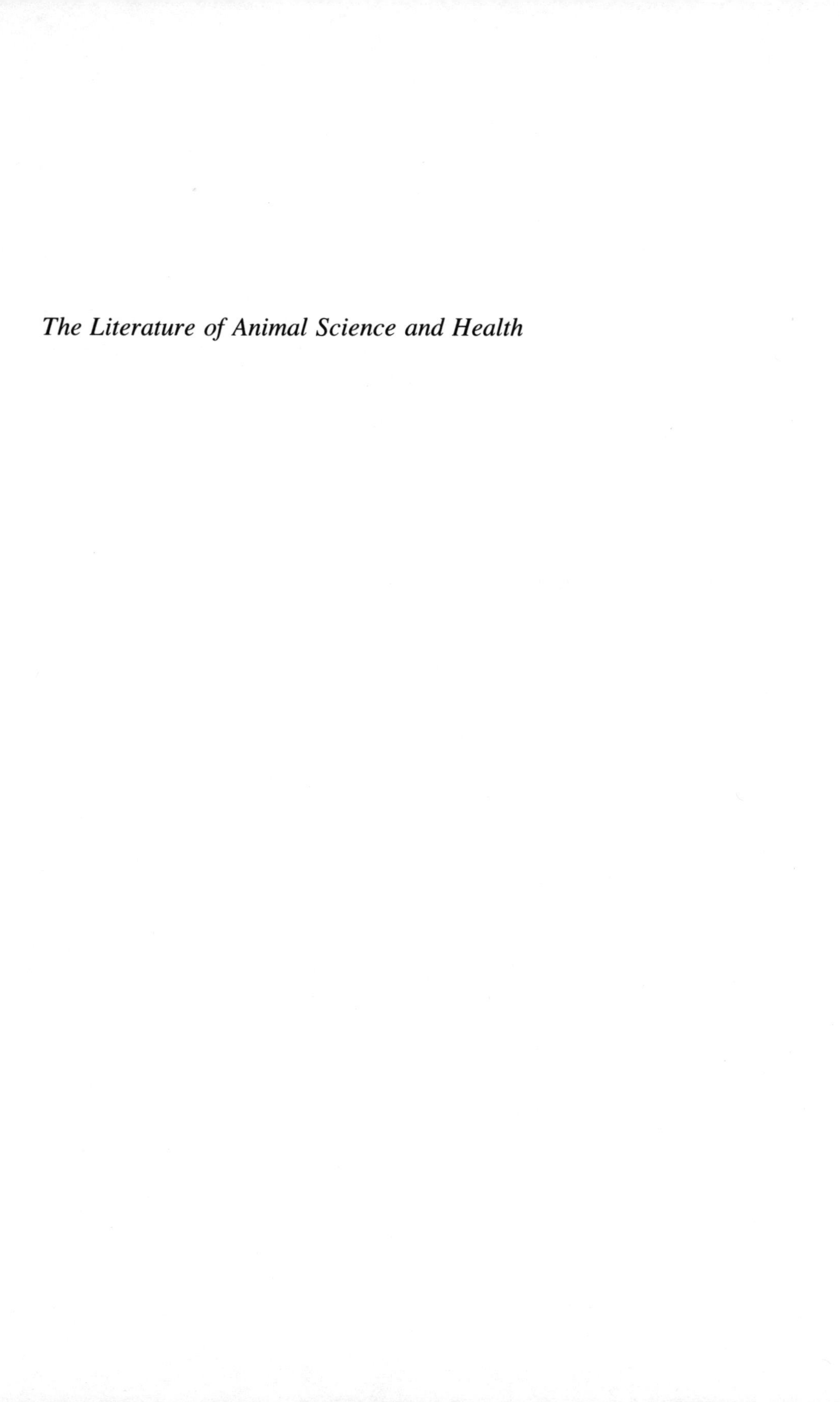

The Literature of Animal Science and Health

A volume in the series

The Literature of the Agricultural Sciences

WALLACE C. OLSEN, series editor

Agricultural Economics and Rural Sociology: The Contemporary Core Literature
  By Wallace C. Olsen

The Literature of Agricultural Engineering
  Edited by Carl W. Hall and Wallace C. Olsen

The Literature of Animal Science and Health
  Edited by Wallace C. Olsen

THE LITERATURE OF ANIMAL SCIENCE AND HEALTH

EDITED BY

Wallace C. Olsen

Cornell University Press

ITHACA AND LONDON

This book was typeset from disks supplied by the staff of the Core Agricultural Literature Project, Albert R. Mann Library, Cornell University. Jane Hunt prepared the machine-readable text and Nicole Kasmer Kresock made final corrections. The research was financially supported by Cornell Agricultural Experiment Station; National Agricultural Library, United States Department of Agriculture; and the Rockefeller Foundation.

First published 1993 by Cornell University Press.

International Standard Book Number 0–8014–2886–6
Library of Congress Catalog Card Number 93–7801
Printed in the United States of America
Librarians: Library of Congress cataloging information
appears on the last page of the book.

♾ The paper in this book meets the minimum requirements of the
American National Standard for Information Sciences—
Permanence of Paper for Printed Library Materials, ANSI Z39.48-1984.

Contents

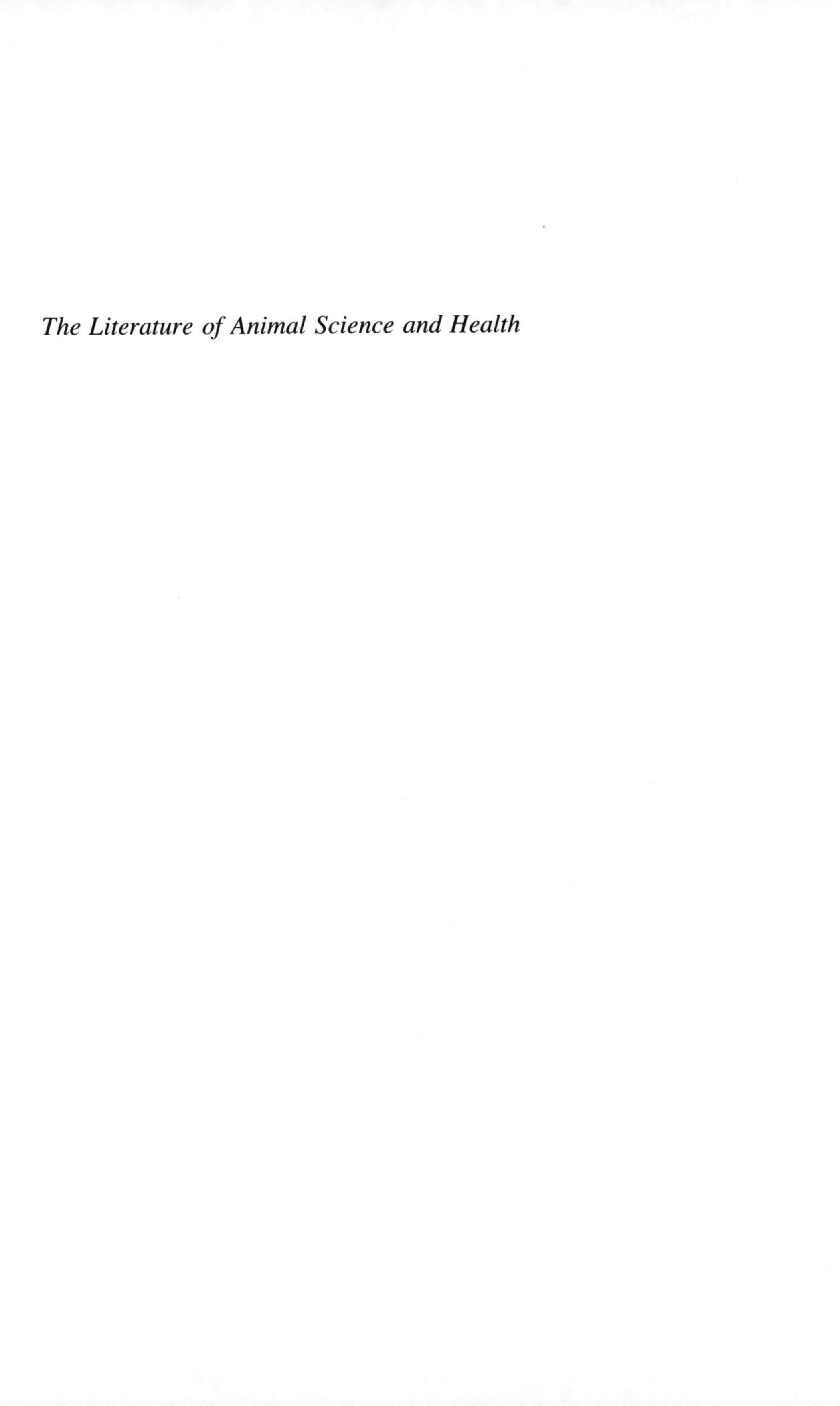

The Literature of Animal Science and Health

1. Development of Animal Science in the United States

RICHARD L. WILLHAM

Department of Animal Science, Iowa State University

> Yet to admire our successes as if they had no past would make a caricature of knowledge.
>
> —J. Brownowski, *The Ascent of Man*

About two million years ago, some hominoids became omnivorous. Animal products from the kill contributed in important ways to the behavioral changes that led to the rapid cultural evolution of humans. Meat eating allowed time for social interaction and made tool development necessary.[1] Both these changes aided humans in the transition to settled agriculture that included the domestication of plants and animals after the last ice age. But it was the ox, when yoked to the scratch plow, that gained for humans the surplus food necessary to create civilization.

The purpose of this chapter is to examine the history of animal science as a discipline of agriculture and the factors that influenced the building of animal science as a profession. The ramifications of the contributions of both husbandmen and scientists to the livestock world are many. This chapter centers on the last two centuries, the industrial and information ages, and concerns primarily events within the United States. During the earlier part of this period the United States was itself a developing nation, whereas the nations of Europe integrated animal science into a developed agricultural structure.

A. Beginnings

Greek and Roman literature on agriculture, written by elder statesmen in their villas, provides a record of the art of husbandry in classical times.[2]

---

1. J. Brownowski, *The Ascent of Man* (Boston: Little, Brown, 1973).
2. F. Harrison, *Roman Farm Management* (New York: Macmillan, 1917).

1

These works were later used by the Cistercian order of monks, who, by extending the knowledge of sheep husbandry in Europe, became the first extension agents.[3] Edward III, the royal wool merchant, laid the foundation for England's "Empire of Wool," which gave the English the experience to precipitate the agricultural and then the industrial revolution of later times.[4] Country gentlemen in Britain developed the pedigree breeding system and formed breeds of livestock complete with herdbooks, in response to the markets of the industrial revolution.[5] In the meantime much had transpired in the colonization of America, both Spanish and British.

Land ownership in Europe was for most an impossible dream.[6] This was one reason to venture the Atlantic as a colonist. By 1800, the people of a new nation were spilling westward over the Cumberland Gap to the American Midwest. Cotton plantations began to spread from the coastal South farther west, and institution-builders followed on the heels of the stump-corn-hog pioneers of the old Northwest.[7] Before Ohio was surveyed in square miles, Jefferson surprised Congress with the purchase of the Louisiana Territory. Abundant land was the decisive factor in the development of American agriculture until the end of the frontier.[8]

Agricultural supply was linked to demand by an expanding transportation network during the first half of the nineteenth century. Construction of roads and bridges was followed by the building of the Erie Canal in 1825. After 1830, steel rails began to lace together the United States.[9] Cincinnati became "porkopolis," but it was William Ogden, a hustler, who saw Chicago as the hub of American agriculture.[10] And the bountiful harvests of the Corn Belt made it so.[11]

European travelers in America were shocked by the inefficiency of early United States agriculture.[12] Britain, before the Industrial Revolution, had

3. R. L. Willham, "The Crown and the Mesta" in F. H. Baker and M. E. Miller, eds., *Sheep and Goat Handbook*, Vol. 4 (Boulder, Colo.: A Winrock International Project published by Westview Press, 1984).

4. M. L. Ryder, *Sheep and Man* (London: Duckworth, 1983).

5. H. C. Pawson, *Robert Bakewell* (London: Crosby Lockwood & Sons, 1957).

6. A. Cooke, *America* (New York: Knopf, 1975).

7. J. W. Thompson, *A History of Livestock Raising in the United States, 1607–1860* (Washington, D.C.: U.S. Dept. of Agriculture, 1942 [*Agricultural History Series* no. 5]).

8. W. W. Cochrane, *The Development of American Agriculture: A Historical Analysis* (Minneapolis: University of Minnesota Press, 1979).

9. R. L. Willham, *The Legacy of the Stockman* (Conway, Ark.: Winrock International and Iowa State University, Conway Printers, 1985).

10. Cooke, *America*.

11. (a) P. W. Gates, *The Farmers' Age: Agriculture 1815–1860*, Vol. III—*The Economic History of the United States* (White Plains, N.Y.: M. E. Sharpe, 1960). (b) G. C. Fite, *The Farmers' Frontier 1865–1900* (Albuquerque, N. Mex.: University of New Mexico Press, 1974).

12. Thompson, *History of Livestock Raising*.

seen an agricultural revolution, a self-conscious movement toward livestock improvement, which began with Robert Bakewell's management of the Dishley estate, Leicestershire, from 1760 to 1795.[13] After gathering stock during extensive trips on horseback, Bakewell welded them into a breed through intense inbreeding and established the Dishley Society to protect the purity of breeds.[14] His imitators developed the British breeds of livestock and established the pedigree breeding system. Stock breeders still subscribe to the principle of pedigree allied to the use of eye judgment for securing adherence to formalized breed type as the basis of successful breeding.[15] The United States imported the system and herdsmen familiar with it along with the stock.

In the early eighteenth century livestock diets were mysterious, but science was beginning to be applied to problems in Europe. The chemist Lavoisier, before losing his head to the guillotine during the French Revolution, concluded after experimentation that nutrition was in fact chemistry. One of the first animal feeding trials was conducted by François Magendie in 1816. In 1827, William Prout in England classified the essential organic nutrients as protein, carbohydrate, and fat. Justus von Liebig was the agricultural chemist destined to keep Germany from starvation in the 1840s who wrote a much-used book on the applications of chemistry to farming.[16] Nutrition work at the British experiment station at Rothamstead began in 1843, and results were published in 1859 by J. H. Gilbert and J. B. Lawes, the same year as Darwin's *Origin of Species*. In 1866 Gregor Mendel published the paper that became the basis for modern genetics. Louis Pasteur developed his germ theory and Nicolas Appert introduced canning of food in France. Clearly, Europe had seen science help solve some pressing problems. Scientific societies began to proliferate; in the United States, the American Association for the Advancement of Science was founded in 1846.

Agricultural education in the United States was an important issue, and progress was made during the 1860s. From 1830 to 1862, there had been efforts made in the U.S. Congress to promote the idea of public support for

13. S. Wright, *Principles of Livestock Breeding* (Washington, D.C.: U.S. Dept. of Agriculture, 1920 [*USDA Bulletin* no. 905]).

14. Pawson, *Robert Bakewell*.

15. I. M. Lerner and H. P. Donald, *Modern Developments in Animal Breeding* (New York: Academic Press, 1966).

16. (a) Justus von Liebig, *Die Organische Chemie in Ihrer Anwendung auf Physiologie und Pathologie*; Later eds. known as *Die Thier-Chemie* . . . (Braunschweig: Verlag von Friedreich Vieweg & Sohn, 1842). (b) Justus von Liebig, 1st American ed. as *Organic Chemistry in Its Applications to Agriculture and Physiology* . . . edited by Lyon Playfair (Cambridge, Mass.: J. Owen, 1841). (c) Referenced in L. A. Maynard, J. K. Loosli, H. F. Hintz and R. G. Warner, *Animal Nutrition* (New York: McGraw-Hill, 1979).

higher education, including agricultural.[17] In 1862, the Morrill Act was passed, establishing the land-grant colleges, the U.S. Department of Agriculture (USDA) was formed, and a new Homestead Act passed.[18] But at the same time the country was immersed in civil war, which devastated parts of the South agriculturally. Reconstruction and the need for food lost by the war brought about the beginning of animal husbandry in the Upper Midwest.[19] In 1865, as the Civil War ended, the Union Stock Yard of Chicago opened for business.[20]

B. Agricultural Colleges

At mid-century agriculture was still largely an art resting on traditions; there was no science save chemistry as noted by Davenport. "What a basis this, on which to found a college to predicate success in agricultural education."[21] Farmers were still pioneers. "Times were not propitious for serious study of a serious problem about a matter that seemed so simple that any fool could farm."[22] The prophets, again, were born ahead of their time!

The Michigan Agricultural College opened in 1855. It was hard to find agricultural teachers; agriculture was not an academic discipline. After the land was cleared the attempt was made to lug in British agriculture wholesale. Turnips failed, but the pedigree breeding system came to stay. The professors of agriculture who succeeded were Levi Stockbridge of Massachusetts, Isaac P. Roberts of Cornell, Manly Miles of Michigan, Norton S. Townshend of Ohio, George E. Morrow of Illinois, and Seaman A. Knapp of Iowa.[23] Michigan was home to the most vigorous and able exponents of science west of Harvard. But science found its early place in the "new education" (land-grant colleges) based on the facts of nature rather than the dicta of human creations.

During the nineteenth century, state fairs became a regular part of agriculture, and livestock markets became centralized to meet the needs of the industrializing East.[24] For the first time in world history, meat for the mil-

17. E. D. Ross, *A History of the Iowa State College* (Ames: Iowa State College Press, 1942).
18. M. S. Smith, *Chronological Landmarks in American Agriculture* (Washington, D.C.: U.S. Dept. of Agriculture, 1979 [*Agricultural Information Bulletin* no. 425]).
19. J. T. Schlebecker, *Whereby We Thrive* (Ames: Iowa State University Press, 1975).
20. W. J. Grand, *Illustrated History of the Union Stockyards* (W. J. Grand, 1986).
21. E. Davenport, "Early Trials of the Agricultural Colleges and Experiment Stations," *American Society of Animal Production, Record of Proceedings of Annual Meeting* (Dec. 1924): 196.
22. Ibid, p. 208.
23. C. S. Plumb, "Address of Professor Charles S. Plumb," *American Society of Animal Production, Record of Proceedings of Annual Meeting*, Dec. 1923: 166–171.
24. B. B. Fowler, *Men, Meat, and Miracles* (New York: Julian Messner, 1952).

lions was a reality.[25] This was the era of longhorn trail drives, cattle barons, and that American folk legend, the cowboy,[26] as well as the empire period back East in oil, steel, railroading, and finance. In 1870, Pasteur conquered anthrax. In 1873, refrigerated rail cars made by the packers moved chilled meat east, a step much opposed by butchers, a scenario repeated with boxed beef a century later.

The founding of the Atlantic and Pacific Tea Company in 1875 marked the beginning of chain retail grocery stores. The same year, the Connecticut Agricultural Experiment Station began innovative research into agricultural problems.[27] The United States celebrated its first 100 years with optimism, and the first modern graduate school was founded at Johns Hopkins University. A year later, Custer made his last stand way out west, and in 1878, the telephone, invented by a sheep enthusiast, Alexander Graham Bell, was employed in commercial use. Willy Kuhne defined enzymes, and the compound microscope made its debut.

During the 1880s, Sir Francis Galton invented the regression coefficient to describe the fact that offspring of extreme parents tended to regress back toward the average. In 1880, Henry P. Armsby published his manual on cattle feeding and the following year J. H. Sanders of Chicago began publishing *The Breeders' Gazette*, which became the Bible for importers and stockmen. In 1882, the first course in animal husbandry was taught, signaling the division of agriculture into disciplines.[28] In 1883, W. H. Henry started the Wisconsin Agricultural Experiment Station, J. Kjeldahl developed his procedure for nitrogen determination, and H. Tappeiner recognized the digestion of cellulose by ruminal microorganisms.[29] Several newly formed American breed associations opened national offices in the livestock records building near the entrance to the world's largest stockyards in Chicago. In 1884, Theobald Smith, a pathologist with the USDA, unraveled the secrets of Texas cattle fever, raising the stature of USDA research.[30] Pharmaceutical houses important to animal raising began in 1886.

After years of effort, the agricultural colleges got what they so desperately needed to foster scientific education: state agricultural experiment stations created by the Hatch Act in 1887. Government put science to work for agriculture. "From that day, colleges of agriculture went definitely on

25. R. Tannahill, *Food in History* (New York: Stein & Day, 1973).

26. C. W. Towne and E. N. Wentworth, *Cattle and Men* (Norman: University of Oklahoma Press, 1955).

27. A. C. True, *A History of Agricultural Experimentation and Research in the United States, 1607–1925* (Washington, D.C.: U.S. Dept. of Agriculture, 1937 [*USDA Misc. Publ.* no. 251]).

28. Plumb, "Address."

29. E. V. McCollum, *A History of Nutrition* (Boston: Houghton Mifflin, 1957).

30. Smith, *Chronological Landmarks*.

a scientific basis, and from that day forward they began to succeed."[31] "Farmers began to feel that the college man must know something and has ways of finding out things not possessed by the man in the corn rows or the feedlot. . . . agrigulture is really teachablee, but from the standpoint of the science involved, not of an art to be practiced by traditional methods." Thus began the slow and often devious change from husbandry to science.[32]

1890 was a red letter year. Scientists joined inventors in the research laboratories of industry. S. M. Babcock developed the simple butterfat test; and big business was decimated by the Sherman Anti-Trust Act, just as the cattle empires had been by the winters of 1886-1887. J. A. Craig started the first animal husbandry department, at the Univerity of Wisconsin. Charles S. Plumb noted that the field of animal husbandry was first made attractive by Craig, who introduced laboratory work in judging and was the father of student judging contests.[33] The first intercollegiate contest was held in 1898 at Omaha, Nebraska. During the 1890s, feed companies came into being, usually because a by-product became available for animal feed.[34] Sweet-feeds originated as a by-product of the protective lining made for Teddy Roosevelt's battleships. Proximate analysis of feedstuffs was perfected by 1895, and the Wolfe-Lehman feed standards were developed in 1897, the same year that cattlemen at Denver founded the American National Cattlemen's Association. In 1898, W. H. Henry, Dean at the University of Wisconsin, published *Feeds and Feeding*. In 1899, W. O. Atwater of Connecticut published caloric values.[35] W. A. Craft spoke of the big three research entrepreneurs: W. H. Henry of Wisconsin, Eugene Davenport of Illinois, and Eugene W. Hilgard of California.[36] By 1900, there was no longer any need to travel to Europe for graduate study in the sciences.

C. A New Century

The Victorian Age saw the twentieth century dawn with great optimism. Geneticists were busy with the rediscovery of Mendel's paper. But the important event in the livestock industry was the 1900 opening of the International Live Stock Exposition in Chicago, the premier livestock exposition of

31. Davenport, "Early Trials of the Agricultural Colleges," p. 200.
32. Ibid, pp. 200–201.
33. Plumb, "Address."
34. L. Wherry, *The Golden Anniversary of Scientific Feeding* (Milwaukee: Business Press, 1947).
35. McCollum, *A History of Nutrition.*
36. W. A. Craft, "The Change from Animal Husbandry to Animal Science" (Presented to Animal Science Staff at Iowa State University, Mimeograph, 1962).

the world. The reasoning for the show was, as one chronicler put it, that "farmers must be taught the difference in profit between a scrub and an animal that is thrifty and well-bred, on the one hand, and, on the other, between old and wasteful methods of feeding and new and improved methods of maturing and preparing animals for market."[37] The exposition sprang into an astonishing existence, drawing on the livestock of a continent. Secretary of Agriculture "Tama Jim" Wilson (who served as secretary for sixteen years under three presidents) said, at the 1902 opening, "The most interesting feature of this exhibit to me, gentlemen, is the presence of these college boys. . . . As for the education of farmers and farmers' sons . . . we have more money at Washington than Harvard, Yale, the University of Chicago, and Stanford combined. We are trying to help the man everywhere in every part of the United States who raises things out of the ground."[38]

After 1900, many farmers graduated from the emerging land-grant colleges. Many participated in the purebred industry as prominent judges and developed purebred herds for education and breeding, which were prime examples of the breeder's art. Students could work with the best of the newly imported germ plasm and learn from Scottish herdsmen who had crossed the Atlantic with the stock. Grand champions and winning judging teams advertised the colleges.

During the early years of the twentieth century, many state colleges that had given students a broad liberal education were confronted with problems of definition. President William M. Beardshear of Iowa State College succinctly summed up the intent of the colleges in 1900: "The theory is that young agriculturists or industrialists must aspire to a liberal education that will make them the peers of any educated or professional man in life."[39] Livestock interests in the states, however, wanted more technical agriculture, and most land-grant colleges rapidly developed into science-based institutions.

The mechanization of farming required the speed of the horse to turn the ground wheels of the new implements. The railroads linked the nation, but it was still the dray teams that delivered within the cities. Draft horses were of major importance.

The Jungle by Upton Sinclair was published in 1905. This vivid descrip-

37. M. F. Horine, "A Bit of Exposition History" in *The Review of the International Live Stock Exposition of 1913* (Chicago: Published by the International Live Stock Exposition, 1913).

38. W. D. Rasmussen, *Men and Milestones in American Agriculture.* Print of 89th Congress, 2d Session, Agriculture Committee (Washington, D.C.: U.S. Govt. Print. Off., Oct. 1966), p. 56.

39. E. D. Ross, *The Land-Grant Idea at Iowa State College* (Ames: Iowa State College Press, 1958), p. 9.

tion of the packing industry in Chicago produced the Food and Drug Act of 1906 and the formation of the American Meat Packers' Association. But ultimately the most important event for agriculture was that the Model T automobile came off Henry Ford's assembly line. This truly changed American livestock agriculture in profound ways. S. M. Babcock demonstrated the salt requirement, and Charles S. Plumb published *Types and Breeds of Livestock*, which established the teaching of livestock breeding as the history of the master breeders.

In 1906, the American Dairy Science Association was formed, and the Poultry Science Association started in 1908. Researchers in animal nutrition, at a meeting called during the 1908 International Live Stock Exposition, formed the American Society of Animal Nutrition.[40] In 1915, teaching, breeding, and management were included, and the name changed to the American Society of Animal Production.[41]

The fruits of science for livestock agriculture became clear as the University of Wisconsin began its synergistic research under Dean W. H. Henry and later Dean Harry L. Russell. By 1911, the purified diet idea had developed from the legendary corn-wheat experiment of Babcock origin. The discovery of Vitamin A by Elmer V. McCollum and M. Davis in 1913 began a long line of advances in the application of science by Edwin B. Hart, Gustav Bohstedt, C. A. Elvehjem, H. Steenbock, and Frank B. Morrison. What developed the synergism among departments was the tireless efforts of C. G. Humphrey, Head of Animal Husbandry.[42]

The USDA research facility at Beltsville, Maryland, opened in 1910, and A. Boss developed the first meat laboratory at the University of Minnesota. F. H. A. Marshall and J. Hammond made Cambridge, England, famous for research in animal reproductive physiology. T. H. Morgan was putting Mendelian genetics to the test with *Drosophila* at Columbia University, and L. J. Cole, a noted geneticist, moved to the University of Wisconsin from Yale.

In 1913, the American Feed Manufacturers Association was formed to help organize the growing number of feed companies. In 1914, the Smith-Lever Act was passed, establishing the Cooperative Extension Service in

40. (a) H. M. Briggs, "Fifty Years of Growth and Progress," *Journal of Animal Science* 17 (1958): 911. (b) R. R. Oltjen, "Significant Milestones in the 75-Year History of the American Society of Animal Science," *Journal of Animal Science* 57 (Suppl. 2, 1983): 1.

41. C. S. Plumb, *History of the Society* (American Society of Animal Producers, 1932 [*ASAP* no. 377]).

42. Gustav Bohstedt, *Early History of Animal Husbandry and Related Departments of the University of Wisconsin-Madison* (Madison: University of Wisconsin Publication, 1958).

the United States.[43] The extension agents were to interpret and take the research results from the agricultural experiment stations directly to the farmers. Researchers had long interacted with farmers, but now there was a structure. The agents worked among the people, working models like the Cistercian monks of old.

Alvin H. Sanders was the editor of the *Breeders' Gazette*, the breeders' Bible, and wrote many books on livestock history, including the breed history of the Shorthorn, Aberdeen-Angus, and Hereford cattle, and of the Percheron horse. In 1915, his book *At the Sign of the Stock Yard Inn* summarized the era of importation of livestock breeds into the United States.[44]

When United States entered World War I, American farmers rose to the occasion and produced food both for their own country and for Europe. During this period, Sir Ronald Fisher published a paper that united population genetics to Mendelian theory; Henry P. Armsby published *The Nutrition of Farm Animals*, in which phosphorus was shown to be essential; Thomas B. Osborn and Lafayette B. Mendel published on the nutritive value of feeds; Henry W. Vaughan published his text *Types and Market Classes of Livestock*. In 1919, with help from colleges and the Extension Service, the USDA launched a national program called "Better Sires: Better Stock," which promoted the use of purebred sires to improve American livestock.[45] The concept has lasted.

The year 1920 saw the start of an agricultural depression that continued on through the bad weather of the 1930s. But science had made great strides in the first two decades of the twentieth century.

D. The Second Twenty Years

The nation reacted to realities of a world war. The optimism with which the century had opened was shattered, and the United States was not ready for international leadership.

43. (a) W. G. Kammlade, "Fifty Years of Progress in Livestock Extension Teaching," *Journal of Animal Science* 17 (1958): 1088. (b) W. G. Zmolek and J. R. Foster, "Extension Animal Science: Past Accomplishments—Future Challenges," *Journal of Animal Science* 57 (Suppl. 2, 1983): 197.

44. (a) A. H. Sanders, *At the Sign of the Stock Yard Inn* (Chicago: Breeders' Gazette Print, 1915). (b) Sanders, *A History of Aberdeen-Angus Cattle* (Chicago: The New Breeders' Gazette, 1928). (c) Sanders, *A History of the Percheron Horse* (Chicago: Breeders' Gazette Print, 1917). (d) Sanders, *Red, White and Roan* (Chicago: American Shorthorn Breeders' Assoc., 1936). (e) Sanders, *Shorthorn Cattle* (Chicago: Sanders Publ. Co., 1918). (f) Sanders, *The Story of the Herefords* (Chicago: Breeders' Gazette Print, 1914).

45. Smith, *Chronological Landmarks*.

The American Society of Animal Production meetings were held at the Sherman House in Chicago at the time of the International Live Stock Exposition from 1920 to 1961. Graduate education was achieving success with the codification of separate disciplines with increasingly diverse jargons. As James Burke noted, "The more the knowledge in a certain field increases, the more esoteric become the languages."[46]

The tractor began to replace horse teams in the Corn Belt, black leg was controlled with a bacterin, and in 1921 the Packer and Stockyards Act was passed to establish standards and control in the industry. Sewall Wright published on systems of mating and introduced the inbreeding coefficient that quantified what the pedigree breeder was doing. Frederick G. Hopkins discovered the amino acid tryptophan to be essential for monogastric nutrition. Both kind and amount of protein became important in poultry and swine diets.

The National Livestock and Meat Board was formed under the leadership of R. C. Pollack, to promote meat products and the entire livestock industry. The Purnell Act of 1925 aided meat research by providing funds for livestock products study. Intercollegiate meat judging contests were begun in 1926, as was federal beef grading. Maurice D. Helser, Fred Beard, Sleeter Bull, Percival Ziegler, William J. Loeffel, David L. McIntosh, and O. G. Hankins established meat science as a discipline.

In 1921, A. F. Schalk of North Dakota State College fistulated cattle for use in nutrition studies, and reported that the procedure had been used in the 1800s by researchers in Europe. The Holstein-Friesian Association commissioned an artist to create a sculpture and presented colleges with cast-iron, painted models of the "true type cow and bull" in 1923. The 4-H clubs began animal projects in the 1920s that involved showing the stock.[47] Poultry breeding companies came into being but had little impact on the industry for a time.[48] Henry A. Wallace set up a hybrid corn company to put the work of E. H. East, G. H. Shell, and D. F. Jones into practice. Hybrid corn began to demonstrate its food potential in commercial livestock production. Ronald A. Fisher published *Statistical Methods for Research Workers*; Hermann J. Muller found that X-rays produced mutations; Vitamin B was discovered; James B. Sumner purified enzymes; and F. F. McKinsey took over extensive and valuable reproductive physiology studies at the University of Missouri. In 1928, Alexander Fleming discovered penicillin. Pro-

46. J. Burke, *Connections* (Boston: Little, Brown, 1978), p. 292.
47. T. Wessel and M. Wessel, *4-H: An American Idea 1900–1980* (Chevy Chase, Md.: National 4-H Council, 1982).
48. O. A. Hanke, ed., *American Poultry History, 1823–1973* (Madison, Wis.: American Printing and Pub., 1974).

gesterone and testosterone were identified in 1929. In California, H. H. Cole and Hart began investigations with pregnant mare serum. In 1930, Jay L. Lush began herdbook research studies after he moved to Iowa State College. The USDA range station in Montana was initiated at Fort Keough. The Warner-Bratzler shear was developed, and H. H. Mitchell reported on the biological value of protein. In 1934, the Chicago stockyards were destroyed by fire, but they were rebuilt in time for the International show.

A cooperative regional swine breeding laboratory was started in 1937 at Iowa State University.[49] Leonard A. Maynard published *Animal Nutrition*; George W. Snedecor, *Statistical Methods*; and Jay L. Lush, *Animal Breeding Plans*. Also, H. A. Krebs defined the cycle that bears his name. An artificial insemination bull stud was started by L. J. Cole, and M. R. Irwin initiated blood typing at the University of Wisconsin. Sulfonamides were used to control animal diseases, and twenty amino acids were clearly identified.

E. The Third Twenty Years

Animal science classrooms in most colleges were vacant during the Second World War. In ruminant diets, Gustav Bohstedt and E. B. Hart showed that urea could be substituted for natural protein. The *Journal of Animal Science* became the new title of the *Proceedings of the American Society of Animal Production* in 1942; L. N. Hazel and J. L. Lush published on the selection index; and between 1942 and 1944, the National Research Council developed dietary standards for livestock.

World War II ended with the atomic bomb and the dawn of a new age, but with little recession in agriculture. This heavily oil-based industry initiated the use of anhydrous ammonia fertilizer which enhanced feed-grain production and grassland farming in the South.[50] The Research and Marketing Act of 1946 provided for the development of regional projects.[51] Samuel Brody published *Bioenergetics and Growth* in 1945, and Sydney A. Asdell published *Patterns of Mammalian Reproduction* in 1946. In 1947, the National Association of Animal Breeders, an organization of breeders of bull

---

49. R. L. Willham, *Contributions of the Regional Swine Breeding Laboratory during the Past 25 Years* (Ames, Iowa: Annual Report of 1962 for the Conference of Collaborators, 1962).

50. Schlebecker, *Whereby We Thrive*.

51. R. L. Willham, "University Animal Breeding Research," Presented at the Breeding and Genetics Symposium on Foundations of Tomorrow at the American Society of Animal Science Meetings, Fort Collins, Colo., *Journal of Animal Science* 44 (1975): 303.

studs, was formed.[52] During this period, the use of isotopes became an integral part of animal science research.[53] In 1947, E. L. Ricks discovered vitamin B_{12}, and in 1949 E. L. R. Stokstad and T. H. Jukes introduced antibiotics into animal rations.[54] Concepts of linear programming were developed in agricultural economics with extensive applications to animal science. There was a surge of research effort in the colleges and university departments. Many returning servicemen took advantage of graduate training with federal assistance under the G. I. Bill.

The National Science Foundation and National Institutes of Health started to fund basic research in 1950. Because of USDA funding already provided, agriculture had difficulty obtaining a share; however, good proposals with broad application were funded. Peter Van Soest noted that, had agriculture become a part of the old universities, as had happened in Europe, the entire scientific community would have been more aware of agricultural problems.[55] In 1950, bull semen was frozen at Cambridge University, and frozen semen was in active use by 1952;[56] Frederick Sanger identified the structure of insulin and Jonas Salk developed polio vaccine, while W. Burroughs demonstrated the growth-promoting effect of feeding defined levels of stilbestrol. The first successful embryo transplant resulted from a cooperative effort between the research arm of the American Breeders Service (E. L. Willett) and the University of Wisconsin (L. E. Casida). H. E. Huxley and Jean Hansen produced a sliding filament theory of contraction for myofibrilla protein, and in 1953 James Watson and Francis Crick published on the structure of DNA (deoxyribonucleic acid), opening a floodgate of research in molecular biology that turned biochemists into geneticists forthwith.

The inexpensive metal backfat probe for swine in 1953 did what the Babcock simple butterfat test had done for the dairy industry—it promoted performance testing. The genes for dwarfism decimated the beef industry, but as a result geneticists were able to introduce perfomance testing.[57] By 1955, fast-food chains were a reality, interstate highway construction subsi-

52. H. A. Herman, *Improving Cattle by the Millions* (Columbia: University of Missouri Press, 1981).

53. J. R. Campbell and J. F. Lasley, *The Science of Animals That Serve Humanity* (New York: McGraw-Hill, 1985).

54. C. M. McCay, *Notes on the History of Nutrition Research* (Bern, Switzerland: Hans Huber, 1973).

55. P. J. Van Soest, *Nutritional Ecology of the Ruminant* (Corvallis, Oreg.: O & A Books, 1982).

56. Herman, *Improving Cattle*.

57. (a) T. J. Marlow, "Evidence of Selection for the Snorter Dwarf Gene in Cattle," *Journal of Animal Science* 23 (1964): 454. (b) L. P. McCann, *The Battle of Bull Runts* (Columbus, Ohio: L. P. McCann, 1974).

dized trucking just as the grants of land had done for the railroads, and massive decentralization of livestock marketing was under way.[58] Jet air transportation became the rule. Land-grant colleges became universities in name as well as function and increased their international dimension.[59]

Then in 1957, Sputnik hurtled across the skies of America. The United States was technologically behind the Soviet Union! Massive interest in all phases of research and science was awakened, and animal science benefited especially in the surge of development of scientific instrumentation. Interferons were discovered the same year.

The fiftieth anniversary of the American Society of Animal Production (ASAP) was celebrated in 1958 with a series of review papers in which disciplines were clearly recognized, but individual species were still paramount. The apologetic paper on livestock judging by A. E. Darlow indicated that a fair number of people were still concerned with stock shows.[60] As he noted, "Each of these men who walked into the classroom of the arena, for all the world to see, has proven to be a master teacher." These men had a profound effect on the purebred industry.

Techniques and Procedures in Animal Production Research was published in 1959 by ASAP. Computers were rapidly developing. In 1960, Walt Harvey presented an analysis of data with unequal numbers and later developed computer programs to analyze such data. After this, much research in animal science became a part of the growing volume of literature in the disciplines.

F. The Fourth Twenty Years

In 1961, the American Society of Animal Production became the American Society of Animal Science.[61] The sixty years of transition from husbandry to science was clearly at an end. The cover of the 1962 *Journal of Animal Science* carried a stylized new ASAS logo that reflected the bronze bull symbol from the International Live Stock Exposition. It is a fitting logo that echoes back across the centuries to a time when the bull was worshipped by ancient herdsmen.[62] A person appears to be guiding the bull,

58. B. C. Breidenstein and Z. L. Carpenter, "The Red Meat Industry: Product and Consumerism," *Journal of Animal Science* 57 (Suppl. 2, 1983): 119.

59. N. S. Raun and K. L. Turk, "International Animal Agriculture: History and Perspectives," *Journal of Animal Science* 57 (Suppl. 2, 1983): 156.

60. A. E. Darlow, "Fifty Years of Livestock Judging," *Journal of Animal Science* 17 (1958): 1063.

61. Oltjen, "Significant Milestones."

62. A. Fraser, *The Bull* (New York: Charles Scribner's Sons, 1972).

suggesting the role of animal science moving into the future. The Society meetings were moved from Chicago to different university campuses beginning in 1963.

The 1960s saw technology invade traditional agriculture.[63] Giant feedlot empires developed in the southwestern United States; a fortified corn-soybean meal diet for swine became commonplace; USDA research on sire-predicted differences brought about a genetic change in milk production; breed association computers printed three-generation pedigrees on registration certificates, which ended pedigree worship;[64] beef breeds from continental Europe were introduced by way of Canada because of United States restrictions; the Roman L. Hruska U.S. Meat Animal Research Center, at Clay Center, Nebraska, was founded and the Beef Improvement Federation was formed.[65] The net energy system for beef was developed.

The 1970s saw management research put into practice in confinement production of livestock.[66] The Texas experiment station introduced the concepts of systems analysis,[67] and the University of California developed modeling ideas, which both revealed great gaps in knowledge. Animal behavior study came into its own,[68] while fiber became important in monogastric nutrition. Recombinant DNA techniques were worked out. Improvements in prediction of genetic values (Best Linear Unbiased Predictors) were made at Cornell University,[69] and embryo transfer came of age. Microcomputers were used in livestock management and decision making. The academic quadrathalon to test the concepts of academic teaching was begun,[70] and beef sire evaluation came of age.[71] The American Society of Animal Science affiliated with the Council for Agricultural Science and Technology in

63. Cochrane, *Development of American Agriculture*.

64. R. L. Willham, "Genetic Improvement of Beef Cattle in the United States," *Journal of Animal Science* 54 (1982): 659.

65. F. H. Baker, "The Beef Improvement Federation," *World Review of Animal Producers* 11 (Sept.-Dec. 1975).

66. H. T. Fredeen and B. G. Harmon, "The Swine Industry: Changes and Challenges," *Journal of Animal Science* 57 (Suppl. 2, 1983): 100.

67. C. R. Long, T. C. Cartwright, and H. F. Fitzhugh, Jr., "Systems Analysis of Sources of Genetic and Environmental Variation in Efficiency of Beef Production: Cow Size and Herd Management," *Journal of Animal Science* 40 (1975): 409.

68. S. E. Curtis and K. A. Houpt, "Animal Ethology: Its Emergence in Animal Science," *Journal of Animal Science* 57 (Suppl. 2, 1983): 234.

69. C. R. Henderson, "Sire Evaluation and Genetic Trends," in *Proceedings of the American Breeding and Genetics Symposium in Honor of Jay L. Lush* (Champaign, Ill.: American Society of Animal Science, 1973).

70. R. E. Taylor and R. G. Kauffman, "Teaching Animal Science: Changes and Challenges," *Journal of Animal Science* 57 (Suppl. 2, 1983): 171.

71. R. L. Willham, "Evaluation and Direction of Beef National Sire Evaluation," Presented at the Beef Symposium at the American Society of Animal Science Meetings, *Journal of Animal Science* 49 (1978): 592.

Iowa in 1971. The American Registry of Certified Animal Scientists granted certification to professional consultants in 1973. Leading animal scientists projected research needs for the twenty-first century.[72]

G. Today

In the 1980s, DNA sequencing became a reality, and supermouse made headlines in *Science*.[73] The Diamond Jubilee papers in the *Journal of Animal Science* reflect the extent of subdiscipline formation within animal science. Diet-health issues are under critical study.[74] The extent of scientific instrumentation now being used in the laboratories of animal science research groups reflects the increasingly basic nature of the research as hormone control comes under examination. Researchers find that retraining is a part of their lives; teachers constantly discard old theories as new ones replace them; and Extension becomes more specialized to service its shrinking but increasingly specialized clientele.

The livestock industry is in transformation. Funds for research are questioned. Agriculture can no longer claim to occupy a special position based on a traditional ethic that is forgotten. The current emphasis is on the total food system, not just livestock production.[75] The food system has quietly become one of the largest high-tech businesses in America, in part due to research in animal science. Those working in livestock agriculture must consider what business we are really in.[76]

Recently, research funding has come from numerous organizations including the USDA and industry organizations with vested interests in research results. Many departments test products and report the results to producers. But the academic freedom of researchers is now more contingent on available funding sources than it was, and the reliance on grants to fund projects has produced a system in which the choice of research topics is defined by administrators rather than scientists, especially in basic studies.

72. W. G. Pond, R. A. Merkel, L. D. McGillaird, and V. J. Rhodes, *Animal Agriculture: Research to Meet Human Needs in the 21st Century* (Boulder, Colo.: Westview Press, 1980).

73. (a) J. S. F. Barker, K. Hammond, and A. E. McClintock, eds., *Future Developments in the Genetic Improvement of Animals* (New York: Academic Press, 1982). (b) J. J. Rutledge and G. E. Seidel, Jr., "Genetic Engineering and Animal Production," *Journal of Animal Science* 57 (Suppl. 2, 1983): 265.

74. C. E. Allen, "New Horizons in Animal Agriculture: Future Challenges for Animal Scientists," *Journal of Animal Science* 57 (Suppl. 2, 1983): 16.

75. T. Urban, "Challenge to Agriculture: Look Ahead, Not Back," *Des Moines Register*, May 6, 1984.

76. J. Naisbitt, *Megatrends* (New York: Warner Books, 1982).

The next step, working on cooperative ventures with industry where the results of the research are proprietary, presents a dilemma for state experiment station researchers in animal science. At best, public information is delayed, which could result in a real time lag in putting results to work.

This portion of the story has the difficulty of not yet being history, which in reality is the record of human activity passed through the filter of time to bring out the relevant issues. Change is now so fast that it is continually taking us by surprise, but one is forced to observe from where one is.

H. Summary

The chunk of meat carved with a flint knife, broiled, and eaten with symbolic relish had profound ramifications for the cultural evolution of human clans. No less is our understanding of cholesterol important to the lightning transition from the industrial to the information age as our new sedentary life style reverberates through our biology, which is still genetically adapted to the opportunities of 20,000 years ago.[77] Cultural evolution is so much faster than biological.

The transition from animal husbandry to animal science was a step in the building of a new and unique social infrastructure, the land-grant system, which continues to contribute to the development of American agriculture. The first segment of the system was the founding of publicly supported colleges to educate the masses. The second was the establishment of agricultural experiment stations to generate scientific knowledge applicable to problems confronting American agriculture. And the third was the organization of the Cooperative Extension Service to apply the new knowledge.

With the formation of the first animal husbandry department at the University of Wisconsin in 1890, the judging of livestock as a laboratory exercise in animal husbandry quickly became the focus of interest for students. The agricultural colleges promoted their expertise by winning judging contests and grand championships at the major expositions. It is ironic that at Wisconsin both the art of judging and the application of science to livestock first appeared!

After the turn of the present century, the second generation of animal husbandry professors made their debut, the product of graduate education provided by researchers of the agricultural experiment stations. These scientists, by the 1920s, were the new breed who defined what higher education

77. G. L. Stebbins, *Darwin to DNA, Molecules to Humanity* (San Francisco: W. H. Freeman, 1982).

for animal agriculture was all about. They made the disciplines, did the creative research, and trained the future generations of animal scientists.

After the traumas of the Great Depression and the Second World War, animal husbandry departments were as ready to change their name to reflect their activity as the colleges were to become universities. Research funds were forthcoming, and livestock producers were ready to adopt new technology. This transition occurred while the departments continued to maintain a degree of rapport with the livestock industry. The whole transition was highly idiosyncratic, branching and diversifying in unique ways in various places to create a wonderland of departments, each serving the perceived needs of its state.

At least ten interdependent factors affected the transition from husbandry to science. They are the explosion of science, the development of American agriculture, the participation in our national experience, the creation of land-grant colleges, the establishment of agricultural experiment stations, the organization of graduate education, the generation of educated producers, the growth of the means to communicate, the founding of a society and journal, and the innovation of industry organizations.

The creation of a field of science within a nation interacts with the developmental stage of that nation. Appropriate technology becomes the key in dealing with the social change that results. Such is true even for developed nations.

2. Literature Patterns
and Trends

WALLACE C. OLSEN
Mann Library, Cornell University

The field of animal science is fairly clearly delineated as that part of agriculture concerned with animals used commercially for meat and other products. Whether it should also be considered to comprise such categories as animals in the wild including fish is open to debate. The intention of Core Agricultural Literature Project of Mann Library, Cornell University, which served as the coordinator for this volume, was to concentrate on those animals and their products closely associated with world agriculture and extensively used by humans. Thus some areas were excluded from investigation, the best example being commercial ocean culture and fishing, which are not standard trades in agriculture although in many countries they are closely allied to it. Farm fish culture, inland and in brackish waters, was included since in most countries this tends to be considered a farming operation. Animals raised for fur, which are not closely allied with agriculture or food, were excluded. These general delineations apply throughout this book.

A major component of the Core Agricultural Literature Project was identification and analysis of the primary literature of value to Third World countries. Animal science presented a particular challenge since those countries and several developed countries merge animal science and veterinary science in one educational or research unit. To respond to this combined approach, the Third World investigations had to include standard animal science along with veterinary medicine. Therefore, a distinction exists, between the developed countries literature of animal science and that of the Third World, in that the latter also includes veterinary medicine. Within the United States, however, operational activities of these two fields have been merged in some cases. An academic example is the joining of animal science and veterinary medicine in a single library, which has been done at the

18

University of California, Davis, at Virginia Polytechnic Institute and State University, and, in a more expanded manner, at the University of Tennessee, Knoxville, where all of agriculture is merged with veterinary sciences in one library facility.

In this book the veterinary or clinical aspects of animal diseases are not included in the consideration of developed countries' literature, but are included in discussions of Third World literature. The overlap of more general health and disease literature with that of animal science in developed countries is nonetheless sizable since the cause and effect process is important to both groups. Therefore, such literature is included for both groups.

These distinctions and the difficulty of dealing with them are exemplified by two of the more substantive guides to the literature of veterinary and comparative medicine.[1] Both sources were useful in the preparation of this book. A diagramatic, proportional representation of the literature from the veterinary medicine point of reference, prepared by H. Broadauf and colleagues, shows overlaps with medicine, agriculture, biology, nutrition, chemistry, and physics.[2] The diagram is reproduced in Gibbs's recent book.[3]

A. Animal Science and Health in Agriculture

Three large databases concentrate on agriculture: AGRICOLA (produced by the U.S. National Agricultural Library), AGRIS (produced by the Food and Agriculture Organization), and CAB ABSTRACTS (produced by CAB International). All database information appears as digitized tapes or compact disks, as well as printed abstracting or indexing publications. All aim to cover the world literature of the agricultural sciences in all subject areas prior to 1985. In 1985–1986, AGRICOLA altered its coverage of journals indexing and began to concentrate on U.S.-published titles. "Many foreign journals previously indexed are no longer indexed because of cooperation with the International Information System for the Agricultural Sciences and

---

1. (a) Ann E. Kerker and Henry T. Murphy, compilers, *Comparative and Veterinary Medicine: A Guide to the Resource Literature* (Madison: University of Wisconsin, 1973). (b) Mike Gibbs, *Keyguide to Information Sources in Veterinary Medicine* (London and New York: Mansell Pub., 1990).

2. H. Brodauf, W. D. Hoffman, and J. H. T. Klawiter-Pommer, *Searching the Veterinary Literature Retrospectively: A Comparative Study of Results from 10 Data Bases Covering the Period January 1972 to December 1974* (Oxford: Oxford Microform Publications for the Commission of the European Communities, 1977). 56p. + 4 microfiche. (EUR 5886). Summary report in *Veterinary Record* 101 (1977): 461–463.

3. Gibbs, *Keyguide to Information Sources . . .* , p. 10.

Technology (AGRIS)."[4] AGRICOLA and CAB ABSTRACTS are selective of citations which they include based on the nature, subject, and value of the individual pieces or articles of literature. CAB ABSTRACTS and AGRIS add about 100,000 citations a year while AGRICOLA has been providing fewer entries each of the past five years and in 1989 entered only 69,720. AGRIS is an international cooperative effort accepting citations on a geographic basis from food and agricultural organizations around the world, and makes few judgments on the value of the literature indexed. It is more representative of Third World literature than the other two files, although prior to 1985 the difference was not great. Earlier studies of the major bibliographic databases indicate that about 20% of each database, is comprised of items not in either of the others.[5]

For a picture of the total numbers of articles, books, proceedings titles, patents, and dissertations in the agricultural sciences, there are no other readily accessible sources than these large bibliographic databases. These must be used to identify the universe of publishing for agriculture and its sub-disciplines. The head of the AGRIS Coordinating Centre reported that 23.2% of that database was made up of animal-related citations in 1978, 23.1% in 1979. Fisheries as a subject was covered separately in the report, and no separate listing was provided for animal diseases or veterinary medicine. Therefore, one must assume that these percentages include animal diseases, which is not the case in Table 2.1.[6] CAB ABSTRACTS reported in 1989 that 13% of its database covered animal science, again excluding veterinary sciences.[7]

B. Subject Concentrations

In the AGRICOLA bibliographic database thirty-three major subject categories relate to the total scope of this study. Only a limited number of these were used for the comparison shown in Table 2.1 (Category codes L000 thru L823; L850 and L851). These thirty-three subject categories were

4. *List of Journals Indexed in AGRICOLA, 1989* (Beltsville, Md.: National Agricultural Library, 1990). Quote is from the "Introduction."

5. Norbert Deselaers, "The Necessity for Closer Cooperation among Secondary Agricultural Information Services: An Analysis of AGRICOLA, AGRIS, and CAB," *Quarterly Bulletin of the International Association of Agricultural Librarians and Documentalists* 31 (1) (1986): 19–26.

6. Abe Liebowitz, "AGRIS since the First Technical Consultation," *Agricultural Libraries Information Notes* 6 (9/10) (1980): 5–7.

7. *CAB Abstracts Online Manual, 1989 Edition* (Wallingford: CAB International, 1989), p. 6.

Table 2.1. Animal science (exclusive of diseases) as a part of all agriculture, derived from online files

	AGRICOLA[a]	CAB ABSTRACTS online[b]
Animal science	396,995	162,186
Total agricultural database	1,376,933	1,086,609
Animal science as % of total database	28.4%	14.9%

[a]For 1980–1990; for subjects included see Table 2.2.
[b]For years 1980, 1983, 1985–1990; for subjects included see Table 2.3.

searched online for numbers of citations for each. The category codes (e.g., L821, M220) are assigned at the time of indexing as an indication of the subject matter of the citation, whether an article, chapter, report or book. More than one subject category in animal science and diseases can be assigned depending on the subject coverage of the item. This is a standard procedure in bibliographic databases in order to allow more than one subject access when two broad subjects are involved in the document. Two or more category codes are registered against most citations. A random sample was drawn from the data in Table 2.2 and used to derive an average of 1.2 animal science category codes per citation. This means that about 20% of the citations are duplicated throughout Table 2.2. It must be remembered that AGRICOLA is a database aimed at serving U.S. agriculture in its college education, research, and government needs. There are few records added to the database unless closely linked to agriculture. Animals in these categories excluded non-edible animals, wildlife, and pets; this is also true of data used from the other two bibliographic databases.

By the subject codes assigned to articles and books in AGRICOLA, one can identify where the greater literature emphases are in animal science and diseases. The major subjects can be compared, with some regrouping into composite categories:

Animal diseases	81,030
Entomology- related	63,678
Genetics and reproduction	57,640
Physiology and biochemistry	55,688
Pests of animals	46,438
Animal nutrition	45,722
Animal production	28,105

Table 2.2. Subject categories and indexed items in animal science and diseases in the AGRICOLA database

Category code and subject	1980	1985	1990	Eleven-year period Total	Yearly average
L000 ANIMAL SCIENCE, general	334	68	54	1,961	178
L001 Entomology-related	6,155	4,225	3,127	63,678	5,789
L002 Apiculture-related	1,529	517	253	9,345	850
L003 Sericulture-related	235	79	64	1,625	148
L100 Animal production	3,538	1,365	981	28,105	2,555
L200 Animal genetics	3,543	1,964	1,508	31,383	2,853
L210 Animal reproduction	2,759	1,745	1,160	26,257	2,387
L300 Animal ecology	1,977	1,638	1,049	22,986	2,089
L400 Animal structure & cytology	1,504	864	647	16,741	1,522
L500 Animal nutrition	5,585	2,721	1,835	45,722	4,157
L600 Animal physiology & biochemistry	4,840	3,859	2,810	55,688	5,063
L700 Animal taxonomy & geography	2,948	1,530	883	26,732	2,430
L820 Pests of animals—gen. & misc.	427	164	72	2,318	211
L821 Pests of animals—insects	2,386	1,668	1,091	22,928	2,084
L822 Pests of animals—helminths	1,640	1,027	390	17,341	1,576
L823 Pests of animals—protozoa	72	726	330	6,169	560
L830 Animal diseases—general	771	450	111	5,414	492
L831 Animal diseases—fungal	225	119	69	1,897	172
L832 Animal diseases—bacterial	2,649	1,982	842	22,810	2,074
L833 Animal diseases—viral	3,522	2,159	895	23,736	2,158
L840 Animal diseases—physiological	1,984	1,644	1,027	19,538	1,776
L841 Misc. animal disorders	1,510	364	0	7,635	694
L850 Protection of stored animal products—gen. & misc.	15	5	2	126	11
L851 Protection of stored animal products—insects	38	16	15	255	23
Primary animal science				460,390	41,854
M000 AQUATIC SCIENCES & FISHERIES, general	57	16	12	450	41
M001 Aquaculture-related	2,700	476	800	26,903	2,446
M100 Aquaculture & fisheries	77	1	0	407	37
M110 Fisheries production	219	84	30	1,741	158
M120 Animal aquaculture	373	143	115	3,065	279
M200 Fisheries & aquaculture management—gen.	38	2	0	195	18
M220 Aquaculture management	41	19	28	377	34
M300 Aquatic biology & ecology—gen.	157	72	68	1,635	149
M310 Aquatic biology & ecology—animals	759	99	83	6,681	607

The entomology-related category is something of a misnomer since it is a catchall for all entomology literature, including taxonomic works where the insects are associated with or have an affect on animals. Most of these 63,000 items will be taxonomic and geographic distribution rather than directly related to diseases or pests of animals.

An effort to see how close the AGRICOLA animal science subject emphases mirror those of AGRIS was attempted. AGRICOLA and AGRIS in the late 1970s reworked their subject coding systems so that they were in agreement. However, in 1985–1986, AGRIS again adjusted its codes so that matches between the two files were not exact. Both basically still use the category L (see Table 2.2) for animal science and in ten of these category codes the matches and definitions are still the same. Select L categories in AGRICOLA in Table 2.2 were used, and 15 AGRIS category codes matching AGRICOLA were searched to coincide with 21 categories in AGRICOLA for four dispersed years: 1975, 1980, 1985 and 1990. Data extracted from AGRIS compact disks showed an average of 2,689 citations a year as opposed to 2,176 for AGRICOLA, all of which were merged into AGRIS. This means that AGRIS adds only about 500–800 animal science citations a year from publications outside the United States. Since 1985 the AGRICOLA file has been reducing its non-United States imprints indexed. A spot check of AGRICOLA citations during the 1985 and 1990 publishing years returns only about 10% from outside the United States, which does not account for the difference in the databases. This low variation leaves some doubts about the inclusiveness of AGRIS as to animal science literature from around the world. There is a close mirroring of the numbers and literature of importance between the two files in only four subjects. In descending significance they are: (1) Animal physiology and biochemistry; (2) Animal diseases; (3) Animal nutrition; (4) Animal genetics and breeding.

The British point of view on subject organization of animal science literature is very different as represented in the CABI abstracting services and the digitized databases. Although the articles and books are put into subject categories similarly, the relationships and subdivisions within a subject are very different. In fact, efforts to arrive at numbers in these subjects which could be matched with the AGRICOLA data proved exceedingly difficult and statistically invalid. It is possible, however, to search the database and identify the citations which are assigned to the various abstracting files, e.g., *Animal Breeding Abstracts*. This method was used to obtain a view of the subject coverage by CAB ABSTRACTS. The citation entries for seven years were counted for five abstracting services coded in the database. Each is listed in Table 2.3 except for *Poultry Abstracts*, which has no data online

Table 2.3. Abstracting publication subject categories in the
CAB ABSTRACTS database

Year	Animal Breeding Abstracts	Dairy Science Abstracts	Herbage Abstracts	Nutrition Abstracts & Reviews, B.
1990	6,307	6,165	2,165	3,489
1989	7,593	6,205	3,862	5,389
1988	7,417	6,364	3,643	5,257
1987	7,265	6,849	3,198	5,332
1986	7,557	6,962	4,456	6,544
1983	6,619	8,130	4,726	5,417
1980	6,907	7,968	3,871	6,549
Total	49,665	48,643	25,921	37,957
Yearly average	7,095	6,949	3,703	5,422

prior to 1983. *Poultry Abstracts*, after 1983 showed a 50% duplication of citations with the other four databases, and was removed from Table 2.3.[8] As with the AGRICOLA file, an article may be assigned to more than one subject category or, in the case of CABI, appear in more than one abstracting file. Thus the duplication rate among them is rather high. Duplicates were not removed from the AGRICOLA data in Table 2.2, but were removed from the CABI information in Table 2.3. An analysis was made of the four CAB ABSTRACTS files to determine the duplication rate within its files, and the gross numbers reduced accordingly. The rate of duplication ranged from 7.3–8.9% in the 1990 citations, and 9.7–9.8% in the 1980 and 1983 citations. A CABI reviewer notes that the online duplication rate from 1984 to the present "is extremely low." Whereas, "a recent analysis has shown that approximately 54% of all the records added to CAB ABSTRACTS database in 1991 were published in one journal only. The balance were published twice or more in hard copy."[9]

The four abstracting journals in Table 2.3 represent the major thrusts of CABI abstracting in animal science, although extensive veterinary medicine literature is also abstracted and published in a separate abstract publication. A direct comparison with the AGRICOLA database is difficult. Table 2.3

8. Personal communication, June 1992, A CABI reviewer of this chapter noted that the 50% duplication in *Poultry Science* "is almost entirely referable to *Animal Breeding Abstracts* and *Nutrition Abstracts (B)*. Virtually all the other 50% in *Poultry Abstracts* are from the veterinary subfile of CAB ABSTRACTS."

9. Ibid.

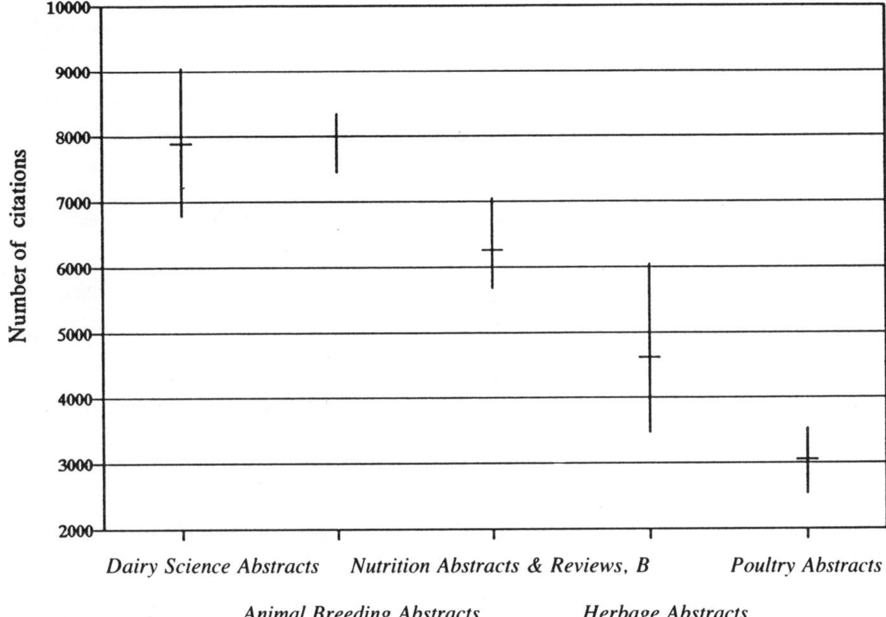

Figure 2.1. Range and median of citations in five CABI abstracting publications, 1980, 1983, 1986–1990.

does provide some general guidelines on the emphases in the literature, which in general follow the data from AGRICOLA.

Some additional data were gathered from five of the abstracting publications of CABI, as represented in Figure 2.1. The number of citations published in the abstracting journals of CABI do not correspond directly to the online data. No duplicates were removed from these numbers.

Another analysis was made to reach a better understanding of the subject differentiation in the animal science field. The primary journal with worldwide influence is the *Journal of Animal Science*, published by the American Society of Animal Science. The Society attempts to represent most aspects of animal science in this journal, the current most critical topics, and research emphasis. The major variation is that little poultry literature has been included in the past ten years, only an estimated 1% of all entries. The 1988 issues of the *Journal of Animal Science* were analyzed following the subject groupings within the *Journal*. These are represented in Table 2.4, with ruminant and nonruminant nutrition merged, although they are separated in the *Journal*, with the nonruminant registering only 7.2% of all technical

Table 2.4. Comparison of subject interests and literature in animal science

Subject	1988 *Journal of Animal Science*	1989 ASAS discipline choice of membership	AGRICOLA (1980–1990)
Nutrition	40.2%	37.0%	17.7%
Physiology & endocrinology	14.4	14.0	21.6
Breeding & genetics	12.7	11.0	22.3
Applied animal science	9.3	24.0	10.9
Growth & development	8.3	5.0	6.5
Environment & behavior	5.5	2.0	8.9
Meat science	5.2	4.0	
Pharmacology & toxicology	2.5		12.1
All others	4.4	3.0	

papers. The 1988 *Journal* issues had 3,421 papers, of which 3,221 were technical papers. The total number of technical articles was 363, averaging 8.7 pages per article. The 4,095 members of the American Society of Animal Science indicated their primary discipline interest upon registration in 1989. Paul V. Malven, Purdue University, obtained a copy of the membership list with this discipline information and provided the information in the center column of Table 2.4. The *Journal* subject orientation and that of the membership are relatively close, with the exception of applied animal science. These are probably individuals who consider themselves generalists but write on specific subjects. It would appear that those working in physiology, endocrinology, breeding, genetics, and reproduction are the most prolific writers per capita. Again, poultry scientists have low representation in ASAS, which may affect the validity of the comparisons for poultry scientists.

C. Language Concentrations

The worldwide scope and subject inclusiveness of the agricultural bibliographic databases provide the best source for information on the languages most heavily used in animal science and health literature. Table 2.5 contains these data and a comparison with the language coverage for all citations in two databases. The AGRICOLA file concentrates on United States imprints and, since 1985, has systematically reduced its non-English language coverage. Therefore, it is likely that the CABI data on language distribution is more representative of worldwide publishing today in animal

Table 2.5. Languages of animal science literature in AGRICOLA and CAB ABSTRACTS

	AGRICOLA		CAB ABSTRACTS	
	Animal science[a]	Total file[b]	Animal science[c]	Total file[d]
English	73.0%	88.4%	67.0%	70.9%
German	4.9	2.8	7.1	5.5
French	2.7	1.6	3.6	3.7
Spanish	1.1	.6	2.4	2.1
Japanese	.6	.6	1.5	1.5
Portuguese	.4	.3	1.0	1.1

[a]AGRICOLA data, 1979–1991. [c]CABI data, 1984–1991.
[b]AGRICOLA data, 1984–1988. [d]CABI data, 1984–1988.

Table 2.6. Percentages of English and non-English literature in three subject areas

Subject	English	Second most common language	
Agricultural Economics and Rural Sociology	87.6%[a]	French	2.5%[a]
	64.1[b]	German	8.0[b]
Agricultural Engineering	88.4[a]	Russian	5.0[a]
	70.9[b]	German	8.9[b]
Animal Science and Health	73.0[a]	German	4.9[a]
	67.0[b]	German	7.1[b]

[a]Data from AGRICOLA online.
[b]Data from CAB ABSTRACTS online.
Sources: Wallace C. Olsen, *Agricultural Economics and Rural Sociology; The Contemporary Core Literature* (Ithaca, N.Y.: Cornell University Press, 1991); Carl W. Hall and Wallace C. Olsen, eds., *The Literature of Agricultural Engineering* (Ithaca, N.Y.: Cornell University Press, 1992).

science and health. In CAB ABSTRACTS "English has steadily increased over the past nine or so years from about 67.5% in 1984 to about 74% currently."[10] The CAB ABSTRACTS searching manual reports, 61% of all documents in the database are in English including all entries going back to 1970.[11]

Two studies of these databases demonstrate a greater inclusion of non-English literature in animal science and health than in the other two subject areas studied, as shown in Table 2.6. The first figures given for each subject area are for AGRICOLA. There appears to be greater agreement be-

10. Ibid.
11. *CAB Abstracts Online Manual*, p. 8.

tween the two databases about the second language of importance in animal science and health than in the other agricultural disciplines.

D. Types of Publications

Both the AGRICOLA and CAB ABSTRACTS databases are encoded with the type of document from which each bibliographic entry emanated, although this is not always precisely done. CAB ABSTRACTS has four format codes: Numbered Parts (journal articles); Numbered Wholes (mostly reports in series); Unnumbered Parts; and Unnumbered Wholes. These last three categories match the definitions of monographs and reports, or parts thereof, as used in the studies in following chapters. Although the AGRI-COLA file uses different descriptions, the divisions may be grouped similarly. The same data from twenty-five categories or subject codes in AGRIS were gathered from a compact disk and are averaged from three dispersed years. Table 2.7 compares these two sources as well as the data from the citation analysis of the Core Agricultural Literature Project detailed in Chapter 5.

Table 2.7. Formats of animal science literature

Source	Journals	Monographs and reports	Dissertations
CAB ABSTRACTS[a]	82.4%	17.6%	
AGRICOLA[b]	93.7	6.3	
AGRIS[c]	76.8	23.2	
Citation analysis data (Chapter 5)	75.0	24.0	1.0%

[a]Data from online file, 1980, 1983, 1986–1990.
[b]Data from online database, 1980–1990.
[c]Data from compact disk datafile, 1980, 1985, 1990.

E. Some Studies of Third World Literature

Discussions have raged for many years over the measurement of literature about Third World topics such as agriculture, as well as about the output and impact of authors from the Third World. Scientific literature has been used as a measure of development and advancement primarily using citation analysis methods. A discussion of citation analysis to measure agriculture economics is provided in an earlier volume.[12] Recently an entire issue (247 pages) of *Scientometrics* (23:1; 1992) included the papers of a 1990 International Conference on Science Indicators for Developing Countries. The reader is referred to this journal to observe the scope of devices used to measure scientific and developmental advancement of which biblometric techniques are the prime tool.

A major study focused on research and publishing trends concerning cattle reproduction in the tropics.[13] This extensive work used 1343 relevant abstracts of documents on bovine reproduction from 1971 through 1985 as included in the CAB ABSTRACTS database. "Search strategies involved the use of general subject codes, as well as more specific terms related to individual reproductive events."[14] Studies include *Bos taurus* cattle, *Bos indicus*, and the crosses between the two. Some of the characteristics of the literature and study results are worth noting:

Asia provided 38% of the publications from seven countries.
Latin America and the United States accounted for 35% of all publications.
African countries (sixteen) produced 18%.
Europe (ten countries) produced 4%.

The most productive countries were: India, 33.5% of all citations; Brazil, 9.5%; Cuba, 7.5%; Venezuela, 5.6%; and South Africa, 5.1%. Of the fifty-six countries represented, the top twenty produced 87.5% of all citations.

The formats of publication were: research journal article, 65.4%; proceedings of meeting, 14.2%; technical and review articles, 10.8%; annual bulletins and reports, 6.9%; and theses, 2.7%. Over the fifteen years, journal articles were never under 50%.

English was used for 67% of all the literature; Spanish for 19%; and Portugese for 9%. French, German, Afrikaans and Czech were also represented by only seven abstracts.

The paper also quantifies the subject concentrations, breeds and reproductive events of this reproduction literature.

12. Wallace C. Olsen, *Agricultural Economics and Rural Sociology; The Contemporary Core Literature* (Ithaca, N.Y.: Cornell University Press, 1991).
13. C. S. Galina and J. M. Russell, "Research and Publishing Trends in Cattle Reproduction in the Tropics: Part 1. A Global Analysis" in *Animal Breeding Abstracts* 55 (10) (Oct. 1987). "Part 2: A Third World Prerogative" by Russell and Galina was published in issue no. 11, Nov. 1987.
14. Galina and Russell, Part 1, p. 744.

In the second paper by Russell and Galina they further analyze, characterize, contrast the literature and make a strong case that tropical countries' literature comes from tropical countries. The list of primary journals cited from the top ten countries demonstrates the lack of commonality among them and a great insularity. Only four titles are listed as major cited publication in two or more countries:

International Journal of Biometerology, among the top five for South Africa and
the United States
Proc. Asociacion Latino Americana de Produccion Animal, highly cited by Brazil,
Cuba, Venezuela, Mexico, United States
Theriogenology, cited by Mexico, Zimbabwe, Nigeria, and United States
Tropical Animal Production, cited by Venezuela and Nigeria.

Some questions exist about subject skews,inclusiveness of the CAB ABSTRACTS, and techniques and applications to animals outside the tropics which will eventually also be appropriate for the tropics. The study underlines some standard points about agricultural literature:

(1) The animal reproduction literature for the tropics is largely localized which does not mean that it is the most valuable literature on a longer time frame. Most of this literature is site-specific and may have little application across country boundaries or have regional significance.
(2) Today's local literature tends to be more heavily represented as reports, workshops, ephemeral, and proceedings volumes.
(3) The shift to English language is clear although for locally-intended literature, local language plays a dynamic role.

A remarkable project originated by the International Livestock Centre for Africa has provided a wealth of information about publishing of the last twenty years on animal science concerning several African countries.

The management of the International Livestock Centre for Africa has an extensive information program which includes a selective dissemination literature service for Third World institutions and network cooperators. They have worked extensively with the International Development Research Centre (Canada) in this and related bibliographic and information services. One of the more interesting projects has been to send teams around sub-Saharan Africa to identify and microfiche non-conventional local literature and make this information and the fiche readily available. These summary listings have been published:

Index to Livestock Literature Microfiched by the ILCA/IDRC Team in Sudan, 1981,
Part II. Issued by ILCA, 1982. 107p.

Index to Livestock Literature Microfiched by the ILCA/IDRC Team in Botswana. Issued by ILCA, 1985. 146p.

Index to Livestock Literature Microfiched in Zimbabwe, compiled by Tesfai Berhane and Negussie Akalework. Issued by ILCA, 1986. 235p.

Index to Livestock Literature Microfiched by the ILCA/IDRC Team in The Gambia, compiled by Tesfai Berhane and Getachew Bulfeta. Issued by ILCA, 1987. 41p.

Index to Livestock Literature Microfiched by the ILCA/IDRC Team in Kenya, compiled by Tesfai Berhane and Sirak Teklu. Issued by ILCA, 1988. 303p.

Index to Livestock Literature Microfiched in Ethiopia, compiled by Mekonnen Assefa. Issued by ILCA, 1990. 237p.

Index to Livestock Literature on Nigeria, compiled by Sirak Teklu. Issued by ILCA, 1992. 279p. 2,066 records.

Index to Livestock Literature Microfiched in Uganda, compiled by Mekonnen Assefa. Issued by ILCA, 1992. 83p. 652 records.

The thousands of records from this elaborate project have been incorporated into the bibliographic database of the Library and Documentation Services of ILCA. Individual copies of the documents may be requested in microfiche if the document is not of restricted distribution. Recent listings have included more literature from conventional sources, such as European and American journals, resulting in listing and indexing centered on the animal science of an African country. Subject indexes are provided with the volumes, as well as author indexes in some issuances.

A brief analysis was made of the *Index* concerned with the livestock literature of Nigeria, compiled by Sirak Teklu. The citations appear to be rather complete from a scouring of databases and sources in Nigeria and ILCA. There are 2,066 entries dispersed under fifty-three subject groupings which include headings such as legislation, soil chemistry and physics, and forestry production all as related to livestock in Nigeria. This inclusiveness makes the collection quite valuable. No indication of a qualitative screen is mentioned and it must be assumed that any item related that could be found was entered in the *Index.*

An analysis was made of one of the large subject groups (20% of all entries) titled "Animal Production." These characteristics emerged:

Monograph items including reports accounted for 63.9 % of all citations, journal articles, 34.4 %, and dissertations 1.7% which were all from the University of Ibadan. The International Livestock Centre for Africa had an office in Ibadan for several years. The International Livestock Centre monographs and reports constituted the greatest number of citations from a single publisher with imprints both from Nigeria and Ethiopia. Several units of the Nigerian government together accounted for the second largest group of publications, followed at some distance by the University of Ibadan and

Ahmadu Bello University. Twenty-six additional publishers are identified although they account for under 30% of all citations. Of the 145 monographic items, ninety-five were published in Nigeria, seventeen in Ethiopia, followed by seven from Great Britain, and six each from Italy and the United States. Eighty percent of the monographs were complete in themselves; that is, they were not cited as IN citations.

Similarly in the same animal production section of the index, thirty of the seventy-eight journal citations were published in Nigeria; fifteen were from Great Britain; and nine each from Italy and Kenya. The rest were of minor influence although only twelve different countries of publication for journals were listed. The most often cited journals in descending order were:

World Review of Animal Production
Nigerian Journal of Animal Production
OAU/STRC Bulletin of Animal Health & Production in Africa
Nigerian Society of Animal Production Proceedings.

All of these are numerically close together. The difficulty with journals in developing countries is their tendency to have a very short life or years of cessation which is the case with the last three titles here. It must be re-emphasized that these numbers do not represent a qualitative value, but do indicate the abundance of locally-produced, and often site-specific literature.

3. Publishing of Major Societies

I. The American Society of Animal Science

FREDRIC N. OWENS

Animal Science Department, Oklahoma State University

With a note by
DENNIS M. HALLFORD

Animal Science Department, New Mexico State University

A. Note on the American Society of Animal Science

The American Society of Animal Nutrition was founded in 1908 by a group of nutritionists from agricultural experiment stations and the United States Department of Agriculture. To broaden the scope of the society, the term "nutrition" was changed to "production" in 1912. To reflect increasing interest in research, the term "production" was changed to "science" in 1961. The size and scope of topics covered by the American Society of Animal Science has expanded greatly. In 1983, for the 75th anniversary of the society, thirty-two invited papers reviewed the history of ASAS and scientific progress in animal science. These were published as Supplement 2 of the Diamond Jubilee Issue of the *Journal of Animal Science*, July 1983.

The stated mission of ASAS is to foster communication and collaboration among those associated with animal science research, education, industry and government. For fulfilling this mission, two primary activities of ASAS are publishing the *Journal of Animal Science* (*JAS*) and sponsoring an annual (national) meeting at which research data and invited symposia are presented. For its first fifty-four years, the annual meeting was held in

Part I of this chapter is also Article 6090 of the Agricultural Experiment Station, Oklahoma State University, 74078.

33

Chicago following Thanksgiving and the National Livestock Exposition. Since 1963, national meetings have been held during the summer months on various university campuses or convention centers rotating among the four geographic sections. These four sections (Northeast, Southern, Midwestern and Western) also hold annual meetings for presentation of research. Abstracts from sectional and national meetings are compiled and published annually. Abstracts were incorporated directly into *JAS* until 1977. Since then, abstracts have been published as a supplement to *JAS*.

B. History of the *Journal of Animal Science*

Before 1940, each secretary of ASAS prepared a proceedings following the annual meetings which, together with the abstracts, was published as the Proceedings of the American Society of Animal Production. On the recommendation of an editorial committee, quarterly publication of *JAS* began in 1942. The first *JAS* editor, Dr. R. W. Phillips, subsequently worked with the FAO in Rome and has provided insight into the early history of *JAS*, as reviewed by R. R. Oltjen.[1] *JAS* began publishing bimonthly in 1967 and monthly in 1969. The founding of *JAS* marked a time at which focus of ASAS was re-directed from practical aspects of animal husbandry to the application of science to improving animal production.

The ASAS business office, membership services, the *JAS* technical editors and *JAS* typesetting are housed in Champaign, Illinois (309 West Clark St., 61820; 217-356-3182) in association headquarters owned by the American Dairy Science Association. Formal contracts indicating the type and cost of services are negotiated yearly by the executive committee of ASAS. For the first time in 1990, editors for four publications typeset in the same office (*JAS, J. Dairy Sci., J. Nutr., Poultry Sci.*) met and discussed topics of similar interest in an attempt to standardize the style and form of these journals to simplify technical editing and typesetting. *JAS* was printed and mailed for many years by Boyd Printing Co., Albany, New York, but since 1990 printing has been handled by Imperial Printing, St. Joseph, Michigan. Being more central in the United States, this location has reduced mailing time to subscribers. Before 1991, *JAS* was 7 x 10 inches in size, but it was enlarged to 8-½ x 11 inches in 1992 to accommodate advertisers.

1. R. R. Oltjen, "Significant Milestones in the 75-Year History of the American Society of Animal Science," *Journal of Animal Science* 57 (Suppl. 2): 1.

C. The Review Process

Since its inception, *JAS* has been a peer-reviewed journal with an editorial board selected by its editors and approved by the ASAS Board of Directors. The editorial board, which consists of reviewers, section editors and the editor-in-chief, reviews submitted manuscripts, and establishes and implements editorial policy. Appointed to the editorial board for three years, members are chosen for their expertise in a specialty field. Members and section editors are chosen from all regions of the United States, Canada and Europe, and come from academic, industrial or governmental institutions. Currently, about 11% of the papers submitted to *JAS* come from non-U.S. institutions, primarily Canada. Scientists from other countries have served on the editorial board, but the delays in communication and incomplete information about the expertise of researchers in other countries has restricted their involvement in the *JAS* review process. Electronic manuscript transmission and increased international contact should alleviate these problems and increase international exchange of information. Currently, association presidents and several symposia speakers from ASAS and the European Association of Animal Production attend each other's annual national meetings. However, an increased rate of publication by non-U.S. authors in *JAS* is not expected, because governments in many countries subsidize their journals to encourage publication.

Currently (1991), eleven section editors supervise review of manuscripts in their fields. Reviews are conducted by society members, primarily by the eighty-nine individuals who serve on the *JAS* Editorial Board. Revised papers are forwarded to the editor-in-chief and the technical editor for final editing, typesetting, proofing and compiling into monthly issues. The editor-in-chief, selected by the ASAS Board of Directors from among active researchers with past service as a section editor, is partially supported by the Society, but is expected to maintain an active research program during a three-year term. The editor-in-chief is an appointed member of the ASAS Board of Directors. Typically, the editor-in-chief is chosen to represent a field of expertise different from that of his predecessor. With advice from section editors and the ASAS Board of Directors, the editor-in-chief is responsible for recruiting replacements for section editors and editorial board members whose terms are completed. Among the 7,000 recipients of *JAS* are 3,856 society members, 933 student affiliates (who pay half the normal membership fee) and 1,797 institutional affiliates.

About 500 papers are published annually in *JAS*, with an average length of 8.7 printed pages. Over the past ten years, the number of pages and papers published in *JAS* has increased by 44 to 55%. Although over 90% of these papers present new research findings, *JAS* publishes review papers from symposia presented by invited speakers at annual or sectional meetings. A new type of article, "Technical Notes," was added in 1989. These are short articles reporting on a new method, technique or procedure employed in research or data analysis. Unsolicited review papers are no longer accepted for publication. The "Style and Form" for publication is revised every three years by the retiring editor-in-chief, with input from the editorial board and the ASAS Board of Directors. The style and form follows the general format recommended by the Council of Biology Editors (CBE). Recent changes in the style and form that deviate from CBE include the addition of an "Implications" section to each article for the author to outline briefly the practical and biological significance of their data, inclusion of many acronyms specific to Animal Science (also listed on the inside cover of each issue), and greatly increased emphasis on statistical anslysis and presentation of data. The style and form is published in *JAS* every three years, and a manuscript submission form is included in each issue.

D. Journal Sections

Until 1967, when *JAS* first exceeded 1,500 pages, the editor worked with up to five associate editors to review manuscripts. Currently, *JAS* is divided into ten sections with eleven section editors (two from Ruminant Nutrition, one dealing with Roughages and Forages and the second with Digestion and Metabolism). The year these sections were formed, which shows the evolution of topics being covered, and the mean percentage of papers in each topic area over a five-year period are presented in Table 3.1. In several cases, sections were separated only after some years as part of another section. For example, "Growth and Developmental Biology" was handled by section editors in "Meat Science" and "Physiology and Endocrinology" from 1981 until 1985, when its own section editor was appointed. Section editors now have full responsibility for review of manuscripts assigned to them. Only in very rare instances (five of the last 1,200 papers) is a section editor's decision to accept a paper questioned.

In addition to research, JAS includes annual society reports, "News and Notes," and job announcements, which comprise about 4% of the total pages of *JAS*. Detailed statistical analysis must be included in all research presented in *JAS*. This requirement probably evolved from the eminent statisticians and biometricians who have conducted research in Animal Science (G. W. Snedecor, W. R. Harvey, C. W. Henderson) and the extensive use of statistics in genetic selection of animals.

Table 3.1. Journal of Animal Science sections, formation date, and size

Section	Year formed	Fraction of papers[a]
Ruminant Nutrition	1967	23%
Physiology and Endocrinology	1967	15%
Breeding and Genetics	1967	14%
Nonruminant Nutrition	1967	10%
Meat Science[b]	1967	6%
Applied Animal Science[c]	1969	13%
Pharmacology and Toxicology	1981	3%
Growth and Developmental Biology	1982	8%
Environment and Behavior[d]	1987	4%
Biography	1987	1%

[a]Mean percentage of papers in each topic area from 1985 to 1990.

[b]Called "Meats" until 1968, and "Meat Science and Muscle Biology" until 1981.

[c]Called "Extension and Teaching" until 1973, and "Applied Animal Science and Teaching" until 1976.

[d]A section called "Behavior" was part of the "Breeding and Genetics" section in 1983–1984.

[e]Provides condensed life stories of six past ASAS members each year.

During recent years, *JAS* has attempted to speed the review process so that the time from receipt to acceptance can average less than 160 days, and from acceptance to publication less than 160 days. This 320-day time lapse from submission until distribution of the article is longer for *JAS* than for several other journals (Table 3.2). Direct comparison with other journals with different review systems is hazardous due to differences in the thoroughness and length of articles, and of the review process. For ease of discussion, it is convenient to divide the total publication time into a first portion, from submission to acceptance, and a second portion, from acceptance until the issue containing the paper is received by the subscriber. Note that review time varies widely from minimum to maximum. If papers require more time for review, author revision, and editing, publication will be delayed. Hence, the minimums rather than the averages should be more meaningful with respect to timeliness. Almost half of the time from submission to printing is between acceptance by the editor-in-chief and mailing to the subscriber.

In an attempt to streamline and speed the publication process, a second technical editor was hired at the typesetting office in Champaign, Illinois, in 1990 and computerized typesetting is being used, as well as FAX transmission for some manuscripts.

Table 3.2. Publication times (days) for various journals in 1989

Journals	Review days[a]			Printing days[b]			Total	
	Average	Minimum	Maximum	Average	Minimum	Maximum	Average	Minimum
J. Anim. Sci.	181	56	413	152	111	248	333	200
J. Dairy Sci.	155	68	340	161	98	201	316	222
J. Nutr.	200	90	421	141	119	179	341	215
FASEB	73	33	110	100	68	130	173	128
Science	82	17	179	71	35	103	153	57
Nature	81	8	242	73	48	105	155	82

[a]Time from manuscript submission until acceptance by the editor-in-chief.
[b]Time from acceptance for publication until receipt by the subscriber.

E. Manuscript Revision and Acceptance Rate

During the past seven years, an average of 72% of the submitted manuscripts were published; the rest were rejected or withdrawn. Acceptance rate often is used by administrators as an index of journal quality. Such a view seems invalid because authors do not submit weak manuscripts to journals with a critical review process. Further, an acceptance rate does not reflect the extent of manuscript revision involved prior to acceptance for publication. Rather than rejecting marginal papers outright, most *JAS* section editors painstakingly indicate to authors what revisions are necessary to improve a paper. In many cases, second and third revisions are required before a paper is accepted. During the past three years, only two of the 1,200 submitted papers were accepted by section editors without any revisions, and these two were revised prior to publication, based on concerns raised by the editor-in-chief. Most accepted papers are revised quite extensively prior to publication.

F. Indexing

Keywords selected by the author from the *CAB Thesaurus* are included at the beginning of every paper. *JAS* publishes an index based on authors and on these keywords at the end of each volume, which consists of either six-month (1969–1987) or one-year (1942–1968, and after 1987) periods. Both abstracts and full-length articles are indexed. Cumulative indexes were published in 1965, 1972, and 1976. In addition, a computer-based reference retrieval system to search 12,300 *JAS* references from 1942 to 1991 for full-length articles by author, keyword or title word was developed at New Mexico State University and is being marketed by ASAS ($250).[2] Authors, keywords and title words also are indexed by various abstracting services. According to one source, *JAS* is indexed in *Biological Abstracts, Biological and Agricultural Index, Chemical Abstracts, Current Contents* ("Agriculture and Veterinary Medicine" section), *Excerpta Medica, Index Medicus, Nutrition Abstracts and Reviews Series B, Science Citation Index, Animal Breeding Abstracts, Current Advances in Biochemistry, Current Advances in Genetics and Molecular Biology, Current Packaging Abstracts, Dairy Science Abstracts, Farm and Garden Index, Field Crop Abstracts, Food Science and Technology Abstracts, Environmental Periodicals Bibliography, Helminthology Abstracts, Index to Science Reviews, Index Veteri-*

2. D. M. Hallford, personal communication.

narius, Maize Abstracts, Nutrition Research Newsletter, Protozoological Abstracts, Pig News and Information, Plant Growth Regulator Abstracts, Sorghum and Millets Abstracts, Rural Recreation and Tourism Abstracts, Soils and Fertilizers, Soybean Abstracts, Triticale Abstracts, Tropical Oil Seeds Abstracts, Veterinary Bulletin, and *World Agricultural Economics and Rural Sociology Abstracts.*[3] *JAS* is also indexed by the National Agricultural Library in the AGRICOLA database, and is available on microfilm from UMI.

An annual membership directory and handbook is also published by ASAS. Mailing lists of members can be prepared by location, affiliation and by section, as well as by species and research specialty.[4]

G. Publication Cost

ASAS income is derived from membership dues ($65/year), institutional subscriptions to *JAS* ($160/year), sales of past publications, page charges ($85/page for ASAS members, $170/page for others) and donations. In addition, the ASAS Board of Directors is progressing with plans to sell advertising space in *JAS* to further defray the cost of publication. Dues have been increased haltingly following inflation rates. To hire a second technical editor to speed publication, in 1991 ASAS increased all charges except page charges to authors. The ASAS Board of Directors has struggled to balance the cost of publishing among authors, members, and institutional (library) subscribers. It seems logical that members should pay a minimum of the pro-rated cost of journal printing and mailing, and that income from institutional subscribers should be applied fully to the cost of publication, because the sole benefit of ASAS to institutions is the journal. But the relative fraction of the cost that should be borne by institutions, often operating with very limited bidgets, versus authors, also with limited funds, is a difficult decision. This decision is further complicated by competing journals. For journals not associated with a society, individual and library subscriptions are often extremely expensive. In turn, the page charge assessed to authors by such journals is often nil; this attracts authors to submit manuscripts. These journals also encourage scientists to request that their libraries subscribe to their publications. Societies with journals must closely monitor the

3. *Ulrich's International Periodicals Directory* (New York: R. R. Bowker Division of Reed Pub., 1991).

4. *Handbook and Membership Directory* (Champaign, Ill.: American Society of Animal Science, 1989).

page charges of such competing journals because if authors are attracted away, society members will be deprived of pertinent and meaningful information.

A subscription to *JAS* accompanies each ASAS membership, although members can choose not to receive *JAS*. Subscribers can also request that their copy be distributed in a program supervised by the Rockefeller Foundation. In this program, ASAS provides a minimum of fifty copies of *JAS* each month free of charge for placement in university and governmental libraries of developing African countries.

H. Non-Journal Publications

Many scientific societies produce a large number of publications each year. In contrast, ASAS has no publications except *JAS*, plus two or more separate supplements to *JAS*, every year. These supplements are available at an additional cost, but are not provided to all subscribers of *JAS*. Attendees receive their *JAS* Supplement at or after the conference or meeting. The Abstracts, summaries of oral or poster presentations at regional or national meetings, form Supplement 1 of *JAS* each year. In addition, one supplement is produced annually from an ancillary symposia (the Biennial Growth Symposia or the Biennial Reproduction Symposia) held preceding each national ASAS meeting on alternating years. Separate non-profit budgets (including registration fees and supporting industry donations) to conduct these conferences and publish proceedings are scrutinized by the ASAS Board of Directors to be certain that the cost of publication will be recovered. Review and typesetting of manuscripts for these supplements are managed by an ad hoc editor, often the chairperson of the conference. Finally, reports from additional symposia (Diet/Health, Antibiotics, Computer Use, Undergraduate Teaching) or select committees (Care of Animals Used in Research and Teaching) have been published recently as *JAS* Supplements.

The low number of ASAS publications beyond these supplements may be related partly to a limited need of ASAS members. Most of the papers from symposia sponsored by ASAS and presented at regional or national meetings already are reviewed and published as part of *JAS*. If papers in a symposium will not meet the scientific scrutiny of review for publication in *JAS* or if more rapid publication is imperative, a conference coordinator may request that the ASAS Board of Directors publish the proceedings as a *JAS* Supplement. The number of added publications also my be low because of limited experience and encouragement to expand publishing. The editor-in-chief, as a research scientist, is not appointed permanently to stimulate publication by ASAS; ad hoc editors are appointed only temporarily to supervise the supplemental publications. Although certain groups, e.g., the Biennial Grazing Conference, have requested that ASAS publish additional proceedings in *JAS* or as a supplement, the ASAS Board of Directors has discouraged involvement with additional groups unless the conference is co-sponsored by ASAS and the topics and speakers are approved in advance by the ASAS Board of Directors. As an alternative to ASAS publishing, local university publishing units already publish proceedings from state conferences; they usually can publish local and regional information faster (photo-duplicating rather than typesetting) and at a lower cost than ASAS. Such units are ideally suited for non-technical editing and publishing, especially for reports with limited interest either geographically, temporally or scientifically.

I. Other Reviewed Animal Agriculture Journals

Many other journals are available for publishing general or specialized animal science research, as listed in Table 3.3. A recent agreement between ASAS and the American Registry of Professional Animal Scientists will permit ASAS members who are not certified by the Registry to publish in their journal, the *Professional Animal Scientist*. This should substitute for

Table 3.3. Publications presenting topics included in the *Journal of Animal Science*

Section	Alternative journals
Applied Animal Science	Anim. Prod.; Profess. Anim. Sci.; J. Prod. Agric.; Livest. Prod. Sci.; Can. J. Anim. Sci.; J. Agric. Sci.
Breeding and Genetics	Anim. Breed. Abstr.; Genetics; Genetic Res.
Environment and Behavior	Appl. Anim. Behav.; Appl. Anim. Ethol.; Anim. Behav.; Physiol. & Behav.
Growth and Development	Growth, Metabolism
Meat Science	Meat Sci.; J. Agr. Food Chem.; J. Food Sci. Techn.; J. Food Biochem.; J. Sci. Food Agric.
Nutrition	J. Dairy Sci.; Br. J. Nutr.; J. Range Manage.; J. Nutr.; Nutr. Res.; Anim. Feed Sci. Technol.; J. Nutr. Biochem.
Pharmacology and Toxicology	Toxicol.; Xenobiotica; Residue Rev.
Physiology and Endocrinology	Biol. Reprod.; Domest. Anim. Endocrinol.; J. Endocrinol.; Theriogenology; J. Reprod. Fertil.; Repro. Nutr. Dev.; Am. J. Physiol.

enlarging the scope of the Applied Animal Science section of *JAS* to increase communication among the many ASAS members involved with teaching and extension.

J. Nonreviewed Animal Agriculture Publications

Nearly every agricultural experiment station maintains a publishing unit for publicizing results of experiments with agricultural animals. At some stations, this consists of an annual summary by species, such as a Feeders' Day Report. At other stations, results are compiled and presented in the form of a miscellaneous publication or a symposium with local and outside specialists reviewing specific topics in a nutrition conference (e.g., Cornell, Georgia, Minnesota Nutrition Conferences). In addition, symposia on selected topics pertinent to a particular region or species are often held, and conference proceedings are published. Topic reviews are also published in many monthly trade publications, including *Feedstuffs, Beef Magazine, Feedlot Management, The Renderers, Animal Health and Nutrition,* etc. Because such data and reviews have not been routinely indexed, retrieval of such buried information has depended primarily on the memory of scientists. With support from USDA, extension specialists from Kansas State University have prepared a computerized index by state, year, author and title word for experiment station publications from 1985 to 1990.[5] This should aid in information retrieval and avoid duplication of research efforts. In addition, CRIS reports of USDA-supported pending and completed research are updated annually with computer records maintained by the USDA.

K. Appraisal of *JAS* by ASAS Members

A survey of ASAS members regarding effectiveness of *JAS* was conducted in 1987 by the ASAS Board of Directors. This was published in 1988.[6] Over 30% of ASAS members responded to the survey. Of the respondents, over 93% were professional members. Over 95% of the respondents considered *JAS* a prestigious journal, and over 73% indicated that *JAS*

---

5. D. D. Sims, personal communication.

6. D. M. Hallford, D. J. Meisinger, and D. G. Spruill, "Effectiveness of the *Journal of Animal Science* in Meeting Membership Needs: Results of a Survey," *Journal of Animal Science* 67 (1988): 1848.

contained information useful in their professional work. The majority of respondents suggested that *JAS* should add a teaching/extension section, as well as a "Notes" section. (A "Technical Notes" section was added in 1989). Some respondents indicated that authors should be encouraged to enlarge their discussion of the practical and biological significance of their data. A section entitled "Implications" has been included in each manuscript submitted after 1989. Placement information and announcements of upcoming meetings and publications are also included in each issue.

L. Appraisal of *JAS* by ASAS Members Publishing in Other Journals

During 1989, a telephone survey of ASAS members was conducted with fifty-three individuals who had published articles during 1989 in research journals other than *JAS* based on a search to match randomly selected names of ASAS members with authors listed by AGRICOLA. This survey was conducted by the Minnesota Center for Survey Research to determine why authors selected a journal other than *JAS* for publishing their research results.[7] Usable responses were obtained from fifty of these individuals. Journals with more than a single paper from an ASAS member included the *J. Dairy Sci.* (9), *Nutr. Rep. Int.* (now *J. Nutr. Biochem.*) and *J. Reprod. Fertil.* (4 each), *Biol. Reprod.* (3), and *Br. Poultry Sci.* (2). Of the respondents, 37% had considered the possibility of publication of their research in *JAS*, but had decided primarily (>51%) based on appropriateness of either the audience or the topic to publish elsewhere. As a second reason, 27% indicated that their paper was not scientific or statistical enough for publication in *JAS*. Lower prestige of *JAS* was a factor in only 16% of the decisions to publish elsewhere. Other advantages for alternative journals that were mentioned included faster publication (35%), lower page charges (22%), a more satisfactory review process (22%), more satisfactory style and form (12%) and more satisfactory printing format (12%). Some 69% indicated that page charges were included in their research budget, but with decreased funding of research, high page charges may restrict publication in the future.

M. Appraisal of *JAS* by Citation Incidence

The impact of various journals is ranked annually within various topic categories by *SCI Journal Citation Reports*, based on the number of times

---

7. J. E. Pettigrew, personal communication.

Table 3.4. Ranking of journals by impact factor in the agriculture, dairy, and animal science category[a]

Rank	Journal	Impact factor
1	Journal of Animal Science	1.364
2	Journal of Dairy Science	1.254
3	Journal of Dairy Research	1.190
4	Animal Production	.970
5	British Poultry Science	.757
6	Applied Animal Behavior Science	.710
7	Livestock Production Science	.680
8	Poultry Science	.642
9	Génétique, sélection, évolution	.618
10	Canadian Journal of Animal Science	.546
11	Archiv für Geflugelkunde	.472
12	Journal of Range Management	.471
13	Animal Feed and Science Technology	.430
14	Australian Journal of Experimental Agriculture	.398
15	Journal of Animal Breeding and Genetics	.389
16	World Poultry Science Journal	.381
17	Archiv für Tierernährung	.374
18	Zuchtungskunde	.321
19	New Zealand Journal of Dairy Science	.304
20	Annales Zootechnie	.250
21	Agricultural Practice	.229
22	Archiv für Tierzucht	.102
23	Australian Journal of Dairy Technology	.100
24	Zivočišná výroba	.020
25	Indian Journal of Animal Science	.019
26	Wool Technology and Sheep Breeding	.000

[a]As modified from *SCI Journal Citation Reports* (1989).

articles from each journal are cited in journals worldwide. Impact factor is thus defined: "When a journal, as opposed to a single article, is being measured, the total number of items published by the journal influences the number of times it is cited; the more it publishes, the greater the number of opportunities it has to be cited. Given a large and small journal of equal quality, the large one will be cited more frequently than the small one. The impact factor discounts this advantage of large journals by showing the average citation rate per published item. This is done by dividing the number of times the journal has been cited by the number of items it has published."[8] The latest printed data available ranked *J. Anim. Sci.* as having the

8. Eugene Garfield, *Citation Indexing—Its Theory and Application in Science, Technology, and Humanities* (Philadelphia: ISI Press, 1979), p. 24.

greatest impact among the twenty-six different journals in the Agriculture, Dairy and Animal Science category, as presented in Table 3.4.[9] The impact factor for *JAS* was also higher than for any of the 163 journals in other agriculture categories (*Agricultural Ecomonics & Policy; Agricultural Experiment Station Reports; Agriculture; Agriculture, Soil Science*). This statistic attests to the high standards maintained by the *JAS* Editorial Board and by authors submitting manuscripts to be published in *JAS*. Certain alternative journals in topic categories other than agriculture to which ASAS members might submit articles have higher citation records than *JAS* (1.36). These include the *J. Nutr.* (1.72) and *Anim. Behav.* (1.81). Such journals have a higher citation incidence because they are widely cited in the life sciences literature beyond agriculture.

N. Anticipated Changes in *JAS*

Many other agricultural research societies publish more than one journal; these differ in scientific complexity and target audience. Although sentiment for a second ASAS journal emphasizing teaching and extension efforts has been expressed by certain ASAS members, the ASAS Board of Directors and the *JAS* Editorial Board have questioned the financial feasibility of a second publication when other outlets (*Nat. Assoc. College Teachers of America J., Profess. Anim. Sci.*, and many trade publications) are available. Nevertheless, the board of directors must remain alert to the needs and desires of ASAS members. Stringent and critical peer review of articles published in *JAS* must be maintained so that its credibility and reputation remain high. However, an additional, more applied journal may be developed to serve ASAS members. Alternatively, considering its size and breadth, *JAS* could be subdivided into individual journals covering closely related topic areas.

An enlarged editorial staff may be required in the future. *JAS* may need to employ an editor-elect to assist the editor-in-chief with final manuscript revisions in certain topic areas and to maintain continuity among all the articles published in *JAS*. Alternatively, a retired ASAS member could serve as the editor-in-chief to coordinate publication of manuscripts forwarded by section editors, if critical review and editing at this final stage were abandoned. Finally, distribution of *JAS* to subscribers on computer diskette in addition to hard-copy has been proposed. This would speed distribution and retrieval of manuscripts based on searched word combinations.

9. *SCI Journal Citation Reports, An Interdisciplinary Index to the Literature of Science, Medicine, Agriculture, Technology and the Behavioral Sciences* (Philadelphia: Institute for Scientific Information, 1989).

Strong commitment to quality by the ASAS and the *JAS* Editorial Board has established and will help maintain the unmatched reputation of the *Journal of Animal Science*.

EDITOR'S NOTE: Dr. Owens provided a brief summary of the *Journal* at the end of his editorship: *Journal of Animal Science* 70:3649–3650 (Dec. 1992)

Journal of Animal Science Reference Retrieval System

Dennis M. Hallford
Animal Science Department, New Mexico State University

In a survey conducted in 1987 by the American Society of Animal Science Board of Directors to evaluate *JAS* effectiveness, a number of respondents indicated a need for a computer-based retrieval system for the *Journal of Animal Science*.[10] Therefore, a database was developed in 1988–1989 and is currently available through ASAS. Yearly updates will also be provided. The database was prepared using a commercially available software package (compiled BASIC) that is supplied with the reference file. The system currently includes over 12,300 references encompassing the entire *Journal of Animal Science* vol. 1–69 (1942–1991). Only full-length articles are indexed along with selected manuscripts from *Reproduction and Growth Symposia*. A second file is in preparation that will contain all abstracts published in *JAS*.

The retrieval system operates on fixed-drive IBM-compatible microcomputers and is capable of searching by author and keyword, including main word in the title. Using modern equipment, author searches run at about 6,000 references per minute, compared with 3,000 per minute for keyword searches. The *JAS* began requiring that authors provide keywords with manuscripts in July 1975 (vol. 41, no. 1). Articles published before 1975 were keyworded by a single individual, who also added additional words after 1975 to maintain consistency for searching purposes. The menu-driven software package allows users to add new references, edit the database and print reference lists in a variety of ways. In addition, lists can be alphabetized by first author or ordered by a file number. The system also maintains alphabetical lists of all authors and keywords (contains author and keyword files in addition to the datafile). This feature allows users to print a list of all keywords used in *JAS* (currently about 8,000) for prior examination before searches are intitiated.

10. Hallford, et al., "Effectiveness of the *Journal of Animal Science*."

The *JAS* Retrieval System is available from: American Society of Animal Science, 309 West Clark Street, Champaign, Illinois, 61820.

II. Influence of the *Journal of Dairy Science* and *Poultry Science*

BARBARA A. DISALVO
Mann Library, Cornell University

The citation analysis of the Core Agricultural Literature Project showed three current journals to be pre-eminent in ranking (see Table 3.5). Therefore, the framework and impact of the journals published by the American Dairy Science Association (ASDA) and the Poultry Science Association (PSA) were investigated. The membership of the three primary associations is very different, without overlap between the ASDA and PSA, but with some distinctions in membership, differing subject concentration and the importance of each of the journals, this analysis seemed essential.

The *Journal of Dairy Science* was established as the official bimonthly publication of the American Dairy Science Association in 1917. In 1934, the *Journal of Dairy Science* began publishing monthly in order to serve better the needs of Association members and the animal science industry.

Table 3.5. Ranking by Core Agricultural Literature Project and *SCI Journal Citation Reports*

	Core Analysis[a]	SCI[b]	Overall[c]
Journal of Animal Science	1	1	1
Journal of Dairy Science	2	2	2
Poultry Science	3	8	3
Journal of Dairy Research[d]	35	3	34

[a]Cf. Chap. 6, pp. 193–94.
[b]Cf. Table 3.4.
[c]Cf. Table 6.1.
[d]By computing impact factor rather than rank, quarterly publications like *Journal of Dairy Research* achieve higher rating.

The history of the *Journal of Dairy Science* has been well documented in three excellent articles by former ADSA historian G. Malcolm Trout.[11] Since the last of the histories in 1981, the *Journal of Dairy Science* has continued to grow in size and importance. In addition to research papers in four broad subject areas, the journal contains industry and Association news and information, and the abstracts of the annual ADSA meeting published as a supplementary issue.

In 1980, 267 papers covering 2,424 pages were published in the research section of the *Journal of Dairy Science*. By 1990, after a steady ten-year increase, 433 papers covering 3,906 pages were published, an increase of 61.1% for pages and 62.2% for papers. As with other peer-reviewed journals, an increase in the time from submission to acceptance to publication combined with an increase in the number of papers submitted had resulted in a backlog of unpublished papers. Technical and research editors introduced lag-time reduction measures which included creation of a standard abbreviations list for authors (1986) and the breakdown of the two subjects areas, "Dairy Foods" and "Dairy Production," into four areas in 1988: "Dairy Foods," "Physiology & Management," "Nutrition, Feeding & Calves," "Genetics & Breeding." An increase in the number of editors and review boards has reduced time from submission to publication to the shortest of the three top journals.

Statistics of two years are available on the number of papers and pages devoted to each of the four new subject areas. These break down:

	1990		1991	
	Papers	Pages	Papers	Pages
Dairy Foods	116	965	128	1,008
Physiology & Management	88	682	93	763
Nutrition, Feeding & Calves	133	1,115	171	1,593
Genetics & Breeding	60	562	59	529

"Nutrition, Feeding & Calves" made up the largest category with an average 35.9% all papers. "Dairy Foods" accounted for 28.8%, and "Physiology & Management" for 21.3%. "Genetics & Breeding," with 14.0%, is the smallest and the only area which showed a slight decrease in papers.

Future plans for *Journal of Dairy Science* include a full text CD-ROM

11. (a) G. M. Trout, "Fifty Years of the American Dairy Science Association," *Journal of Dairy Science* 39 (1956): 625–633. (b) G. M. Trout, "The *Journal of Dairy Science* and Its Editors: A Review," *Journal of Dairy Science* 58 (1975): 272–286. (c) G. M. Trout, "The American Dairy Science Association," *Journal of Dairy Science* 64 (1981): 876–899.

database of all sections. In recent years, the full text of the *Journal of Dairy Science* has been stored on magnetic tapes which may facilitate migration to compact disk.

Poultry Science celebrated its 75th year of publishing in 1986. This monthly publication of the Poultry Science Association consists of eight subject areas of research papers, sections titled "Research Notes," and "Association Notes," information on administrative business, and book reviews. A supplementary volume containing abstracts of the annual meetings of the Poultry Science Association and the Southern Poultry Science Society is also published. Two categories of research papers, "Immunology" and "Molecular Biology," were added in 1988 to the existing six sections: "Breeding & Genetics," "Education & Production," "Environment & Health," "Marketing & Production," "Metabolism & Nutrition," and "Physiology & Reproduction." "Marketing & Production" was changed to "Processing & Production" in 1990. Papers for each section are reviewed by the section editor and a board of associate editors. Blind review of submitted papers was instituted in 1988.

The area of "Metabolism & Nutrition" accounted for the greatest number of research papers accepted for publication, 28.9% on average in the three years preceding the addition of the two new areas in 1988, and 32% for 1988–1990. An overall average for each section is difficult to determine for recent publication years since the impact of adding two categories has not yet been established. A total of 38 papers was published in the two new sections for 1988–1990. For 1985–1987, "Education & Production" followed at 16.5%, then "Physiology & Reproduction" at 16.0%, "Environment & Health" at 15.2%, "Marketing & Production" with 12.5%, and, finally, "Breeding & Genetics" with 11.3%.

The total number of papers published increased by 12.6%, from 341 in 1985 to 384 in 1990. A dropoff in the number of accepted papers occurred during 1987–1989, the result of an increase in page charges and a greater number of rejections. The rejection rate was a direct result of concern on the part of many reviewers that a significant number of experiments lacked sufficient controls. An informal survey of Association membership conducted in 1989 addressed the concerns of the reviewers and resulted in the establishment of a new journal, published privately, by those members whose research results had been rejected.[12] A new title began in 1992, *Journal of Applied Poultry Research* but it is too early to determine the impact on *Poultry Science*. Following the survey, an ad hoc committee was formed to make recommendations on guidelines for submission of papers.

---

12. Personal communications with Karl Nestor and Robert Ringer, August 1992.

As a service to PSA members, former journal editor John F. Stephens and others at Ohio State University created a reference retrieval system containing 14,137 citations to papers published in *Poultry Science* from 1941 to 1991. The database is for use on an IBM or compatible computer. Features include menu-driven searching by author, keyword or title word, secondary searches, and the ability to save retrieved records as a separate database. Keywords are those assigned in the journal since 1980. Appropriate keywords were assigned to papers published earlier. The database complete with software is available from the Poultry Science Association, 309 West Clark Street, Champaign, Illinois, 61820.

Table 3.6 compares the number of pages and papers in the research sections of the three association journals for 1990.

Table 3.6. Societal membership and journal data

	Members[a]	Pages	Papers
ASAS	4,588	4,540	491
ADSA	3,200	3,324	397
PSA	3,000	2,344	347

[a]*Encyclopedia of Associations*, 27th ed., 1993.

Fredric Owens reported earlier in this chapter that the number of pages and papers published in *Journal of Animal Science* increased by 44% to 55% over the past ten years. Similarly, the *Journal of Dairy Science* realized an increase of 51.4% in the number of pages and a 52.8% increase in the number of papers published from 1980 to 1990. *Poultry Science* decreased in both the number of pages and papers for the same period, due to an increasing rejection rate of from 17 to 29% over the same ten years. The 29% rejection rate occurred in 1987 concurrent with the peak of reviewers' concerns with the quality of experiments reported in submitted papers. With the restructuring of guidelines for papers to *Poultry Science*, the 1991 figure of 372 papers accepted again returned to a level comparable to that of the 445 of 1980. The average number of papers published annually in *Journal of Animal Science* is 500, averaging 8.7 pages each. In 1991, the *Journal of Dairy Science* published 500 papers, averaging 8.8 pages each. For *Poultry Science*, the average number of pages is 6.7.

4. Statistics and Databanks
in Animal Science

GEORGE R. WIGGANS

Agricultural Research Service, U.S. Department of Agriculture

ROBERT E. McDOWELL

Department of Animal Science, North Carolina State University

Numbers constitute the world's most common language. Animal numbers or kilograms of grains are universally understood. Quantitative statistics are widely employed in the agricultural sector. They serve as a basis for quantifying world food supplies and developing national policies on production, marketing, and world trade, serve as guides to producers on pricing, and are used to monitor health problems for humans and animals.

In animal agriculture, the prediction of future production levels and international trade requires knowledge of historical production of animal populations. Many groups collect data on animals for numerous purposes, from international organizations, most notably the Food and Agricultural Organization (FAO), national governments, to species or breed organizations which use data as part of improvement programs to individual owners and for management purposes. With the advent of computers, records were transferred to electronic databanks. Animal science was an early user of computers and databanks, and remains one of the heaviest in agriculture. The most recent illustration is an advanced computer application meeting at INFORMART in Dallas, Texas, in 1992 with support from the American Farm Bureau, Elanco Products Co., and the U.S. Department of Agriculture. The three day meeting provided twenty-seven papers, plus displays, panels and discussions.[1] Outside government, many organizations maintain data for their own needs, reporting periodically, and in some cases providing data for research.

---

1. *Proceedings of the Advanced Computer Applications in Animal Agriculture*, Feb. 1992, Dallas, Texas (Ithaca, N.Y., ACAAA Conference and Department of Animal Science, Cornell University, 1992).

A. Statistics

The FAO was established in 1946 with its main mission to monitor the world's agriculture and animal production as well to develop estimates of available foods and the nutritional status of humans. The *FAO Production Yearbook*, published annually, has become the main source of statistics used in planning global strategies. It shows livestock numbers, animal product commodities from all reporting countries, numbers of horses, mules, asses, buffaloes, camels, cattle, goats, pigs, sheep, chickens, ducks, and turkeys. It also gives data on certain animal products, such as meat, milk and milk products, wool, hides and skins, and fats.

The World Bank and the International Monetary Fund also have become collectors and users of statistics gathered globally. For instance, a popular annual publication from the World Bank, the *World Bank Atlas*, includes information on human population in all countries and territories: gross national product (GNP) per capita, population growth rate, GNP per capita growth rate, the share of agriculture in gross domestic product (GDP), estimated daily calorie supply per capita, life expectancy, total fertility rate, and literacy rate. These statistics are critical for planning economic strategies. Of almost equal value are the Internal Monetary Fund's statistics, used to guide governments and warn them of overdrafts in trade balances and borrowing.

The U.S. Department of Agriculture and similar organizations in countries of Europe and Oceania collect statistical information on national and international livestock production and marketing. These statistics are vital for producers, marketers, processors and other parties with interest in the animal industries. The summations are issued at brief intervals and/or annually. No official statistics are yet published on the numbers or production of horses, pet animals, domesticated rabbits or minor livestock groups.

In the United States, the Economic Research Service, U.S. Department of Agriculture, uses assembled statistics to conduct economic research in order to provide economic intelligence on the livestock production situation and outlook for producers as related to the national and international economy.

A number of countries now have marketing services to provide market news through the public media to facilitate the marketing and distribution of animal commodities. An example is the Foreign Agricultural Service (FAS) of the U.S. Department of Agriculture, which gathers statistics to monitor the world livestock situation. These data are used to estimate potential export markets for all livestock products. The reports also issue warnings to U.S. producers and exporters about likely sources of competition in foreign markets. These projections are reported to animal producer organizations through FAS's *Circular Series*. For intensive systems of production in poultry and swine, the forecasting can be critical.

The U.S. Department of Agriculture publishes guidelines on developing methods for statistical surveys and how these statistics can be used in estimation procedures.[2]

The gathering of statistics on animal production and diseases is vital to national governments in development of policies and is a necessity to researchers in identifying problems and setting guidelines for improving efficiency of animals. Statistics and their interpretation bring together governments, scientists, and producers. Use of one or more of the computerized abstracting services can be quite useful in identifying some of the many ways that statistics have been used in the fields of animal production and health. Thus regional, national, and global planning relies on agricultural statistics of which animal agriculture is an important part. Prediction of future production levels and flows of international trade require data on historical production and animal populations. The commodities market is driven by forecasts based on production statistics.

B. Use of Data

Statistics of animal numbers and characteristics of animals when accumulated over time can constitute a databank. Development of computers with large storage capacity has become of immense value in animal agriculture. Many are in existence and the number is expanding. For example, all animal and poultry breed societies in the United States have databanks to help their members make breeding selections with an emphasis on economic value.

Producers rely on information from databanks to manage and improve livestock. Knowledge of an animal's reproductive status, production, and health are necessary for effective management on farms. Measurement of productive performance has been important historically. Programs for recording production details, such as the amount of milk produced by a cow, have been initiated in nearly all the developed countries and are now gaining popularity in the developing countries. Milk recording in cattle is most

---

2. (a) USDA, *Hog and Pig Reports: A Handbook on Surveying and Estimating Procedures* (Washington, D.C.: USDA Economics, Statistics and Cooperative Service, ESCS-66, 1979b). (b) USDA, *Cattle Reports: A Handbook on Surveying and Estimating Procedures* (Washington, D.C.: USDA Statistical Reporting Service, ESS-13, 1981). (c) USDA, *Agricultural Statistics Board Catalog: 1990 Releases* (Washington, D.C.: USDA National Agricultural Statistics Service, 1989).

widespread, with some databanks being developed on buffaloes, sheep, goats, and poultry. The first purpose of production recording is to produce information for management decisions. Performance information on a herd or flock provides a basis for effective communication between field agents and producers. A longer-term benefit is to serve as a basis for genetic improvement through selection. With the development of computer capabilities and methods for analysis of data (statistical procedures), the study of populations of animals and implementation of national programs of genetic improvement have become possible. Genetic improvement programs rely on performance records. Through analysis, production is apportioned to genetic and environmental causes. Increased accuracy in analysis has resulted from more completely accounting for the genetic and environmental factors affecting animal performance.

Statistical procedures play a fundamental role in research, and are relied on to determine whether treatment differences can be explained by chance or reflect true differences between the treatments. Modelling biological processes has been an important application of statistical procedures for fifty years. Accurate models of livestock enterprises, or parts of them, allow prediction of consequences of various policies without the expense of field testing.

C. An Exemplary Data Collection Program

The Dairy Herd Improvement (DHI) program in the United States illustrates the organization, development, and functions of a national data collection program. This program was initiated in 1905 to encourage farmers to improve efficiency of their herds. Milk yield and other traits, such as the fat content of milk, were recorded. The methods have been modified and refined many times since the program began. Computers replaced hand calculations in the 1950s and moved onto the farms in the 1980s. Testing of milk samples on the farm was replaced by centralized laboratories using electronic fat, protein and somatic cell testing equipment.

Records from the farms are processed in nine regional United States centers. Completed and in progress lactation records are calculated and returned to the farms within a few days of submission. Lactation information is sent periodically to the U.S. Department of Agriculture. Individual cow lactation records are used to produce national evaluations of sires and cows.

Coordination at the national level is required to ensure uniformity and accuracy of data. This is handled through a twelve-member policy board consisting of five member farmers, a representative from the Purebred

Dairy Cattle Association, one from the National Association of Animal Breeders (representing AI organizations), and two Extension dairy specialists from land-grant universities.

The objectives of DHI are to: (1) provide useful data for dairy farmers to aid in improving efficiency of their operations; (2) maintain uniformity and high integrity in record keeping; and (3) provide data for use in research and education.

The DHI system has successfully included an increasing proportion of farms in the program. Presently, 46% of the dairy cattle in the United States are recorded in DHI programs. A range of programs have been developed to meet the needs of producers. Low cost programs rely on producer collected data. For plans where a DHI employee records the production data, many options are available, including recording only one milking per month AM or PM (AM/PM testing), instead of two or three milkings on test day. To reduce costs, plans with less frequent DHI visits are being investigated. Based on analysis of data, some of these arrangements will become accepted testing plans. The range of programs allows selecting that program which produces the information at the least cost. DHI types of programs in Mexico, Puerto Rico, Columbia, and Taiwan have been the main force in dairy development in these countries.

D. Databanks in Genetic Evaluation

Data are stored to support routine evaluation systems. All genetic evaluation systems depend on animal genealogy information. Breed associations and performance recording agencies collect data and maintain the files. Pedigree information is shared with those doing evaluations. There has been an historical understanding that progeny inherit characteristics from their parents. Mendel's work began the science of modern genetics by determining the genetic mechanisms of inheritance of specific traits. The dilemma of understanding quantitative traits within the framework that Mendel proposed has been a challenge to both animal and plant breeders.

Sewall Wright provided the basis for quantifying relatedness in 1922.[3] He proposed a relationship matrix that indicated the fraction of genes that animals are expected to have in common due to common ancestors. He also laid the groundwork for understanding inbreeding, which may depress pro-

---

3. Sewall Wright, "Coefficients of Inbreeding and Relationship," *American Naturalist* 56 (1922): 330.

duction and fitness traits. His relationship matrix is the basis for current evaluation techniques that use information observed on one animal to predict genetic merit of other animals.

J. L. Lush developed the selection index concept.[4] His insight addressed the problem of differing amounts of information on candidates for selection. Without some accounting for the variability of the information, the most extreme individuals could usually be those with the least information. Selection index provides a mechanism for shrinking estimates of genetic merit based on their variability. His *Animal Breeding Plans* remains an important monograph today.

C. R. Henderson extended selection index concepts mathematically.[5] His mixed model equations allowed simultaneous estimation of fixed effects and prediction of genetic values. This was an advance over the selection index concept in which environmental influences were assumed to be known. Henderson introduced Best Linear Unbiased Prediction (BLUP). This concept has become the basis for genetic evaluation worldwide.

In addition to inventing the mixed model equations that make BLUP computationally feasible for a large class of problems, Henderson developed a simple method to derive the inverse of the numerator relationship matrix.[6] He determined that the inverse could be constructed from a list of animals and their parents, and was much easier to generate than the relationship matrix itself. This rapid method has been the basis of recent implementations of animal models where the animal producing the record is the focus of the model, not her sire as in sire models. The inverse of the relationship matrix makes possible the inclusion of ancestors without records themselves in the equations.

Genetic evaluation is based on the statistical concept of a model that describes the factors affecting yield. The model also specifies the portion of variability ascribed to each factor. A system of equations is constructed and then solved to determine the estimated value of each level of each factor in the model. Over the last forty years with the increase in computer capabilities, models have become more realistic; fewer approximations have been necessary in order to solve the equations. Currently, all relationships among animals can be considered in an evaluation.

4. J. L. Lush, *Animal Breeding Plans*, 3d ed. (Ames: Iowa State College Press, 1945).

5. C. R. Henderson, "Estimation of General, Specific, and Maternal Abilities" (Ph.D. diss., Iowa State University, 1948).

6. C. R. Henderson, "A Simple Method for Computing the Inverse of a Numerator Relationship Matrix Used in Prediction of Breeding Values," *Biometrics* 32 (1976): 69.

E. Genetic Evaluation Procedures

Genetic evaluation efforts have included methods of comparison of animals with contemporaries and parents. A daughter-dam comparison was used in the United States, but suffered in accuracy by failing to account for differing environmental factors affecting production of the daughter and her dam. In 1961, a herdmate comparison was introduced. This procedure compared production of cows to that of other cows milking at the same time. In this way, environmental influences could be considered, but the procedure was less effective in comparison of animals over time and in accounting for a differing genetic level of competition.

Various improvements were made to correct problems thus identified. In 1974, the Modified Contemporary Comparison (MCC) was introduced into the DHI program.[7] This procedure introduced the concept of a fixed genetic base, and accounting for the merit of the competition. The focus was on bull evaluation, but evaluations for cows were computed using the results from bulls. The concept underlying the MCC was to consider the variability of each type of information and combine information appropriately. The MCC was an approximation of BLUP that could be calculated within the existing computer constraints. L. D. Van Vleck and E. J. Pollak[8] and A. E. Freeman[9] provide a more complete history of evaluation procedures.

In 1989, an animal model was adopted for genetic assessments in the DHI program.[10] With this procedure, cows and bulls are evaluated simultaneously, so that the evaluation of each animal can contribute to the evaluation of every other animal. The procedure uses repeated calculation of the evaluations to allow information on one animal to spread to all affected animals. Through this consideration of all relationships, progeny contribute to a cow's evaluation, and the merit of the mates of a bull can be considered when computing his evaluation. Unknown parents are accounted for by forming groups as presented by R. L. Quaas.[11] This procedure gives every animal a parent, either known parent or an unknown parent group.

7. F. N. Dickinson et al., "Procedures Used to Calculate the USDA-DHIA Modified Contemporary Comparison," in *USDA Prod. Res. Rep.* no. 165 (Washington, D.C.: USDA, 1976), p. 18.

8. L. D. Van Vleck and E. J. Pollak, *Sire Evaluation Methods: Past Present, and Future; Proceedings of the National Invitational Workshop on Genetic Improvement of Dairy Cattle, Milwaukee, Wis.* (Ithaca, N.Y.: Cornell University, 1984).

9. A. E. Freeman, "C. R. Henderson Contributions to the Dairy Industry," *Journal of Dairy Science* 74 (1991): 4045.

10. (a) G. R. Wiggans and P. M. VanRaden, *USDA-DHIA Animal Model for Genetic Evaluations* (Washington, D.C.: National Cooperative Dairy Herd Improvement Program Handbook, Fact Sheet H-2, 1989). (b) G. R. Wiggans and P. M. VanRaden, "Method and Effect of Adjustment for Heterogeneous Variance," *Journal of Dairy Science* 74 (1991): 4350.

11. R. L. Quaas, "Additive Genetic Model with Groups and Relationships," *Journal of Dairy Science* 71 (1988): 1338.

Further refinements are under development, including accounting for inbreeding and developing methods to include data from other countries. Inclusion of data from the country where a bull was first evaluated improves his evaluation in the importing country.

In addition to the national evaluation system for milk yield traits, a similar animal model system is applied to type conformation traits. With type there are linear traits that describe specific characteristics of the cow as well as a final composite score. Collection of data on calving difficulty is coordinated by the National Association of Animal Breeders. These data are analyzed with a categorical model where the likelihood of various levels of calving difficulty are predicted. A categorical analysis is the appropriate analysis for data where the observation is an indication of which group the animal was assigned to such as easy or difficult calving. Wiggans provides greater detail on the various genetic evaluation programs in dairy cattle.[12]

Using dairy records to predict the performance of subsequent generations of cows and bulls has been of great economic value. Careful assessments of bulls and cows permit matings among highly selected cows and bulls to produce bulls with a high probability of contribution to breed improvement.

Currently, accurate methods of genetic evaluation for yields of milk have been developed and utilized in nearly all major dairying countries. Use of these procedures has resulted in intense selection of bulls and their wide use in artificial insemination. In the United States, the increase in genetic merit of cows born each successive year is over 160 kg of milk per lactation. This trend appears to be accelerating.

F. Variance Components

When considering how to improve performance of livestock, a fundamental question is if the trait of interest is inherited. No progress can be made genetically on traits that are determined only by environmental factors. Estimation of variance is the process of assigning the observed variation components to genetic and environmental causes. Heritability is the fraction of the variation that is assigned to genetics. Rapid genetic progress can be made in highly heritable traits. Variance component estimation is complicated by the extremely unbalanced nature of field data. Animals are represented in only a few of the environment categories, and bulls have daughters in the same environment as only a few other sires. Henderson

12. G. R. Wiggans, "National Genetic Improvement Programs for Dairy Cattle in the United States," *Journal of Animal Science* 69 (1991): 3853.

provided early methods of variance component estimation that have been widely used.[13] They were an extension of methods appropriate for balanced data. Henderson provides a comprehensive development of BLUP evaluation concepts and variance component estimation methods.[14] Since 1971, restricted maximum likelihood (REML) has gained favor.[15] The Expectation-Maximization algorithm of Dempster et al. has been a widely used method of doing the computations.[16] REML is computationally intensive and iterative. Techniques that would enable REML to be applied to large data sets are being developed. Searle reviewed the development of variance component estimation in 1991.[17]

G. Marker-Assisted Selection

In selection, animals are ranked according to genetic evaluations derived from phenotypic observations on the animal and its relatives. Because heritability is not 100%, evaluations are only approximate. Recent advances in molecular genetic techniques have enabled the determination of characteristics of individual chromosomes. Gelderman et al. provided an early report on the application of markers to milk yield.[18] A collection of probes which match with specific segments of DNA have been developed. With these tools, it can be determined if an animal has a specific sequence of DNA. These probes can be used to develop markers, identifiable sites where differences between animals can be detected. By associating markers with productive characteristics of animals, selection decisions can be assisted using the marker information. Typically the marker is not the gene that controls the traits of interest, but it is located in the same region. This association is called linkage. Because of crossing over, this linkage relationship must be verified in each family. Cowan et al. reported on the prolactin gene and its relationship with milk yield in a particular bull family.[19] Weller, et al.,

13. C. R. Henderson, "Estimation of Variance and Covariance Components," *Biometrics* 9 (1953): 226.

14. C. R. Henderson, *Applications of Linear Models in Animal Breeding* (Guelph, Ont.: University of Guelph, 1984).

15. H. D. Patterson and R. Thompson, "Recovery of Inter-Block Information When Block Sizes Are Unequal," *Biometrika* 58 (1971): 545.

16. A. P. Dempster, N. M. Laird, and D. B. Rubin, "Maximum Likelihood from Incomplete data Via the EM Algorithm," *J. R. Stat. Soc. Ser. B* 30 (1977): 1.

17. S. R. Searle, "C. R. Henderson, the Statistician, and His Contributions to Variance Component Estimation," *Journal of Dairy Science* 74 (1991): 4035–4044.

18. H. Gelderman, U. Peiper, and B. Roth, "Effects of Marker Chromosome Sections on Milk Performance in Cattle," *Theor. Applied Genetics* 70 (1985): 138.

19. C. M. Cowan, M. R. Dentine, R. L. Ax, and L. A. Schuler, "Structural Variation around Prolactin Gene Linked to Quantitative Traits in an Elite Holstein Sire Family," *Theor. Applied Genetics* 79 (1990): 577.

presented a method for determining the merit of chromosomes of bulls through the yields of their granddaughters.[20] This proposal is designed to minimize the amount of DNA analysis necessary.

This is an area of extensive research. Work on identifying the location of genes on human, mouse, and fruit fly chromosomes often can be transferred to the study of farm animals because extensive regions of chromosomes are often similar across species. The developing knowledge of gene location derives largely from the ability to manipulate DNA using probes of arbitrary sequences of base pairs. The most promising view of how these tools can be applied is if individual genes of significant economic effect can be located. Then probes can be developed that are essentially for that particular gene. Using these probes, candidates for selection can be evaluated based on which alleles of these important genes they have as soon as a DNA sample can be obtained. If enough such genes are available, genetic merit of bulls can be predicted without conducting a progeny test. Analysis of daughter performance would serve to test the accuracy of the earlier predictions. Success of progeny testing programs will be improved by screening candidate bulls on several genetic markers before individual genes are identified. Bulls with the positive allele have a higher probability of success. Determination of the economic value of the chromosomal regions associated with markers illustrates the synergism of the chromosomal and field data.

As better techniques are developed to characterize bulls for desired genomes, it will become possible to identify sires which transmit specific traits affecting composition of their daughters' milk which are useful to humans such as immunoglobins to control or alleviate certain health problems. Use of selected, fertilized embryos can be used to create transgenic cows—animals genetically altered to manufacture and secrete in their milk large quantities of scarce and biologically important human proteins.

H. Multiple Ovulation and Embryo Transfer (MOET)

Artificial insemination has enabled individual bulls to have a very large impact on populations. Several bulls have more than 50,000 daughters and one bull has 1.6 million granddaughters. The ability of a single bull to have many daughters has enabled intensive selection on the male side of the pedigree. Recent advances in reproductive technology now make possible

20. J. I. Weller, Y. Kashi, and M. Soller, "Power of Daughter and Granddaughter Designs for Determining Linkage between Marker Loci and Quantitative Trait Loci in Dairy Cattle," *Journal of Dairy Science* 73 (1990): 2525.

collecting many ova from cows and transferring them to recipient cows for gestation. Some cows now have more than 100 progeny carried by recipients.

Multiple ovulation is stimulated by hormone injection. Non-surgical techniques for collection of the ova have been developed. The technique is substantially more expensive than collecting bull semen, but has become widespread, particularly with dams of bulls for progeny testing programs.

A landmark study by F. W. Nicholas and C. Smith showed that rates of genetic progress could be increased substantially through the use of MOET and a nucleus herd where outstanding animals were developed and then their genetic merit transferred to the commercial population.[21] Further work in this area has identified the reduction in generation interval as the primary reason for the increasing rate of improvement. For example, bulls are used extensively based on the performance of their sisters instead of daughters.

Two general types of nucleus herds have been proposed, open and closed. With an open scheme, outstanding animals from the general population may be incorporated into the nucleus herd. This option provides access to some additional outstanding animals, but those animals may have incomplete information. Another category is adult versus juvenile schemes. Juvenile schemes (young animals) have the shortest generational interval. Virgin heifers are superovulated to serve as dams for the next generation. With adult schemes, the animal's own performance is used in the selection decisions with an increase in accuracy at the expense of lengthening the generation interval. In estimating the benefits from MOET schemes, analysis must consider the Bulmer effect which describes the reduction in genetic variation expected with selection.[22]

The lessons of MOET schemes have been adapted to some degree in the progeny test programs of AI organizations. Instead of maintaining a single nucleus herd, the nucleus consists of the progeny from planned matings, both male and female. These animals are the primary breeding population. The lesson on the importance of reducing the generation interval is expressed by including in the sampling program sons of first calf heifers and sons of bulls still awaiting their first evaluation. This situation is considered an open dispersed nucleus system. All systems depend on accurate recording of performances and genealogy.

21. F. W. Nicholas and C. Smith, "Increased Rates of Genetic Change in Dairy Cattle by Embryo Transfer and Splitting," *Anim. Prod.* 36 (1983): 341.

22. M. G. Bulmer, "The Effect of Selection on Genetic Variability," *American Naturalist* 105 (1971): 201.

I. Databanks for Other Species

In many developed countries, breed societies for specialized beef breeds have databanks to help their breeders in traits having economic value. Performance records on sires and cows are used to evaluate growth and maternal ability traits. However, the more extensive nature of beef production systems has made improvement programs more difficult to conduct. In particular, low use of artificial insemination (AI) reduces the benefits possible from genetically superior bulls. There has been a recent increase in the use of AI bulls as sires of bulls, and most bull dams are sired by AI bulls. With this trend, AI is having a significant impact.

There are as yet limited numbers of national genetic databanks for poultry and swine, since large commercial companies are most influential in genetics. In both species intensive systems of developing lines, which are frequently synthetics or composites of conventional breeds or types, have been pursued by individual companies. More controlled environments can be imposed for poultry and swine, thereby reducing the variation among individuals. This allows adequate analysis of data with relatively simple procedures and small populations.

Breed associations for swine in the United States have assembled a database which is having an impact, as are databases in Canada, Norway, Sweden, Denmark, Germany, and France. One focus of these databases is to derive assessments of lines recommended for use as sire and maternal lines.

For a long while in the United States, Random Sample Tests were conducted periodically in poultry from national sampling. In these tests, regressed least square means were determined for pens of birds to estimate genetic superiority. The random tests have been discontinued because of high costs and limited desire of commercial companies to have their lines tested by competitors. There are a number of limited databanks being developed by universities. The majority of these collect records for bird health, and support studies of epidemiology, pathology, parasitology, and immunology.

Goat breeders in the United States, countries of Western Europe, and Cyprus have formed dairy record programs similar to DHI for cattle. Summations of performance are used to encourage individual breeders toward better performance efficiency. Use of artificial insemination is as yet quite limited, therefore, few bucks have daughters in many herds. Since there are no standards for carcasses and recommended slaughter weights, databanks on meat from goats have not been established. There are, however, data on standardized grades for meat of lambs which are used in world trade and general monitoring of trends among breeds.

For wool of sheep and mohair from goats important in world trade, databanks are maintained for use in projections of production and price range. Such data have high value in the main producing countries, particularly Australia and New Zealand.[23] These two countries also have national databases for sheep genetic evaluations.

Most horse breed societies maintain databanks of pedigrees. Additionally, these societies store information on winnings of individuals in shows or races. Records from these databanks are employed from time to time to develop predictions directed toward selective breeding and identification of recessive genes.

Rabbit breeders are gradually developing databanks through breed societies for use in developing guidelines for breed improvement through selections.

For laboratory animals, especially mice and rats, numerous selected lines have been developed. In the United States, the National Institutes of Health, which supports much of the research with laboratory animals, maintains a bibliography on the characteristics of these lines to guide researchers on potential sources of lines or strains most appropriate for their research. This bibliography, along with a similar listing in the United Kingdom, is available through computerized abstracting services such as CABI ABSTRACTS.

Breed societies for pets, principally cats and dogs, collect pedigree information and individual winnings in competition shows or exhibits. The breed society for the Greyhound breed of dogs carefully follows the performance of individuals in races. These records are used for planning matings.

In summary, among the objectives of most databanks on animals are: (1) to enable systematic collection of adequate information to rank animals on traits of interest; (2) to motivate members of breed societies toward goals in both phenotypic and genetic changes for improved performance and durability; and (3) to protect the integrity of breeds through identifying the carriers of undesirable recessive genes. The latter is a secondary focus at present, but artificial insemination and embryo transfer damage to a breed could be quite significant if some males were determined to be carriers after widespread use within a breed.

J. Breed Society Functions

Most breed societies or associations around the world periodically issue herd or studbooks for their members. Management of the data and publica-

---

23. USDA, 1989, *Agricultural Statistics Board Catalog: 1990 Releases.*

tion costs are supported through fees derived from registrations by breeders of their animals. The Shorthorn Breed Society in England has been issuing an annual herdbook for well over 100 years. Some associations in the United States, such as the American Jersey Cattle Club and the Holstein Association, have followed suit since the early 1900s. Prior to computers and performance records, the herdbooks mainly included names of breeders, pedigree information, and listings of animals registered with the society each year. Charles S. Plumb, a professor of animal husbandry at Ohio State University, was instrumental in putting together one of the largest collections of herd or stubooks from around the world. He described this genre of literature and provided extensive listing in a book published in 1930. The Ohio State University Library at that time had 4,150 separate herdbook volumes.[24]

Some of the smaller breed associations still use herdbooks, but most societies have computerized animal registrations and performance records. For example, Holstein breeders may select the Remote Computer Access option for easy access to database information for obtaining records of registrations, transfers or sales to other breeders, lactation records of individual cows, type or confirmation scores, cow and bull Predicted Transmitting Abilities (PTA), name and address of owners, and identification of outstanding individual animals in the breed.

In the United States, twelve of the beef breed associations have formed the Beef Improvement Federation to standardize their procedures and make their databases comparable. Through courtesy or small fees, the breed societies will develop tapes or floppy disks from their databases for use by researchers. With the rapidly increasing interest in preservation of animal germplasm, efforts are being made by FAO and scientists in the United States and Europe to encourage the formation of breed societies in developing countries.

K. Databanks in Animal Health

One of the major missions of the World Health Organization (WHO) and FAO is to monitor diseases of humans (WHO) and animals (FAO), as well as to create awareness of possible zoonosis (transmission from animals to humans). As a collaborative action of FAO/WHO/OIE (Office International

---

24. Charles S. Plumb, *Registry Books on Farm Animals; A Comparative Study* (Columbus; Ohio State University Press, 1930). 306p.

of Epizootics), the *Animal Health Yearbook* is issued annually.[25] Identified diseases are listed for each country. As diseases are determined to occur in particular countries, these are added. Additions of newly identified diseases, change in status, or absence of one or more diseases are used to monitor the extent of diseases. Such information is valuable in accessing problems of certain major epizootic diseases such as foot-and-mouth disease or Aftosa, rinderpest, and African swine fever in animals. Scrutiny of the yearbooks is also quite important in determining barriers for world trade of animal products; for example, the United States only permits fresh or frozen meat imports from countries free of foot-and-mouth disease.

In 1979, the U.S. Department of Agriculture sponsored an international symposium on animal health and disease databanks.[26] The objective was to explore cooperation possibilities and to make plans for computerizing abstracts which could be indexed for searches on the epidemiology, pathology, and recommended treatments that can be useful as diagnostic tools and for therapy. One of the few compilations of animal health databanks resulted from this effort.[27]

The Institut d'Elevage et de Medecine Veterinaire des Pays Tropicaux (IEMVT) at Maisons Alfort, France, has established a large literature collection. Merck & Company, Inc., of the United States also maintains a large bibliographic file for use by their staff in the periodic preparation of *The Merck Veterinary Manual*, a handbook of diagnosis and therapy for veterinarians. Certain United States university veterinary colleges are also building banks of abstracts.

The National Animal Health Monitoring System (NAHMS) is an information system created by the U.S. Department of Agriculture designed to collect, analyze, and report on animal health events for most domestic species in the United States. The system is housed in Fort Collins, Colorado. In this system, a stratified, random sample of producers is selected in participating states. These farms keep daily records of all animal health events and report to a central location for entry into the NAHMS database. From this data, reports are prepared to assist in farm management and help veterinarians in prevention and control. The NAHMS was started in 1989, and its success will depend largely on producer cooperation. The next few years should see much more coordination of materials characterizing diseases and general health disorders for a wide array of animal species.

25. *FAO Animal Health Yearbook* (Rome: FAO/WHO/OIE, 1956 +).

26. USDA, *Proceedings of International Symposium on Animal Health and Disease Data Banks* (Washington, D.C.: 1979 [*USDA Misc. Pub.* no. 1381]).

27. National Agricultural Library, *International Directory of Animal Health and Disease Data Banks* (Washington, D.C.: 1980 [*USDA Misc Publ.* no. 1423]). 93p.

L. Databanks in Germplasm Conservation

With expanding recognition that genetic diversity in domesticated animals and fowl is narrowing and numerous breeds or types are endangered, efforts are increasing to conserve existing types. Animal genetic resources are internationally vital to the United States, since nearly all important agricultural crops and all domestic animal species originated outside the Western hemisphere.

There has been a national plant genetic resources program operating in the United States since 1945. A similar system remains in the developing stage for animals. A national committee of scientists submitted a plan to Congress in 1992 as a proposal for the National Animal Germplasm Program. The proposal encompasses collection of data in the United States and internationally on all domestic animals and fowl.[28]

There are national programs underway in Brazil, Germany, India, Russia, and associated republics. Internationally, FAO has initiated databanks on cattle, buffalo, pigs, sheep, and goats, with emphasis on data collection for indigenous types in various developing countries. All nations are being invited to participate. Methodology for data collection and plans for use were published in 1986.[29] The European Association of Animal Production (EAAP) has underway a databank for the region with emphasis on characterizations of more than 100 breeds or types of livestock and fowl nearing extinction.[30] The objectives of the germplasm data collections are to:

(1) catalog the available genetic resources of the world;
(2) facilitate acquisition and characterization of potentially useful animal germplasm;
(3) ensure genetic variation through preservation of selected stocks; and
(4) facilitate utilization of useful germplasm in research and industry.

Foods, non-food goods, and services of domesticated animals are essential to humans throughout the world. Thus the interdependence between humans and animals is high in most societies and will continue to increase in order to meet the needs of human population growth. Similar to the

28. National Animal Germplasm Program Committee, *National Animal Germplasm Program* (Washington, D.C.: U.S. Dept. of Agriculture, 1991).

29. (a) FAO, *Animal Genetic Resources Information* (Rome: FAO, 1986). (b) FAO, *Animal Genetic Resources Databanks: 1. Computer Systems Study for Regional Databanks* (Rome: FAO, 1986). (c) FAO, *Animal Genetic Resources: 2. Description Lists of Cattle, Buffalo, Pigs, Sheep and Goats* (Rome: FAO, 1986).

30. C. Simon, *Data Banks and the Conservation Policy; Proceedings of the 4th World Congress on Genetics Applied to Livestock Production* (Edinburgh: 1990).

situation in plants, the genetic bases are seriously narrowing in the developed countries.

Among the major focuses in animal research of the future will be gene mapping to determine, among other things, those breeds or types with genetic resistance to certain diseases. The identified genetic resistance of the N'Dama cattle, native to the wet areas of West Africa, to the disease trypanosomiases transmitted by the tsetse fly represents an example which will be important for future livestock production in Africa. Data collections are critical to identifying genetic resources for animals; therefore, all those involved with animal agriculture are strongly encouraged to participate in creating international germplasm databanks. Marker-Assisted Selection and Multiple Ovulation and Embryo Transfer are potential beneficiaries of international databanks.

M. Computerized Abstract for Animal Science and Industry

Internationally, each country with a genetic evaluation program has one or more agencies that collect, maintain, and analyze data. Results from these evaluations for a variety of livestock species are printed and distributed. These reports can be acquired for information and guidance in developing research programs.

Before attempting to establish databanks on animal performance, particularly for research or student training, it is recommended that one or more of the computerized abstract collections be surveyed to understand the concepts of data types and some of the analytical methods available.

In Africa, scientists can, for example, contact the International Livestock Center for Africa (ILCA) and request to become a participant in the Selective Dissemination of Information (SDI service) provided by ILCA. Lists of keywords and other indicators of research interest of users are the keys to accessing information stored in the system. The ILCA database of bibliographic data comes directly from CABI and AGRIS database tapes, coupled with data generated by ILCA's research and that gathered from most countries of Africa. Printouts of information befitting the profile of individuals is made quarterly and forwarded to SDI participants.

Computerized abstracts found most useful in animal science are described in Table 4.1.

Table 4.1. Most useful computerized indexes and abstracting services in animal science

	Subject	Producer
Agribusiness U.S.A. Database	Agricultural industry	Pioneer Hi-Bred International, Inc.
AGRICOLA	Agriculture, food, nutrition (emphasis on U.S. agriculture; 1.6 million citations)	U.S. Dept. of Agriculture, National Agricultural Library
AGRINDEX: AGRIS, International Info System for Agricultural Sciences and Technology	Agriculture (1.3 million citations, some abstracts; worldwide on all aspects of agriculture; accumulates 10,000 records per month)	Food and Agriculture Organization of the United Nations
BIOSIS: Biosciences Information Services	Worldwide literature of research in life sciences (plant and animal)	Biological Abstracts
CABI ABSTRACTS: Animal Breeding Abstracts Dairy Science Abstracts Nutrition Abstracts, B.	Reports of research (horses, cattle, buffalo, sheep, goats, pigs, fur bearers, laboratory mammals, other mammals, poultry and other birds, fish and invertebrates in aquaculture, general and theoretical genetics and general reproduction; best for most aspects of animal production)	Commonwealth Bureau of Animal Breeding and Genetics: International Information Services
CRIS (CRIS/USDA): Current Research Information System	Agriculture research in progress	U.S. Dept. of Agriculture, Cooperative States Research Service
Dissertation Abstracts International	Thesis dissertations (citations with abstracts; international since 1961; adds 2,500 records per month)	UMI International
ILCA: International Livestock Centre for Africa	African livestock, forage agronomy, milk and meat processing, livestock policy	International Livestock Centre for Africa
Life Sciences Collection	Life sciences (citations with abstracts; worldwide plant and animal agriculture)	Cambridge Scientific Abstracts
On Line Service: DIALOG	U.S. literature on the business of agriculture; numerous files	DIALOG Information Services, Inc.

5. Citation Analysis and Core Lists of Primary Monographs, Post-1950

WALLACE C. OLSEN

Mann Library, Cornell University

Citation counting and analyses have been used extensively in libraries and scholarship to answer questions or to observe patterns and trends in literature use. Beginning in the 1950s, citation analysis grew dramatically as a result of two major thrusts: (1) the implementation of computing storage and speeds in compilation and analysis, and (2) publication of immense citation databases, *Science Citation Index* and the *Social Science Citation Index*,[1] which index the citations in articles in approximately 5,500 journals. Bibliometric techniques have been used in a variety of applications within the publishing, library, and scholarly communities. They have proven useful in measuring research and education productivity, in determining a scholar's output and impact, and as indicators of social and economic growth.

Readers are referred to a discussion of citation analysis and its applications in the agricultural sciences in a recent publication by the author.[2] To further pursue citation analysis, readers are directed to a comprehensive collection of articles edited by Christine L. Borgman, on bibliometric methods for the study of scholarly communication.[3]

A structured citation database is necessary from which correlations, data, and conclusions can be obtained. This study began by examining the Institute for Scientific Information's print and online tools.[4] It was clear upon

---

1. *Science Citation Index* and *Social Science Citation Index* are products of the Institute for Scientific Information, Philadelphia.

2. Wallace C. Olsen, *Agricultural Economics and Rural Sociology: The Contemporary Core Literature* (Ithaca, N.Y.: Cornell University Press, 1991). 356p.

3. Christine L. Borgman, ed., *Scholarly Communication and Bibliometrics* (Newbury Park, Calif., and London: Sage Publications, 1990). 363p.

4. *Science Citation Index.*

examination, however, that these publications did not adequately include the literature of animal science and, therefore, had limited use. Some useful data from ISI sources concerning the journal literature will be given in the chapter following. One problem with the ISI databases is that they deal with the research literature. Citations at the ends of largely research articles are reflective of the point of view and approach of a researcher. This may or may not reflect the literature used by an educator or applications practitioner, particularly in the agricultural sciences. It was necessary to establish another path for identification of titles and for quantifying what we wanted to know. Findings then had to be related to other studies or databases wherever valid.

A. Purpose and Methods

The primary aim of the study reported here was to determine the core literature of animal science and health of the past forty years which still has impact in academic teaching and research today. A further aim was to determine the relative rank and merit of the titles for the worldwide academic community, but also for the developing or Third World countries if this proved different. This focus required a careful analysis of the tools and citation analysis methods to determine the core literature. As indicated earlier, the research literature analyses are relatively numerous and useful, but they do not measure that literature of greatest value to advanced students and beginning researchers. The aim of this study was to identify the literature in the middle of a continuum from undergraduate college education, through advanced and graduate studies, to post-doctoral research. There is, of course, a large overlap from the center of the continuum into undergraduate and advanced research literature.

A variety of literature tools exist to aid in this process such as specialty abstracting tools, *Animal Breeding Abstracts* being a good illustration.[5] These tools present comparison problems caused by differing subject definitions and groupings, time periods, and formats of coverage. Literature studies already published offer some help, but they are few and tend to concern themselves with journals only, while the aim here was to examine all formats.

Some qualitative literature evaluations by professionals in animal science and health have been done. These are largely literature reviews, but also

5. *Animal Breeding Abstracts* published from 1916 by Commonwealth Agricultural Bureaux International.

selective readings brought together in book form, reserve readings used in academic departments as adjuncts to the classroom, and landmark animal science monographs. This overview literature most clearly met the aims of the project as a valid method to establish a base and to identify literature use-patterns. Overview literature incorporates two desired quality factors: the works are classics in their own right, and they are peer-reviewed. As we surveyed the citations to literature in many monographs and landmark works, it became clear that animal scientists are nearly as closely tied to their literature and citation justification as are the agricultural economists to theirs.

Citation analysis has pitfalls in methods and applications and must be carefully executed within different disciplines, by databases used, and by time periods. These are summarized and discussed in a previous work.[6] Potential problems can be eliminated or minimized through a variety of techniques, some statistical, some empirical. An extensive knowledge of the literature of the field can obviate false starts and misdirection.

An effort was made to locate those monographs and literature reviews which best fit established criteria to eliminate possible skews. This included adequate coverage of different dates of publication, subject scope to match the major areas of animal science in the past forty years, and geographic distribution of publications or authors. Attention was also paid to publishing organizations with heavy influence and credibility in the discipline. This Core Agricultural Literature Project had a particular interest in determining if the developed country literature was oriented differently than that for the Third World. Therefore, this bias was included for the purposes of comparison of these two groups. In this regard, the subject coverage for the two communities could not match since the developed countries generally exclude the clinical or veterinary aspect of the subject from animal science. In the Third World, academic departments of animal science, diseases, and veterinary medicine are merged as one operation for education and research. Therefore, for Third World applications, veterinary literature had to be included in the analysis along with the standard animal science literature. This expanded the scope of the work extensively and resulted in a larger core of monographs for the Third World than animal science monographs for developed countries.

The Core Agricultural Literature Project created a Steering Committee to guide and counsel the project efforts. One of the tasks of this group was to aid in determining the source documents to be used for analysis. The Steering Committee members were:

6. Olsen, *Agricultural Economics and Rural Sociology*, Chapter 4.

Donald M. Kinsman
  University of Connecticut
  Storrs, Connecticut

P. V. Malven
  Purdue University
  West Lafayette, Indiana

Robert E. McDowell
  North Carolina State University
  Raleigh, North Carolina

Linda Sametz de Walerstein
  Universidad Nacional Autonoma
  de Mexico, Mexico City

Richard Warner
  Cornell University
  Ithaca, New York

Nineteen monographic works were identified and approved by the Steering Committee for citation analysis, along with twenty-five journal literature reviews. The project was fortunate to have an editor of literature reviews for *Animal Breeding Abstracts* as a Steering Committee member.

Sources of Citations Analyzed in Animal Science and Health

Asterisked items (*) were not analyzed, but monographs were extracted for inclusion in lists for evaluation.

Monographs

American Society of Animal Science. *Current Concepts of Animal Growth, Vol. I; A Symposium held in Conjunction with the 74th Annual Meeting of ASAS, 1982, University of Guelph.* Champaign, Ill.; ASAS, 1985. (Journal of Animal Science, Vol. 61, Supp. 2)

*Asociacion Mexicana de Educacion Agricola Superior. *Bibliographifia Basica para las Instituciones de Educacion Agricola Superior.* Montecillos, Mexico; Colegio de Postgraduados, 1986. 394p. Section on animal science and health with 335 valid monograph titles were examined and some titles extracted for evaluation.

*Bogart, Ralph, and Robert E. Taylor. *Scientific Farm Animal Production.* 2d ed. Minneapolis; Burgess Pub. Co., 1983. 415p.

*Bundy, Clarence, Ronald V. Diggins and Virgil W. Christensen. *Livestock and Poultry Production.* 5th ed. Englewood Cliffs, N.J.; Prentice-Hall, 1982. (1st ed., 1954.)

Butterworth, Martyn H. *Beef Cattle Nutrition and Tropical Pastures.* London and New York; Longman, 1985. 489p.

*Carles, Alan B. *Sheep Production in the Tropics.* Oxford and New York; Oxford University Press, 1983. 213p.

Child, R. Dennis, and Evert K. Byington, eds. *Potential of the World's Forages for

Ruminant Animal Production. 2d ed. Morrilton, Ark.; Winrock International Livestock Research and Training Center, May 1981. 107p.

Cole, D. J. A., and W. Haresign, eds. *Recent Developments in Poultry Nutrition*. London; Butterworths, 1989. 344p.

Conrad, H. Russell. *NFIA Literature Review on Iron in Animal and Poultry Nutrition: Iron in Ruminant Nutrition*. West Des Moines, Iowa; National Feed Ingredients Assoc., 1980. 31p.

Crotty, Raymond. *Cattle, Economics and Development*. Farnham Royal, U.K.; Commonwealth Agricultural Bureaux, 1980. 253p.

Danfaer, Allan. *A Dynamic Model of Nutrient Digestion and Metabolism in Lactating Dairy Cows* = En dynamisk model af naeringstoffernes fordojelse og omsoetning hos malkekoer. Mit dansk sammendrag. Copenhagen; Trykt i Frederiksberg Bogtrykkeri, 1990. 511p. (Beretning fra Statens Husdryrbrugsforsog no. 671; Report from the National Institute of Animal Science, Denmark)

*Ensminger, M. E. *Animal Science*. 8th ed. Danville, Ill.; Interstate Printers & Publishers, 1983. (1st ed., 1950.)

*Gibbs, Mike. *Keyguide to Information Sources in Veterinary Medicine*. London and New York; Mansell Pub., 1990. 459p.

Hammond, John, ed. *Progress in the Physiology of Farm Animals*. London; Butterworths Scientific Pub., 1954–1957. 3 vols. 9 articles analyzed from vols. 1 and 3.

Haresign, W., and D. J. A. Cole, eds. *Recent Advances in Animal Nutrition, 1988*. London and Boston; Butterworths, 1989. 250p.

International Livestock Centre for Africa. *Livestock Systems Research Manual, Vol. 1: Description and Diagnosis of Livestock Production Systems*. Addis Ababa, Ethiopia; ILCA, 1990. Various paging.

Jainudeen, M. R., and A. R. Omar, eds. 1st ed. *Animal Production and Health in the Tropics; Proceedings, 1st Asian-Australian Animal Science Congress*, Serdang, Sept. 1980, Serdang, Selangor; Penerbit Universiti Pertanian Malaysia, 1982. 482p.

Lawrie, Ralson, ed. *Developments in Meat Science-4*. London and New York; Elsevier Applied Science, 1988. 367p.

Nixey, C., and T. C. Grey, eds. *Recent Advances in Turkey Science; Papers from the 21st Poultry Science Symposium, Harper Adams Agricultural College, Newport, Shropshire, 1987*. London, etc.; Butterworths, 1989. 373p. (Poultry Science Symposium no. 21)

Pond, W. G., and J. H. Maner. *Swine Production and Nutrition*. Westport, Conn.; Avi Pub. Co., 1984. 731p.

Robards, G. E., and R. G. Packham, eds. *Feed Information and Animal Production; Proceeding of the 2d Symposium on the International Network of Feed Information Centres*. Farnham Royal, U.K., and Blacktown, N.S.W., Australia; Commonwealth Agricultural Bureaux and INFIC, 1983. 516p.

Simpson, James R., and Phylo Evangelou, eds. *Livestock Development in Subsaharan Africa: Constraints, Prospects, Policy*. Boulder, Colo.; Westview Press, 1984. 407p.

Smith, A. J., and R. G. Gunn, eds. *Intensive Animal Production in Developing Countries; Proceedings of a Symposium organized by the British Society of Ani-

mal Production, Harrogate, Nov. 1979. Surrey, U.K.; British Society of Animal Production, Thames Ditton, 1981. 481p. (Occasional Publications of BSAP)
*Stufflebeam, Charles E. *Principles of Animal Agriculture*. Englewood Cliffs, N.J.; Prentice-Hall, 1983. 464p.
Verde, Luis S., and Angel Fernandez, eds. *World Conference on Animal Production, 4th*, Buenos Aires, Argentina, Aug. 1978. *Memorias* . . . Buenos Aires; Asociacion Argentina de Produccion Animal, 1980. 2 vols. 724p.
Yousef, Mohamed K., ed. *Animal Production in the Tropics*. Proceedings of a Symposium, Feb. 1981, University of Gezira, Sudan. (200 scientists from 20 countries on 4 continents). New York; Praeger Scientific, 1982. 376p. 24 papers.

Journal Articles

Isaksson, Arni. Salmon Ranching: A World Review. *Aquaculture*, Vol. 75 (1988) 1–33.
Animal Breeding Abstracts. The following literature reviews were analyzed.
>   Vol. 57 (10) 1989. O. L. Bondoc, C. Smith and J. P. Gibson. A Review of Breeding Strategies for Genetic Improvement of Dairy Cattle in Developing Countries.
>   Vol. 57 (7 & 8) 1989. C. S. Galina and G. H. Arthur. Review of Cattle Reproduction in the Tropics. Part 1: Puberty and Age at First Calving. Part 2: Parturition and Calving Intervals.
>   Vol. 56 (11) 1988. A. K. Sheridan. Agreement between Estimated and Realised Genetic Parameters.
>   Vol. 56 (6) 1988. J. Ruane. Review of the Use of Embryo Transfer in the Genetic Improvement of Dairy Cattle.
>   Vol. 56 (2 & 3) 1988. R. A. Mrode. Selection Experiments in Beef Cattle. Part 1: A Review of Design and Analysis. Part 2: A Review Responses and Correlated Responses.
>   Vol. 54 (12) 1986. F. D. Brien. A Review of the Genetic and Physiological Relationships Between Growth and Reproduction in Mammals.
>   Vol. 53 (3) 1985. E. A. Tolley, D. R. Notter and T. J. Marlowe. A Review of the Inheritance of Racing Performance in Horses.
>   Vol. 53 (1) 1985. R. A. Sutherland, A. J. Webb and J. W. B. King. A Survey of World Pig Breeds and Comparisons.
>   Vol. 52 (10) 1984. E. B. Burnside, A. E. McClintock and K. Hammond. Type, Production and Longevity in Dairy Cattle: A Review.
>   Vol. 52 (7) 1984. L. G. Butler and W. M. C. Maxwell. A Review of the Efficiency of Conversion of Feed into Wool.
>   Vol. 52 (5) 1984. W. R. Lamberson and D. L. Thomas. Effects of Inbreeding in Sheep: A Review.
>   Vol. 51 (2) 1983. J. C. McCarthy and P. B. Siegel. A Review of Genetical and Physiological Effects of Selection in Meat-Type Poultry.
>   Vol. 49 (7) 1981. C. J. Thwaites. Development of Ultrasonic Techniques for Pregnancy Diagnosis in the Ewe.

Vol. 49 (3) 1981. A. K. Sheridan. Crossbreeding and Heterosis.

Vol. 48 (12) 1980. E. J. Warwick. Effect of Genetic Factors on the Nutrient composition of Animal Products.

Critical Reviews in Poultry Biology. Vol. 1, no. 1 (1987). Edited by Rodney R. Dietert. 269p. (Two articles analyzed; by Gordon Scanes and Simon H. Shane.

Journal of Animal Science, Vol. 57 (Suppl. 2) 1983: Presentations at the General Session of the 75th Annual Meeting of the American Society of Animal Science.

H. F. Hintz and E. L. Squires. Equine Reproduction and Nutrition: Recent Developments and Opportunities for Future Research. pp. 58–74.

R. T. Berg and L.E. Walters. The Meat Animal: Changes and Challenges. pp. 133–146.

D. R. Ames and D. E. Ray. Environmental Manipulation to Improve Animal Productivity. pp. 209–220.

J. P. Fontenot, L. W. Smith and A. L. Sutton. Alternative Utilization of Animal Wastes. pp. 221–233.

S. E. Curtis and K. A. Houpt. Animal Ethology: Its Emergence in Animal Science. pp. 234–247.

G. E. Dickerson and R. L. Willham. Quantitative Genetic Engineering of More Efficient Animal Production. pp. 248–264.

A. H. Trenkle and D. N. Marple. Growth and Development of Meat Animals.

D. H. Baker and V. C. Speer. Protein-Amino Acid Nutrition of Nonruminant Animals with Emphasis on the Pig: Past, Present and Future. pp. 284–299.

R. W. Seerley and R. C. Ewan. An Overview of Energy Utilization in Swine Nutrition. pp. 300–314.

E. R. Miller and E. T. Kornegay. Mineral and Vitamin Nutrition of Swine. pp. 315–329.

P. J. Dziuk and R. A. Bellows. Management of Reproduction of Beef Cattle, Sheep and Pigs. pp. 355– 379.

R. P. Amann and B. D. Schanbacher. Physiology of Male Reproduction. pp. 380–403.

W. Hansel and E. M. Convey. Physiology of the Estrous Cycle. pp. 404–424.

F. W. Bazer and N. L. First. Pregnancy and Parturition. pp. 425–460.

R. L. Baldwin and M. J. Allison. Rumen Metabolism. pp. 461–477.

W. N. Garrett and D. E. Johnson. Nutritional Energetics of Ruminants. pp. 478–497.

F. N. Owens and W. G. Bergen. Nitrogen Metabolism of Ruminant Animals: Historical Perspective, Current Understanding and Future Implications. pp. 498–518.

C. B. Ammerman and R. D. Goodrich. Advances in Mineral Nutrition in Ruminants. pp. 519–533.

R. L. Reid and T. J. Klopfenstein. Forages and Crop Residues: Quality Evaluation and Systems of Utilization.

Journal of Dairy Science, 1989; Vol. 72

Symposium: Interactions of Nutrition and Reproduction. pp. 747–814. Three papers by six authors.

Symposium: Genetics of Disease Resistance. pp. 1313–1362. Three papers by four authors.

Symposium: Cytogenetics and Cell Biology: Chromosome Preparation and High Resolution Banding Techniques; A Review, by Mogens Ronne. pp. 1363–1377.
Symposium: Mammary Function During Involution: Approaches to the Manipulation of Mammary Involution, by S. P. Oliver and L. M. Sordillo. pp. 1647–1678.
Symposium: Reproductive Immunology. pp. 3353–3380. Three papers by eight authors.
Journal of Dairy Science, 1988; Vol. 71.
Symposium: Health Problems in the Periparturient Cow. pp. 2557–2606. Three paper by six authors.
Symposium: Problems of Pathogenic Bacteria in the Dairy Industry.
Pathogenic Bacteria in Milk—A Review, by P. C. Vasavada. pp. 2809–2816.
Industry Response to the Problems of Pathogenic Bacteria, by T. C. Everson. pp. 2820–2929.
Journal of Dairy Science, Vol. 64(6) June 1981. On the occasion of the American Dairy Science Association: The Third Twenty-Five Years, 1957–1981. 26 of the 53 papers were citation analyzed.

B. Compilation and Citation Analysis

The 25,533 citations in these overview and literature publications were systematically analyzed and the following data gathered:

Title of publication;
Date of publication;
Format of publication (e.g., journal or monograph);
Category of publisher (e.g., commercial press, university, government).

During this process early in the study, the titles of monographs were noted and entered into a computerized list. Each time the same monograph or a chapter in it was cited, a tally was made for that title. Similarly, each time a journal or report series was cited, a tally was made for it. The end result is a systematic count of which journals, report series, and monographs were cited and the numbers of times. Additional select data were gathered which provide the basis for some analysis in this and the following chapter.

Before we examine the results, some definitions must be understood. Distinctions among journals, serial works, and monographs are necessary. Series issues, short works, and books were treated as monographs when they were cited as distinct works with an author or editor, when a title was distinctive, and when the item was complete in itself. Therefore, a work such as an *FAO Animal Production and Health Paper* in which the subject was complete in the issue and distinct from the next issue in the series was counted and identified as a monograph. The same was true of proceedings volumes with distinctive titles which varied from one year to the next. Those with no distinct titles or special subject focus were counted as journals. Journals follow the pattern of having several articles on different and very specific subjects which are usually only a few pages long. Chapters in books were counted as monographic titles. These definitions worked well since they followed the citation patterns of animal science authors.

In the compilation process select materials were excluded:

(1) Very short monographs, fifty pages or fewer, which were cited only once.
(2) Country, State, or Provisional documents of brief pagination, often highly specialized and site specific.
(3) Select, esoteric works when in a difficult to read language, or when very limited in geographic scope.
(4) Specialized geographic materials when not in a national or international context, and which got cited only once.
(5) Early background, technique, and statistical working tools. Some works of this type were kept in the lists based on the number of times cited.
(6) Early editions were combined with the latest edition although information is usually given on both.

These analyses offered some overall patterns of publishing which are briefly noted here.

Format of Literature Cited in Analysis

The purpose of an article or book dictates the nature of the literature cited. Therefore, a journal article reporting the results of research will tend to cite the research literature, supporting methodologies, and overview earlier works. As mentioned, this study has attempted to identify advanced university instructional literature plus the basic research literature. The choice of the literature which was analyzed had to be systematically made. Much of the literature and many state-of-the-art reviews analyzed from the journals are heavily oriented toward latest developments and current research. It is logical to expect citation differences between this journal corpus and that of the monographs. The diversity, however, is not great.

The journal literature cited in both groups ranged from 72.3% in the monographs, to 80.6% in the journals. Citations from the two sources average to 75.0% to journals, 24.0% to monographs, and 1.0% to dissertations. This is very different than the literature percentages from citation analysis in the two earlier studies of this project.[7] Variations are shown in Table 5.1

7. Ibid., p. 60; and Carl Hall and Wallace C. Olsen, eds., *The Literature of Agricultural Engineering* (Ithaca, N.Y.: Cornell University Press, 1992).

Table 5.1. Literature formats of citations analyzed in journals and monographs

	% to journals	% to monographs	% to dissertations, patents, standards
Agricultural Economics and Rural Sociology	54.8%	43.5%	1.7%
Agricultural Engineering	58.1	38.2	3.7
Animal Science and Health	75.0	24.0	1.0

and Figure 5.1. Total citations from journal source documents were 32.6% of all citations analyzed.

Technical report series where each report is on a specific subject and complete in that issue were counted as monographs since these individual items are actually very small monographs. They are put in a report series for convenience of publishing, storage, and distribution. Therefore, the monographs may be subdivided into reports in series and more traditional monographs. These reports amounted to 18.1% of all monographs cited (18.8% in monographic source documents and 16.2% in journal source documents). Reports amount to only 4.4% of the total 25,533 citations analyzed. Their influence is greater than dissertations at 1.0% of all citations.

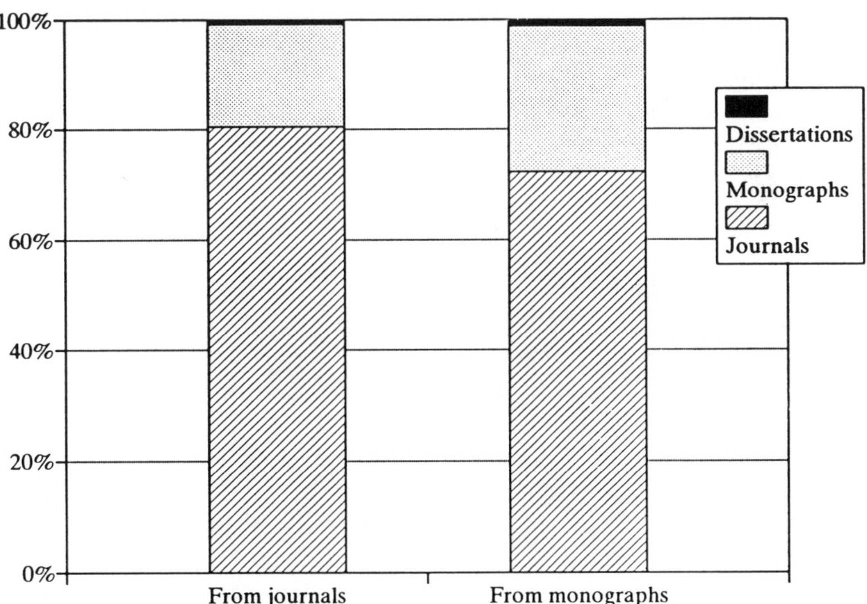

Figure 5.1. Literature formats of citations analyzed in journals and monographs.

C. Monograph Peer Evaluation and Tabulations

The monograph list compiled by citation analyses was examined by the Steering Committee members prior to being sent for peer evaluation. Two animal scientists with extensive experience in developing countries were also asked to look at the list and determine which titles had application for the Third World. Primary feedback on Third World appropriateness came from Facultad de Medicina Veterinaria y Zootecnia, Universidad Nacional Autonoma de Mexico in Mexico City. This assistance continued throughout the process of evaluation with the coordination of the librarian of the university, Linda Sametz de Walerstein, a member of the Steering Committee.

These processes resulted in:

(1) Breaking the master list into two portions, one for the developed countries and a second for the Third World nations. There was extensive overlap between the two.
(2) A developed countries list that included nearly 1,500 titles. Since the next step was to have these titles ranked by animal scientists, the Steering Committee felt that evaluations would be unrealistic unless the titles were placed into subject groups and distributed to specialists in those subjects. This resulted in six subject lists using the basic categories of the *Journal of Animal Science* with an additional general category. The first subject list was sent to all reviewers along with the appropriate list for their subject specialty. Lists were issued in these categories:
    (a) General Agriculture and Animal Science, International Development, Economics, and Animal Welfare;
    (b) Applied Animal Science, Production, Management, and Environment;
    (c) Breeds and Genetics, Reproduction, Behavior, and Ethology;
    (d) Anatomy and Physiology, Growth Biology, and Meat Science;
    (e) Nutrition, Metabolism, Feeds and Feeding;
    (f) Diseases, Pharmacology, Toxicology, and Medicine.

These six lists for developed countries went through several iterations. Titles were dropped and added upon the recommendation of reviewers as well as through the citation analysis process. Approximately 1,500 monograph titles were evaluated in the developed countries list, of which 959 made the final compilation.

In a similar manner a maximum of 1,800 monographs were evaluated in the Third World listing which resulted in a core of 1,033. Instructions to the reviewers carefully discussed the aim of identifying monographs of academic and instructional value for Third World institutions, or those which should be represented in a university library in the developed world. This is a rejection rate of 43% for Third World monographs and 36.5% for developed countries titles.

The rejected titles tended to fall into categories: (1) the work is outdated, although it may have been very good twenty or thirty years before; (2) the language is too difficult for scientists to handle easily, therefore the work is less well known or used than others; (3) the subject matter is acceptable, but the approach is arcane or too application-oriented. Here are some representative titles which did not make the core listing:

Dent, J. B., and J. R. Anderson. Systems Analysis in Agricultural Management. Sydney and New York; J. Wiley, 1971. 394p.

Eibl-Eibesfeldt, Irenaus. The Biology of Peace and War: Men, Animals, and Aggression . . . trans. by Eric Mosbacher. New York; Viking Press, 1979. 294p. (Translation of Krieg und Frieden aus der Sicht der Verhaltensforschung.)

Ewer, T. K. Practical Animal Husbandry. Bristol, U.K., and Littleton, Mass.; Wright Scientechnica, 1982. 257p.

Falesi, Italo C. Solos da Rodovia Transamaz Udio Falesi. Apresentado no Seminoario Internacionales. Bel ria Donorte; 1972. 196p. (Summary in Portuguese and English.)

Food and Agriculture Organization. East African Livestock Survey; Regional: Kenya, Tanzania, Uganda. Rome; United Nations Development Program and FAO, 1967. 3 vols. (FAO/SF no. 21/Reg.)

Food and Agriculture Organization. FAO Agricultural Commodity Projections to 1990. Rome; FAO, 1986. 212p. (FAO Economic and Social Development Paper no. 61)

Food and Agriculture Organization, International Expert Consultation. Dairy Cattle Breeding in the Humid Tropics, 2d, 1979, Hissar, India; Proceedings. . . . Hissar, India; Haryana Agricultural University, 1980. 301p.

Fowler, Stewart H. Beef Production in the South. Modified ed. Danville, Ill.; Interstate, 1979. 934p. (1st ed., 1969. 959p.)

Fox, Michael W. Abnormal Behavior in Animals. Philadelphia; Saunders, 1968. 563p.

Geist, Valerius, and Fritz R. Walther, eds. The Behaviour of Ungulates and Its Relation to Management; Papers of an International Symposium, Nov. 1971. Morges, Switzerland; International Union for Conservation of Nature and Natural Resources, 1974. 2 vols.

Gilliam, Henry C. U.S. Beef Cow-Calf Industry. Washington, D.C.; U.S. Dept. of Agriculture, Economic Research Service, 1984. 60p. (Agricultural Economic Report no. 515)

Golosov, I. M. Mikroklimat Zhivotnovodeheskikh Ferm (Microclimate of the Stock-Raising Farm). Leningrad; Lenizdat, 1974. 118p. (In Russian.)

Lillie, Robert J. Air Pollutants Affecting the Performance of Domestic Animals: A Literature Review. Washington, D.C.; U.S. Dept. of Agriculture, Agricultural Research Service, 1972. 109p. (Revised from 1970 issue.) (USDA Agriculture Handbook no. 380)

Following are the names of reviewers for each type of list.

Developed Countries Animal Science and Health Monograph Reviewers

Jack L. Albright
  Purdue University
F. R. Allaire
  Ohio State University
R. L. Baldwin
  University of California, Davis
Fuller W. Bazer
  University of Florida
J. Boza
  Universidad de Granada
  Spain
Peter J. Brumby
  Waihi, New Zealand
Ted Burnside
  University of Guelph, Canada
Carl E. Coppock
  Texas A & M University
Stanley Curtis
  Pennsylvania State University
Robert T. Duby
  University of Massachusetts,
  Amherst
Zybigniew Duda
  Agriculture University of Wroclaw
  Poland
Dr. and Mrs. Roy S. Emery
  Michigan State University
Gustavo Garcia Delgado
  Universidad Nacional Autonoma de
  Mexico
Upson Garrigus
  University of Illinois
Mike Gibbs
  Hertfordshire, England
Richard D. Goodrich
  University of Minnesota
Ingemar Hansson
  Swedish University of
  Agricultural Sciences
Kálmán Incze
  Hungarian Meat Research Institute
  Budapest
E. Keith Inskeep
  West Virginia University
Richard H. Jacobson
  Cornell University

Donald M. Kinsman
  University of Connecticut
Robert E. McDowell
  North Carolina State University
Travis McGuire
  Washington State University
Elizabeth Oltenacu
  Cornell University
Arthur L. Pope
  University of Wisconsin, Madison
R. L. Preston
  Texas Tech University
W. R. Pritchard
  University of California, Davis
Eero Puolanne
  University of Helsinki, Finland
T. S. Rumsey
  Agricultural Research Service
  U.S. Dept. of Agriculture, Nebraska
John Sabine
  Waite Agricultural Research Institute
  Glen Osmond, South Australia
Dieter Schams
  Technical University of Munich
  Germany
Robert Scholtens
  University of Tennessee
G. Stanley Smith
  New Mexico State University
Watse Sybesma
  Research Institute for Animal
  Production, Netherlands
I. Tasaki
  Nagoya University, Japan
Derek Tribe
  Australian Academy of
  Technological Sciences &
  Engineering
  Parkville, Victoria
W. van der Hel,
  with the assistance of
  Profs. Wiepkema and Zwart
  Wageningen Agricultural University
  Netherlands
Joint Evaluations
Animal and Dairy Science Research

Institute, Republic of South Africa:
  Raymund Naude
  J. H. Hofmeyer
  E. H. Kemm
  J. J. Joubert
Universidad Nacional Autonoma de
  Mexico:
    Rosa Paramo
    Humberto Troncoso
    Hector Sumano
    Luis Zarco
    Rene Rosiles

University of Veterinary Sciences,
  Budapest, Hungary; coordinated by
  Mary Cserey, Central Library:
    Geza Biro
    Simon Ference
    Sandor Fekete
    Ferenc Hajos
    Ference Karsai
    Tibor Kassai
    P. Rafai
    Tuboly Sandor

Third World Animal Science and Health Monograph Reviewers

Kwaku Agyemang
  International Trypanotolerance
  Center, The Gambia
W. S. Alhassan
  Animal Research Institute
  Accra, Ghana
Patricio Berríos-Etchegarsey
  Facultad de Ciencias Veterinarias y
  Pecuarias
  Universidad de Chile
Frank Bryant
  Texas Technical University
Justin K. Cameons
  Asian Development Bank
  Manila, The Philippines
Noël Chabeuf
  Institut d'Elevage et de Médecine
  Vétérinaire des Pays Tropicaux
  Cedex, France
Lucia P. de Vaccaro
  Instituto de Produccion Animal
  University of Central Venezuela
C. Devendra
  Malaysian Agriculture Research and
  Development Institute
  Serdang, Selangor
N. I. Dim
  Ahmadu Bello University
  Zaria, Nigeria
Ramon Fallas
  Escuela Centroamericana de
  Ganadera
  Atenas, Costa Rica
Saul Fernandez-Baca

Food and Agriculture Organization
  Santiago, Chile
Christian F. Gall
  Centre for Agriculture in the Tropics
  and Subtropics
  University of Hohenheim,
    Germany
Gustavo Garcia Delgado
  Facultad de Medicina Veterinaria y
  Zootecnia
  Universidad Nacional Autonoma de
  Mexico, Mexico City
Jane Homan
  University of Wisconsin, Madison
Luis Latrille
  Universidad Austral de Chile
D. A. Little
  International Trypanotolerance
  Centre, The Gambia
J. H. Maner
  Winrock International Institute for
  Agricultural Development
  Morrilton, Arkansas
Robert E. McDowell
  North Carolina State University
R. Nagarcenkar
  National Dairy Research Institute
  Haryana, India
Barry Nestel
  Redhill, Surrey, England
Mark Nicholson
  International Livestock Centre for
  Africa
  Addis Ababa, Ethiopia

Ayn Nour
  Purdue University
P. Nyathi
  Ministry of Land, Agriculture, &
  Rural Settlement, Zimbabwe
Osvaldo Paladines
  Universidad Catolica de Chile
Renato R. Peixoto
  Pelotas, Brazil
James R. Simpson
  University of Florida
E. B. Sonaiya
  Obafemi Awolowo University
  Ile-Ife, Nigeria
Alberto Stephano
  Leon, Guanajuato, Mexico
John Trail
  International Livestock Centre for
  Africa, Nairobi, Kenya
Lucia Vaccaro
  Facultad de Agronomia
  Universidad Central de Venezuela
Achmanu Zakaria
  University of Brawijaya
  Jalan Mayor Jendral Haryono
  Malang, Indonesia

Joint Evaluations
Nigerian Economic Affairs Office
  Lagos:
    K. B. David-West
    Tom Aire
    B. K. Ogunmodede
Universidad Nacional Autonoma de
  Mexico:
    Rosa Paramo
    Humberto Troncoso
    Hector Sumano
    Luis Zarco
    Rene Rosiles
Universiti Pertanian Malaysia,
  Selangor Darul Ehsan, Malaysia:
    M. R. Jainudeen
    Nadzri Salim
    Che Teh Fatimah Nachiar
    Iskandar
    Henry Too Hing Lee
    Abdul Aziz Saharee
    Sheikh Omar Abdul Rahman
University of the Phillipines, Los
  Banos:
    Cledualdo Perez
    Valentino G. Arganosa
    Vicente G. Momongan
    Francisco F. Penalba

Weighting the Monograph Lists

Several elements were used to rank the titles. Numeric scores were assigned to these elements and each title computed. Procedures were as follows:

(1) The data used are counts made each time a monograph or a chapter of a monograph was cited in the Sources of Citations. This element was given the weight of 1 per citing.
(2) Rankings by reviewers were coded for each of the two top rankings. These were graded two and one and multiplied times the number of recommendations in each category. A statistical equalization on the six developed countries lists was required because the first, a general list, was sent to each reviewer resulting in ten times as many evaluations as for the specialty lists.
(3) If a title was reprinted it was given a score of 1.
(4) If a title went through more than one edition, it was given a score of 2.

The equation for the computations is:

$$(\# \text{ Counts} \times 1) + (\# \times 2 + \# \times 1) +$$
$$(\text{Reprint} \times 1) + (\text{Editions} \times 2)$$

This formula was used for both lists of monographs which were ranked separately. By this equation, the peer evaluations accounted for between 83% and 93% of all the scores in the two lists.

Within each list the scores were broken into three logical ranges based on accrued value. Rankings in three categories within each list are provided to aid in making decisions for purchase, preservation, or collection assessment. The fewest titles in both lists are in the first rank or most important titles; the greatest number of titles are in the third rank. Percentages of titles in each list by ranking are:

Developed countries list			Third World list	
No. of titles	Percentage		No. of titles	Percentage
147	15.3%	First rank	148	14.4%
367	38.3	Second rank	438	42.4
445	46.4	Third rank	446	43.2
959	100.0%		1,033	100.0%

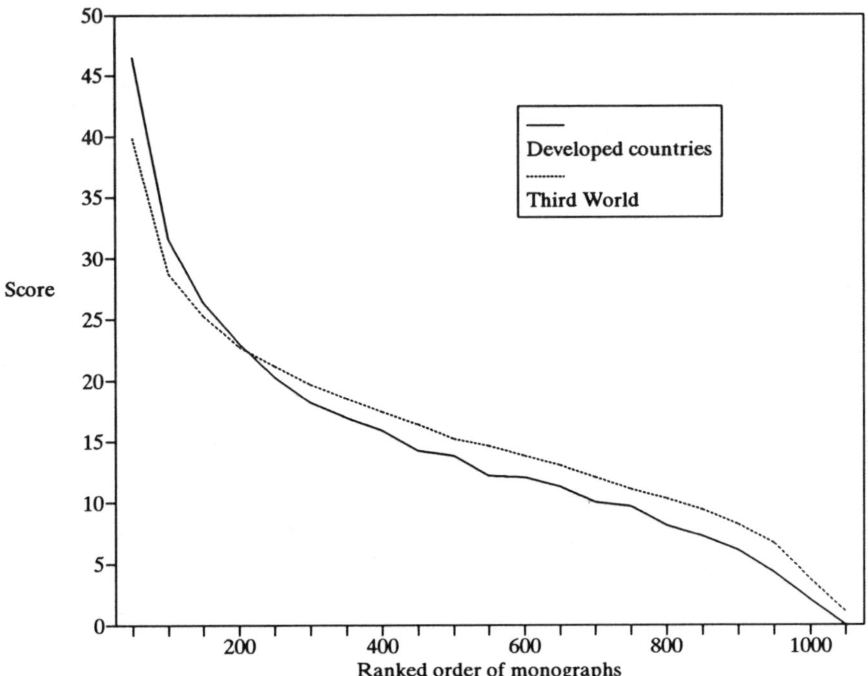

Figure 5.2. Final scoring on monographs.

Readers are reminded that all the titles in this Core List are valuable monographs for instruction and research today. Those which are less valuable were never entered for consideration in many cases, or removed by peer-evaluations with a drop rate of 36.5 to 45%. Therefore, all the titles in the two lists should be viewed as core.

The two lists have been merged in the following compilation. Rankings for a title are within its own listing only, i.e., developed countries or Third World list. Where no ranking is shown, the title is not in that list. There are 1,302 unique titles in the combined list of which 681 are common to both, a 52.3% duplication. These 681 constitute the most valuable core titles because they are highly rated in both groups. Figure 5.2 shows the score on monographs by cumulation.

Core List of Monographs for Developed and Third World Countries, 1950–1990, 1302 titles

Developed countries ranking		Third World ranking
	A	
Second	Acha, Pedro N., and Boris Szyfres. Zoonoses and Communicable Diseases Common to Man and Animal. 2d ed. Washington, D.C.; Pan American Health Organization, Pan American Sanitary Bureau, Regional Office of the World Health Organization, 1987. 963p. (Translation of Zoonoses y Enfermedades Transmisibles Comunes al Hombre y a los Animales. PAHO, 1977. 708p.)	Second
Third	Acharya, R. M. Sheep and Goat Breeds of India. Rome; Food and Agriculture Organization, 1982. 190p. (FAO Animal Production and Health Paper no. 30)	Second
Second	Acker, Duane. Animal Science and Industry. 3d ed. Englewood Cliffs, N.J.; Prentice-Hall, 1983. 658p. (1st ed. Dubuque, Iowa; William C. Brown Co., 1960.)	Second
Second	Adams, Roger L. P., John T. Knowler, and David P. Leader. The Biochemistry of the Nucleic Acids. 10th ed. London and New York; Chapman & Hall, 1986. 526p.	
	Adjare, Stephen O. Beekeeping in Africa. Rome; Food and Agriculture Organization, 1991. 130p. (FAO Agricultural Services Bulletin no. 68/6)	Third
	Adler, Norman T., ed. Neuroendocrinology of Reproduction: Physiology and Behavior. New York; Plenum Press, 1981. 555p.	Third

Developed countries ranking		Third World ranking
Third	Advanced Computer Applications in Animal Agriculture, Proceedings . . . Dallas, Feb. 1992, sponsored by American Farm Bureau, Elanco Products Co., USDA-CSRS. Ithaca, N.Y.; Dept. of Animal Science, Cornell University, 1992. 223p.	
	Agar, N. S., and P. G. Board. Red Blood Cells of Domestic Mammals. Amsterdam and New York; Elsevier, 1983. 420p.	Third
First	Agricultural Research Council (Great Britain). The Nutrient Requirements of Farm Livestock. 2d ed. London; Agricultural Research Council, 1980–1981. 3 vols. (1st ed., 1965–1967.)	First
Third	Agricultural Research Council (Great Britain). The Nutrient Requirements of Pigs: Technical Review. 2d ed. Farnham Royal, U.K.; Commonwealth Agricultural Bureaux, 1981. 307p.	Third
First	Agricultural Research Council (Great Britain). The Nutrient Requirements of Ruminant Livestock: Technical Review. Farnham Royal, U.K.; Commonwealth Agricultural Bureaux, 1980. 351p. (Enlarged ed. of: The Nutrient Requirements of Farm Livestock. No. 2: Ruminants. 1965.)	First
Second	Ainsworth, G. C., and P. K. C. Austwick. Fungal Diseases of Animals. 2d ed., rev. by G. C. Ainsworth. Slough, U.K.; Commonwealth Agricultural Bureaux, 1973. 216p. (1st ed., 1959.)	
Third	Aitkin, Flora C., and R. G. Hankin. Vitamins in Feeds for Livestock. Farnham Royal, U.K.; Commonwealth Agricultural Bureaux, 1970. 230p. (Commonwealth Bureau of Animal Nutrition, Technical Communication no. 25)	
	Akratanakul, Pongthep. Beekeeping in Asia. Rome; Food and Agriculture Organization, 1986. 112p. (FAO Agricultural Services Bulletin no. 68/4)	Third
	Alba, Jorge de. Reproduccion Animal. Mexico; Prensa Medica, 1985. 548p.	Third
Second	Alberts, Bruce, et al. Molecular Biology of the Cell. 2d ed. New York; Garland Pub., 1989. 1219p. (1st ed., 1983.)	Second
Second	Alcock, John. Animal Behavior: An Evolutionary Approach. 4th ed. Sunderland, Mass.; Sinauer Associates, 1989. 596p. (1st ed., 1975.) (Available in Spanish as Comportamiento Animal: Enfoque Evolutivo. Barcelona; Salvat.)	First
Second	Alderson, Lawrence, ed. Genetic Conservation of Domestic Livestock. Wallingford, Oxon, U.K.; CAB International, 1990. 240p.	First
Third	Alexander, G. I., and O. B. Williams. The Pastoral Industries of Australia: Practice and Technology of Sheep and Cattle Production. Sydney; Sydney University Press, 1975. 567p. Reprinted.	Second
Second	Allan, W. H., John E. Lancaster, B. Toth, and W. H. Allan.	

Developed countries ranking		Third World ranking
	Newcastle Disease Vaccines: Their Production and Use. Rome; Food and Agriculture Organization, 1978. 163p. (Rev. ed. of: The Production and Use of Newcastle Disease Vaccines. FAO, 1973.)	
Third	Allan, William. The African Husbandman. New York; Barnes & Noble, 1965. 505p.	Third
Second	Allen, David, and Brian Kilkenny. Planned Beef Production. 2d ed. London and New York; Granada, 1984. 229p.	
Third	Altman, Philip L., and Dorothy S. Dittmer. Metabolism. Bethesda, Md.; Federation of American Societies for Experimental Biology, 1968. 737p. (Rev. and updated ed. of Standard Values in Nutrition and Metabolism, edited by E. C. Albritton.)	
	Alton, G. G., L. M. Jones, and D. E. Pietz. Laboratory Techniques in Brucellosis. 2d ed. Geneva; World Health Organization, 1975. 163p. (World Health Organzation Monograph no. 55) (1st ed., 1963.)	First
Second	Altschul, Aaron M. Processed Plant Protein Foodstuffs. New York; Academic Press, 1958. 955p.	
Second	Altschul, Aaron M., ed. New Protein Foods. New York; Academic Press, 1974–1985. 5 vols. (Vols. 3–5 edited by A. M. Altschul and Harold L. Wilcke.)	Third
	Alves Santiago, Alberto. El Cebu; Ganado Bovino para los Paises Tropicales. Translated from Portuguese. Mexico; Uteha, 1980. 481p. (Earlier ed., 1967.)	Third
Second	American Breeders Service, Inc. A. I. Management Manual. DeForest, Wis.; American Breeders Service, 1983. 199p. (Available in Spanish as Manual para Inseminadores de America Breeders Service: Inseminacion Artificial.)	
Second	American Public Health Association. Standard Methods for the Examination of Dairy Products. 15th ed. edited by Gary H. Richardson. Washington, D.C.; American Public Health Association, 1985. 412p. (1st ed., 1910. Title varies, numerous different editors of editions.)	
	American Rabbit Breeders Association. Standard of Perfection; Standard Bred Rabbits and Cavies. Bloomington, Ill.; American Rabbit Breeders Association, 1986. 206p. (1971 ed., 91p.)	Second
Second	American Society of Agricultural Engineers. Livestock Environment; International Livestock Environment Symposium Proceedings, April 1974, Nebraska Center for Continuing Education, University of Nebraska-Lincoln. St. Joseph, Mich.; American Society of Agricultural Engineers, 1974. 429p. (Cover title: Livestock Environment Affects Production, Reproduction, Health.)	
	American Society of Agronomy. Tropical Forages in Livestock Production Systems; Proceedings of a Symposium . . . Annual	Second

<table>
<tr><td>Developed
countries
ranking</td><td></td><td>Third
World
ranking</td></tr>
</table>

	Meeting of the Amerian Society of Agronomy, Crop Science of America, and Soil Science Society of America, Las Vegas, Nevada, November 1973. Madison; American Society of Agronomy, 1975. 104p. (A.S.A. Spec. Pub. no. 24)	
Second	American Society of Animal Science. Symposium on Use of the Computer in Animal Science Teaching, Research and Extension. Champaign, Ill.; American Society of Animal Science, 1978. 64p. (Cover title: Use of Computer in Animal Science.)	
First	American Society of Animal Science. Techniques and Procedures in Animal Science Research. Rev. ed. Albany, N.Y.; 1969. 274p. (First ed. published as: Techniques and Procedures in Animal Production Research. Beltsville, Md.; 1959.)	First
Third	American Society of Animal Science, American Dairy Science Association, National Research Council (U.S.). Committee on Animal Nutrition. Interactions of Mycotoxins in Animal Production. Proceedings of a Symposium, July 1978, Michigan State University. Washington, D.C.; National Academy of Sciences, 1979. 197p.	Second
Second	Amlacher, Erwin. Textbook for Fish Diseases. Jersey City, N.J.; T. F. H. Publications, 1970. 302p. (Translation of Taschenbuch der Fischkrankheiten, by D. A. Conroy and R. L. Herman. 2d ed. Stuttgart; Fischer, 1972. 378p.) (Available in Spanish as Manual de Enfermedades de los Peces. Zaragoza, Spain; Acribia, 1964.)	
	Amstutz, H. E., ed. Bovine Medicine and Surgery. 2d ed. Santa Barbara, Calif.; American Veterinary Publications, 1980. 2 vols. (1st ed., edited by W. J. Gibbons et al., 1970.)	Second
	Anderson, John J. B., ed. Parturient Hypocalcemia; Proceedings of a Conference on Parturient Paresis in Dairy Animals, 1968, University of Illinois. New York; Academic Press, 1970. 276p.	Second
Second	Anderson, O. Roger. Comparative Protozoology: Ecology, Physiology, Life History. Berlin and New York; Springer-Verlag, 1988. 482p.	Third
	Andrewartha, Herbert G. Introduction to the Study of Animal Populations. 2d ed. London; Chapman & Hall; Chicago; University of Chicago Press, 1971. 283p. (1st ed., 1961.) (Available in Spanish as Introduccion al Estudio de Poblaciones Animales. Madrid; Alhambra, 1973.)	Third
Third	Andrews, A. H. Calf Management and Disease Notes. 1st ed. Harpenden, U.K.; A. H. Andrews, 1983. 284p.	Second
Second	Annison, E. F., and D. Lewis. Metabolism in the Rumen. London and New York; Methuen & J. Wiley Publishers, 1959. 184p. (Available in Spanish as Metabolismo en el Rumen. Mexico; Uteha.)	

Developed countries ranking		Third World ranking
Second	Arnold, G. W., and M. L. Dudzinski. Ethology of Free-Ranging Domestic Animals. Amsterdam and New York; Elsevier, 1978. 198p.	Second
Third	Arrington, Lewis R., and K. C. Kelley. Domestic Rabbit Biology and Production. Gainesville; University Presses of Florida, 1976. 230p. (Available in Spanish as Produccion y Biologia de los Conejos Domesticos. 1st ed. trans. by Ines Pardal. Buenos Aires; Hemisferio Sur, 1984.)	
	Arthur, Geoffrey H., David E. Noakes, and Harold Pearson. Veterinary Reproduction and Obstetrics (Theriogenology). 6th ed. Philadelphia; Bailliere Tindall, 1989. 641p. (Originally published as F. Benesch's Die Geburtshilfe bei Rind und Pferd; trans. in 1938. 2d ed., 1951, as Veterinary Obstetrics.) (Available in Spanish as Tratado de Obstetricia y Ginecologia Veterinaria. Mexico City; Labor, 1965.)	First
Second	Ashdown, Raymond R., Stanley H. Done, and Stephen W. Barnett. The Ruminants. Baltimore, London and New York; University Park Press, Gower Medical Publishing, 1984. 234p.	Second
	Asian Productivity Organization. Livestock and Poultry Industry in Selected Asian Countries; Report of Survey on Diversification of Agriculture, Livestock and Poultry Production, Conducted in Rep. of Korea, Rep. of China, Thailand and Singapore. Tokyo; The Organization, 1975. 129p.	Third
	Aspinall, K. W. First Steps in Veterinary Science. London; Bailliere Tindall, 1976. 213p.	Third
First	Association of Official Analytical Chemists. Official Methods of Analysis of the Association of Official Analytical Chemists. 14th ed. Vol. 1–6: Official and Tentative Methods of Analysis of the Association of Official Agricultural Chemists. Vol. 7–10: Official Methods of Analysis of the Association of Official Agricultural Chemists. Washington, D.C.; Association of Official Analytical Chemists, 1984. 1141p. (10th ed., 1965. 13th ed., 1980. 1018p.)	
First	Atlas, Ronald M. Microbiology: Fundamentals and Applications. 2d ed. New York and London; Macmillan, 1988. 807p. (1st ed., 1984.)	Second
First	Austic, Richard E., and Malden C. Nesheim. Poultry Production. 13th ed. Philadelphia; Lea & Febiger, 1990. 325p. (12th ed., by M. C. Nesheim, R. E. Austic and Leslie E. Card, 1979.)	Second
Second	Austin, B., and D. A. Austin. Bacterial Fish Pathogens: Disease in Farmed and Wild Fish. Chichester, U.K. and New York; Halsted Press, 1987. 364p.	Second
First	Austin, C. R., and Roger V. Short, eds. Reproduction in Mammals. 2d ed. Cambridge and New York; Cambridge University	First

Developed
countries
ranking

Third
World
ranking

Press, 1982–1986. 5 vols. (1st ed., 1972.) (Available in Spanish as Procesos de Reproduccion en los Mamiferos. 1st ed. Mexico; Prensa-Medica, 1982.)

B

Third — Bagenal, Timothy B. Methods for Assessment of Fish Production in Fresh Waters. 3d ed. Oxford; Blackwell Scientific Publications, 1978. 365p. (1st–2d ed., edited by W. T. Ricker.) — Second

Bailey, Allen J., ed. Recent Advances in the Chemistry of Meat; Proceedings of a Symposium . . . ARC Meat Research Institute, Langford, April 1983. Organized by the Food Chemistry Group of the Royal Society of Chemistry and the Food Group of the Society of Chemical Industry. London; Royal Society of Chemistry, 1984. 245p. — Third

Bain, R. V. S., et al. Haemorrhagic Septicaemia. Rome; Food and Agriculture Organization, 1982. 54p. (FAO Animal Production and Health Paper no. 33) (Rev. of FAO Agricultural Studies no. 62, 1963.) — Second

Second — Baker, Frank H., ed. Sheep and Goat Handbook. Boulder, Colo.; Westview Publishing, 1983. 600p. (International Stockmen's School Handbooks no. 3) — First

Third — Baker, James K., and W. J. Greer. Animal Health: A Layman's Guide to Disease Control. Danville, Ill.; Interstate Printers and Publishers, 1980. 402p. — Second

Third — Baker, James K., and Elwood M. Juergenson. Approved Practices in Swine Production. 6th ed. Danville, Ill.; Interstate Printers & Publishers, 1979. 432p.

Third — Baldwin, R. L., ed. Animals, Feed, Food and People: An Analysis of the Role of Animals in Food Production. Boulder, Colo.; Westview Press, 1980. 149p. (AAAS Selected Symposium no. 42) — Second

Second — Balinsky, Boris I. An Introduction to Embryology. 5th ed. Philadelphia; Saunders College Pub., 1981. 768p. (1st ed., 1960. 562p.) (Available in Spanish as Introduccion a la Embriologia. 5th ed., rev. Barcelona; Omega.)

Bard, J., et al. Handbook of Tropical Fish Culture, edited by Order of the Ministry of Foreign Affairs of France. Nogent-sur-Marne, France; Centre Technique Forestier Tropical, 1976. 165p. (Translation of Manuel de Pisciculture Tropicale) — Third

Third — Bardach, John E., John H. Ryther, and William O. McLarney. Aquaculture: The Farming and Husbandry of Freshwater and Marine Organisms. New York; J. Wiley-Interscience, 1972. 868p. (Available in Spanish as Acuacultura. 1st ed. Mexico; Agt, 1986.) — Second

Developed countries ranking		Third World ranking
	Bargai, Uri, John W. Pharr, and Joe P. Morgan. Bovine Radiology. 1st ed. Ames; Iowa State University Press, 1989. 198p.	Third
Second	Barker, J. S. F., Keith Hammond, and A. E. McClintock, eds. Future Developments in the Genetic Improvement of Animals. Sydney and New York; Academic Press, 1982. 228p.	Second
Third	Barnabe, Gilbert, ed. Aquaculture . . . trans. by Lindsay Laird. New York; Ellis Horwood, 1990. 2 vols. (Translation from French.)	Third
Third	Barnett, J. L., ed. Manipulating Pig Production: Proceedings of the Inaugural Conference of the Australasian Pig Science Association, Albury, New South Wales, November 1987. Werribee, Australia; Australasian Pig Science Association, 1987. 242p.	Second
	Barnett, S. F. Ticks and Tick-Borne Disease Control: A Practical Field Manual. Rome; Food and Agriculture Organization, 1984. 2 vols. (621 p.)	First
Third	Barone, Robert. Atlas d'Anatomie du Lapin; Atlas of Rabbit Anatomy. Paris; Masson, 1973. 219p. (French and English.)	Third
	Barrett, M. A., and P. J. Larkin. Milk and Beef Production in the Tropics. London; Oxford University Press, 1974. 245p. (Available in Spanish as Produccion Lechera y de Carne de Res en los Tropicos. Mexico; Diana, 1979.)	Second
	Barron, Norman. Pig Farmer's Vet Book. 10th ed. Alexandria Bay, N.Y.; Diamond Farm Book, 1978. 180p.	Third
	Bartik, Michal, and Alois Piskac. Veterinary Toxicology. Amsterdam and New York; Elsevier, 1981. 346p.	Second
	Bartlett, Harley H. Fire in Relation to Primitive Agriculture and Grazing in the Tropics; Annotated Bibliography. Ann Arbor; University of Michigan, 1955–1957. 2 vols. (Vol. 2 has imprint: Ann Arbor, University of Michigan Dept. of Botany. Vol. 1 is Supplement to Background Paper no. 34, Wenner-Gren Foundation International Symposium, "Man's Role in Changing the Face of the Earth." Princeton, N.J., June 1955. Vol. 2 was presented at the 9th Pacific Science Congress, Bangkok, Thailand, November 1957.)	Third
Second	Barton, R. A., and W. C. Smith, eds. Proceedings of the World Congress on Sheep and Beef Cattle Breeding, 1980, Palmerston North, N.Z. Palmerston North, N.Z.; Dunmore Press, 1982. 2 vols.	
Third	Basu, S. B. Genetic Improvement of Buffaloes. New Delhi; Kalyani Publishers, 1985. 187p.	Second
First	Bath, Donald L., et al. Dairy Cattle: Principles, Practices, Problems, Profits. 3d ed. Philadelphia; Lea & Febiger, 1985. 473p. (1st ed. by R. C. Foley, 1972. 693 p.) (Available in Spanish as Ganado Lechero. 2d ed. Bogota; Interamericana, 1982.)	First

Developed countries ranking		Third World ranking
Third	Battaglia, Richard A., and Vernon B. Mayrose. Handbook of Livestock Management Techniques. Minneapolis; Burgess, 1981. 595p.	Second
Second	Baxter, S. H. Intensive Pig Production: Environmental Management and Design. London and New York; Granada, 1984. 588p.	Second
Second	Baxter, S. H., M. R. Baxter, and J. A. D. MacCormack, eds. Farm Animal Housing and Welfare: A Seminar in the CEC Programme of Coordination of Research on Animal Welfare. Boston; M. Nijhoff, 1983. 343p.	
Second	Bearden, H. Joe, and John W. Fuquay. Applied Animal Reproduction. 2d ed. Reston, Va.; Reston Pub. Co., 1984. 382p. (1st ed., 1980. 337p.) (Available in Spanish as Reproduccion Animal Aplicada . . . trans. by Hector Sumano Lopez and Luis Ocampo Camberos. Mexico; Manual Moderno, 1983.)	Second
Second	Becker, Raymond B. Dairy Cattle Breeds; Origin and Development. Gainesville; University of Florida Press, 1973. 554p.	
	Beetsma, J., and P. Segeren. Beekeeping in the Tropics. Wageningen, Netherlands; Agromisa/Conn.A, 1988. 85p. (Agrodok no. 32)	Third
Third	Beitner, Rivka, ed. Regulation of Carbohydrate Metabolism. Boca Raton, Fla.; CRC Press, 1985. 2 vols.	
First	Bell, D. J., and B. M. Freeman, eds. Physiology and Biochemistry of the Domestic Fowl. London and New York; Academic Press, 1971–1984. 5 vols. (Vol. 4–5 edited by B. M. Freeman.)	Second
Third	Bell, Hershel M. Rangeland Management for Livestock Production. 1st ed. Norman; University of Oklahoma Press, 1973. 303p.	Third
First	Bell, J. C., Stephen R. Palmer, and J. M. Payne. The Zoonoses: Infections Transmitted from Animals to Man. London; Edward Arnold, 1988. 241p.	Third
Second	Belloin, J. C. Milk and Dairy Products: Production and Processing Costs. Rome; Food and Agriculture Organization, 1988. 119p. (FAO Animal Production and Health Paper no. 62)	Second
Second	Belschner, H. G. Sheep Management and Diseases. 10th ed. London; Angus & Robertson, 1976. 838p. (1st ed., Sydney, 1950.)	First
Second	Belschner, H. G., and Marshall J. Edwards. Cattle Diseases. Rev. ed. London; Angus & Robertson, 1984. 378p.	Second
Second	Belschner, H. G., and Robert J. Love. Pig Diseases. Rev. ed. London; Angus & Robertson, 1984. 152p.	Second
Third	Belshaw, R. H. Hastings. Guinea Fowl of the World. Liss, Hampshire, U.K.; Nimrod Book Services, 1985. 192p.	Third
	Berg, J. C. T. van den. Dairy Technology in the Tropics and Subtropics. Wageningen; Pudoc, 1988. 290p.	Third

Developed countries ranking		Third World ranking
Third	Berg, J. C. T. van den. Strategy for Dairy Development in the Tropics and Subtropics. Wageningen; Pudoc, 1990. 192p.	Third
Second	Berg, Roy T., and R. M. Butterfield. New Concepts of Cattle Growth. New York; J. Wiley, 1976. 240p. (Available in Spanish as Nuevos Conceptos en el Desarollo de Ganado Vacuno. Zaragoza; Acribia, 1979.)	Second
First	Bergey, David H., John G. Holt, and Noel R. Krieg. Bergey's Manual of Systematic Bacteriology. 4 vols. Baltimore; Williams & Wilkins, 1984–1989. (1923 ed. by D. H. Bergey. 442p.)	First
Third	Bergmeyer, Hans U., Jurgen Bergmeyer, and Marianne Grassl, eds. Methods of Enzymatic Analysis. 3d ed., rev. and enlarged. Weinheim, Germany; Verlag Chemie, 1983–1986. (1st German edition published in 1962 as Methoden der Enzymatischen Analyse.)	Third
Second	Berrier, H. H. Animal Sanitation and Disease Prevention. 2d ed. Dubuque, Iowa; Kendall/Hunt Pub. Co., 1977. 226p.	Second
	Berruecos, J. M. Mejoramiento Genetico del Cerdo. Mexico City; Arana, 1972. 243p.	Third
Third	Bessei, Werner, ed. Disturbed Behaviour in Farm Animals. Stuttgart; Ulmer, 1982. 199p.	Third
	Best, Charles H. Best and Taylor's Physiological Basis of Medical Practice, edited by John R. Brobeck. 10th ed. Baltimore; Williams & Wilkins, 1979. 1437p. (Available in Spanish as Bases Fisiologicas de la Practica Medica. 1st ed. Buenos Aires; Medica Panamericana, 1986.)	Third
	Beuving, G., C. W. Scheele, and P. C. M. Simons, eds. Quality of Eggs; Proceedings of the First European Symposium, Hotle de Keizerskroon, Apeldoorn, May 1981. Beekbergen, Netherlands; Spelderholt Institute for Poultry Research, 1981. 278p.	Third
Third	Beveridge, Malcolm C. M. Cage and Pen Fish Farming: Carrying Capacity Models and Environmental Impact. Rome; Food and Agriculture Organization, 1984. 131p. (FAO Fisheries Technical Paper no. 255)	Third
	Beverly, J. R., et al. Improving Reproductive Efficiency in Beef Cattle. Bryan, Tex.; Glidwell Printers, 1972.	Second
Third	Birge, Edward A. Bacterial and Bacteriophage Genetics: An Introduction. 2d ed. New York; Springer-Verlag, 1988. 414p. (1st ed., 1981. 359p.)	Third
First	Bisping, Wolfgang, and Gunter Amtsberg. Colour Atlas for the Diagnosis of Bacterial Pathogens in Animals. Berlin; P. Parey Scientific Publishers, 1988. 339p. (Text in English and German.)	Second
Second	Black, J. L., and P. J. Reis, eds. Physiological and Environ-	

<table>
<tr><td>Developed
countries
ranking</td><td></td><td>Third
World
ranking</td></tr>
<tr><td></td><td>mental Limitations to Wool Growth: Proceedings of a National Workshop, Leura, New South Wales, Australia, April 1978. Armidale, Australia; University of New England Publishing Unit, 1979. 405p.</td><td></td></tr>
<tr><td>Third</td><td>Blackwelder, Richard E., and Benjamin A. Shepherd. The Diversity of Animal Reproduction. Boca Raton, Fla.; CRC Press, 1981. 141p.</td><td>Third</td></tr>
<tr><td>Third</td><td>Blake, Philip. Livestock Production. London; Heinemann, 1985. 376p.</td><td></td></tr>
<tr><td>First</td><td>Blakely, James, and David H. Bade. The Science of Animal Husbandry. 5th ed. Englewood Cliffs, N.J.; Prentice-Hall, 1990. 618p. (4th ed., 1985. 683p.)</td><td>Second</td></tr>
<tr><td></td><td>Blanshard, J. M. V., and J. R. Mitchell, eds. Food Structure: Its Creation and Evaluation; Proceedings of the 44th Nottingham Easter School in Agricultural Science. London and Boston; Butterworths, 1988. 504p.</td><td>Third</td></tr>
<tr><td>First</td><td>Blaxter, K. L. Energy Metabolism in Animals and Man. Cambridge, U.K. and New York; Cambridge University Press, 1989. 336p.</td><td>Second</td></tr>
<tr><td>First</td><td>Blaxter, K. L. The Energy Metabolism of Ruminants. Rev. ed. London; Hutchinson, 1967. 332p. (Earlier ed., Thomas Pub., 1962. 329p.) (Available in Spanish as Metabolismo Energetico de los Rumiantes . . . trans. by Gaspar Gonzalez y Gonzalez. Zaragoza; Acribia, 1964.)</td><td>First</td></tr>
<tr><td>Third</td><td>Bligh, John. Temperature Regulation in Mammals and Other Vertebrates. New York and Amsterdam; Elsevier, 1973. 436p.</td><td></td></tr>
<tr><td>Second</td><td>Block, Seymour S., and Carl A. Lawrence. Disinfection, Sterilization, and Preservation. 3d ed. Philadelphia; Lea & Febiger, 1983. (1st ed., by C. A. Lawrence and S. S. Block, 1968.)</td><td>Third</td></tr>
<tr><td>First</td><td>Blood, D. C., and Otto M. Radostits. Veterinary Medicine: A Textbook of the Diseases of Cattle, Sheep, Pigs, Goats and Horses. 7th ed. London and Philadelphia; Bailliere Tindall, 1989. 1502p. (Available in Spanish as Medicina Veterinaria. 5th ed. Bogota; Interamericana, 1982.)</td><td>First</td></tr>
<tr><td>Second</td><td>Bloom, William, and Don W. Fawcett. A Textbook of Histology. 10th ed. Philadelphia; Saunders, 1975. 1033p. (Seven editions as Maximow and Bloom's Textbook of Histology, 1930–1957.)</td><td>Third</td></tr>
<tr><td>Third</td><td>Blowey, R. W. A Veterinary Book for Dairy Farmers. Ipswich, U.K.; Farming Press, 1985. 397p.</td><td>Second</td></tr>
<tr><td>Second</td><td>Blum, Jean-Claude, and J. Wiseman. Feeding of Non-Ruminant Livestock: Collective Edited Work. London and Boston; Butterworths, 1987. 214p. (Translation of L'Alimentation des Animaux Monogastriques.)</td><td>Second</td></tr>
</table>

Developed countries ranking		Third World ranking
Third	Blunt, Michael. The Blood of Sheep: Composition and Function. New York; Springer-Verlag, 1975. 224p.	Third
Third	Boda, K., ed. Physiology of Ruminant Nutrition; Proceedings of the IV International Symposium on Physiology of Ruminant Nutrition, High Tatra, Czechoslovakia. Kosice; Institute of Animal Physiology, Slovak Academy of Sciences, 1987. 551p.	
	Bogan, J. A., P. Lees, and A. T. Yoxall. Pharmacological Basis of Large Animal Medicine. Oxford and Boston; Blackwell Scientific Publications, 1983. 565p. (Available in Spanish as Bases Farmacologicas de la Medicina en Grandes Especies. 1st ed. trans. by L. Ocampo and H. Sumano. Mexico; Cientifica, 1986.)	Second
Second	Bogdan, A. V. Tropical Pasture and Fodder Plants, Grasses, and Legumes. London and New York; Longmans, 1977. 475p.	First
Third	Boggs, D. L., and R. A. Merkel. Live Animal, Carcass Evaluation and Selection Manual. Dubuque, Iowa; Kendall-Hunt Pub. Co., 1979.	
	Bojrab, M. Joseph, ed. Current Techniques in Small Animal Surgery. 3d ed. Philadelphia; Lea & Febiger, 1990. 950p. (1st ed., 1975. 583p.) (Available in Spanish as Medicina y Cirugia en Especies Pequenas. Mexico; CECSA, 1980.)	Second
Second	Bondi, Aron A., and David Drori. Animal Nutrition. Chichester, U.K. and New York; J. Wiley, 1987. 540p. (Translation of Hazanat ba le. . . .)	
Second	Bone, Jesse F. Animal Anatomy and Physiology. 3d ed. Englewood Cliffs, N.J.; Prentice-Hall, 1988. 572p. (1st ed., 1979. 560p.) (Available in Spanish as Fisiologia y Anatomia Animal . . . trans. by Luis Ocampo Camberos. Mexico; Manual Moderno, 1983.)	First
Third	Bonner, John Tyler. The Evolution of Culture in Animals. Princeton; Princeton University Press, 1980. 216p. (Available in Spanish as Evolucion de la Cultura en los Animales . . . trans. by Natividad Sanchez. Madrid; Alianza, 1983.)	
Second	Boorman, K. N., and B. M. Freeman. Food Intake Regulation in Poultry: Proceedings of the 14th Poultry Science Symposium, September 1978. Edinburgh; British Poultry Science, 1979. 469p.	
	Booth, D. A., ed. Hunger Models; Computable Theory of Feeding Control. London and New York; Academic Press, 1978. 478p.	Third
First	Booth, Nicholas H., and Leslie E. McDonald, eds. Veterinary Pharmacology and Therapeutics. 6th ed. Ames; Iowa State University Press, 1988. 1227p. (Earlier eds. by L. McDonald; and L. Meyer Jones, H. Booth and L. McDonald.) (Available in	First

Developed countries ranking		Third World ranking
	Spanish as Farmacologia y Terapeutica Veterinaria. Zaragoza; Acribia, 1987.)	
	Borchert, Alfred. Parasitologia Veterinaria . . . trans. by Miguel Cordero del Campillo. Zaragoza, Spain; Acribia, 1975. 745p. (Translation of Lehrbuch der Parasitologie fur Tierarzte.)	Third
	Boserup, Ester. The Conditions of Agricultural Growth; The Economics of Agrarian Change Under Population Pressure. Chicago; Aldine Pub. Co., 1965. 124p. (Reprinted, 1977.)	Third
Second	Botkin, M. P., R. A. Field, and C. L. Johnson. Sheep and Wool: Science, Production and Management. Englewood Cliffs, N.J.; Prentice-Hall, 1988. 451p.	Second
Second	Bourne, F. J., ed. The Mucosal Immune System: Proceedings of a Seminar in the EEC Programme of Coordination of Agricultural Research on Protection of the Young Animal Against Perinatal Diseases, University of Bristol, School of Veterinary Science, England, September 1980. The Hague and Boston; M. Nijhoff, 1981. 560p.	Third
Third	Bourne, Geoffrey H., ed. The Structure and Function of Muscle. 2d ed. New York; Academic Press, 1972–1973. 4 vols. (1st ed., 1960. 3 vols.)	
Second	Brackett, Benjamin G., George E. Seidel, and Sarah M. Seidel, eds. New Technologies in Animal Breeding; Proceedings . . . OTA Conference on Impacts of Applied Genetics: Animal Breeding, Denver, 1980. New York; Academic Press, 1981. 268p.	First
Second	Bramley, A. J., F. H. Dodd, and T. K. Griffin, eds. Mastitis Control and Herd Management; Proceedings . . . Ayr, Scotland; Hannah Research Institute, 1981. 290p. (National Institute for Research in Dairying Technical Bulletin no. 4)	Second
Third	Brander, George C. Chemicals for Animal Health Control. London and Philadelphia; Taylor & Francis, 1986. 170p.	
Third	Brander, George C., D. M. Pugh, and R. J. Bywater. Veterinary Applied Pharmacology and Therapeutics. 4th ed. London; Bailliere Tindall, 1982. 582p. (1st–2d ed. published by P. W. Daykin.)	Second
Second	Brem, G. Ex Situ Cryoconservation of Genomes and Genes of Endangered Cattle Breeds by Means of Modern Biotechnological Methods. Rome; Food and Agriculture Organization, 1989. 122p. (FAO Animal Production and Health Paper no. 76)	
Third	Bremner, A. S. Poultry Meat Hygiene and Inspection. London; Bailliere Tindall, 1977. 186p. (Available in Spanish as Higiene y Inspeccion de la Carne de Aves. Zaragoza; Acribia, 1980.)	Second
Third	Brent, Gerry. Housing the Pig. Ipswich, U.K.; Farming Press, 1986. 248p.	Second

Developed countries ranking		Third World ranking
Third	Brent, Gerry. The Pigman's Handbook. 2d ed. Ipswich, U.K.; Farming Press, 1987. 244p. (1st ed., 1982.)	
Third	Breymeyer, A. I., and G. M. VanDyne, eds. Grasslands; Systems Analysis and Man. Cambridge, U.K. and New York; Cambridge University Press, 1980. 950p.	Second
First	Briggs, Hilton M., and Dinus M. Briggs. Modern Breeds of Livestock. 4th ed. New York; Macmillan, 1980. 802p. (1st ed., 1949.) (Available in Spanish as Razas Modernas de Animales Domesticos. Zaragoza; Acribia, 1971.)	
Second	Briggs, Michael H., ed. Urea As a Protein Supplement. Oxford and New York; Pergamon Press, 1967. 466p.	Second
Third	Briskey, Ernest J., ed. The Physiology and Biochemistry of Muscle As a Food; Proceedings of an International Symposium, Sponsored by the University of Wisconsin, July 1965, with the support of U.S. Public Health Service Research Grant EF-00727-01, Division of Environmental Engineering and Food Protection, and a Special Grant from the American Meat Institute Foundation. Madison; University of Wisconsin Press, 1966. 437p.	Third
Second	Brock, Thomas D., and Michael T. Madigan. Biology of Microorganisms. 5th ed. Englewood Cliffs, N.J.; Prentice-Hall, 1988. 835p. (4th ed., 1984.) (Available in Spanish as Microbiologia. 1st ed. trans. by Gustavo Lonngi V. and Teresa de Jesus Garza. Naucalpan de Juarez; Prentice-Hall, 1987. 2d ed., rev. as Biologia de los Microorganismos. Barcelona; Omega.)	Second
First	Brody, Samuel. Bioenergetics and Growth, with Special Reference to the Efficiency Complex in Domestic Animals. New York; Van Nostrand Reinhold, 1945. 1023p.	Second
Third	Brooke, C. H., and M. L. Ryder. Declining Breeds of Mediterranean Sheep. Rome; Food and Agriculture Organization, 1973. 68p. (FAO Animal Production and Health Papers no. 8)	Third
Second	Broster, W. H., R. H. Phipps, and Colin L. Johnson. Principles and Practice of Feeding Dairy Cows. Shinfield, U.K.; NIRD, 1986. 322p. (Available in Spanish as Estrategias de Alimentacion para Vacas Lecheras de Alta Produccion. Mexico; AGT.)	Second
	Brown, Arthur M., and Donald W. Stubbs. Medical Physiology. New York; J. Wiley, 1983. 914p.	Third
Third	Brown, M. H., ed. Meat Microbiology. London and New York; Elsevier, 1982. 529p.	Third
	Bulliet, Richard W. The Camel and the Wheel. Cambridge, Mass.; Harvard University Press, 1975. 327p.	Third
Third	Bundy, Clarence, Ronald V. Diggins, and Virgil W. Christensen. Livestock and Poultry Production. 5th ed. Englewood Cliffs, N.J.; Prentice-Hall, 1982. 656p. (1st ed., 1954.) (Avail	Second

Developed countries ranking		Third World ranking
	able in Spanish as Produccion Avicola. Mexico; CECSA, 1981.)	
Second	Bundy, Clarence, Ronald V. Diggins, and Virgil W. Christensen. Swine Production. 5th ed. Englewood Cliffs, N.J.; Prentice-Hall, 1984. 400p. (1st ed., by C. E. Bundy and R. V. Diggins, 1956. 337p.) (Available in Spanish as Produccion Porcina. Mexico; CECSA, 1981.)	Second
	Bureau Europeen en d'Information pour le Developpement de la Sant Animale. Future Production and Productivity in Livestock Farming: Science Versus Politics; Proceedings of a DSA Symposium, Strasbourg, April 1986. Amsterdam and New York; Elsevier, 1986. 254p.	Third
	Bureau Europeen en d'Information pour le Developpement de la Sant Animale. Safety and Quality in Food: Wholesome Food for All: Views of the Animal Health Industries; Proceedings of a DSA Symposium, March 1984. Amsterdam and New York; Elsevier, 1984. 258p. (Text in English, French or German.)	Third
Third	Burnet, Frank M., and David O. White. Natural History of Infectious Disease. 4th ed. Cambridge, U.K.; University Press, 1972. 278p. (1st ed., 1953.) (Available in Spanish as Historia Natural de la Enfermedad Infecciosa. Madrid; Alianza.)	Third
Third	Burns, George W. The Science of Genetics: An Introduction to Heredity. 4th ed. New York; Macmillan, 1980. 608p. (1st ed., 1969. 399p.)	Second
Second	Burny, A., and M. Mammerickx, eds. Enzootic Bovine Leukosis and Bovine Leukemia Virus. Boston; M. Nijhoff, 1987. 283p.	Second
	Burt, R. L., et al., eds. The Role of Centrosema, Desmodium, and Stylosanthes in Improving Tropical Pastures. Boulder, Colo.; Westview Press, 1983. 292p.	Third
First	Butler, G. W., and R. W. Bailey. Chemistry and Biochemistry of Herbage. London and New York; Academic Press, 1973. 3 vols.	Second
Second	Butler, John E., et al., eds. The Ruminant Immune System; Paper of the International Symposium on the Ruminant Immune System, 1980. New York; Plenum Press, 1981. 891p.	Second
Second	Butterworth, M. H. Beef Cattle Nutrition and Tropical Pastures. London and New York; Longmans, 1985. 500p.	First
First	Buttery, P. J., and D. B. Lindsay, eds. Protein Deposition in Animals; 29th Easter School in Agricultural Science. London and Boston; Butterworths, 1980. 305p.	First
First	Buttery, P. J., D. B. Lindsay, and N. Bruce Haynes. Control and Manipulation of Animal Growth; Proceedings of the 43d Nottingham Easter School. London and Boston; Butterworths, 1986. 347p.	Second

Developed countries ranking		Third World ranking

C

Developed countries ranking		Third World ranking
Third	Cairns, John, Gunther S. Stent, and James D. Watson, eds. Phage and the Origins of Molecular Biology: Essays Published on the Occasion of the Sixtieth Birthday of Max Delbruck. Cold Spring Harbor, N.Y.; Cold Spring Harbor Laboratory of Quantitative Biology, 1966. 340p.	
	Caldwell, H. S. The Water Buffalo: A Project. Rome and New York; Food and Agriculture Organization, 1977. 283p. (Abridged version of The Husbandry and Health of the Domestic Buffalo, 1974.)	Second
	Calle Escobar, Rigoberto. Animal Breeding and Production of American Camelids. Lima; Per Ficos de Abril; Mt. Shasta, Calif.; Printed by Talleres Gr 3-R Ranch, 1984. 358p. (Translated from Spanish.)	Second
First	Calnek, B. W., et al., eds. Diseases of Poultry. 9th ed. Ames; Iowa State University Press, 1991. 929p. (1st ed., edited by Harry E. Biester et al., 1943. 1005p.)	First
First	Campbell, John R., and John Foster Lasley. The Science of Animals That Serve Humanity. 3d ed. New York; McGraw-Hill, 1985. 834p. (1st ed., 1969, as The Science of Animals That Serve Mankind. 771p.)	Second
Second	Campbell, John R., and Robert T. Marshall. The Science of Providing Milk for Man. New York; McGraw-Hill, 1975. 801p.	
	Campbell, Terry W. Avian Hematology and Cytology. 1st ed. Ames; Iowa State University Press, 1988. 101p.	Second
Third	Campion, Dennis R., Gary J. Hausman, and Roy J. Martin, eds. Animal Growth Regulation. New York; Plenum Press, 1989. 405p.	
	Camus, E., and N. Barre. Heartwater: A Review. Paris; OIE, 1988. 147p. (Translation of La Cowdriose; Revue Generale des Connaissances. 2d ed. Maisons-Alfort, France; Institut d'Elevage et de Medecine Veterinaire des Pays Tropicaux, 1988. Etudes et Syntheses de l'IEMVT no. 4)	Third
Third	Canadian Council on Animal Care. Guide to the Care and Use of Experimental Animals. 2d ed. Ottawa; The Council, 1980. (1st ed. published as Care of Experimental Animals, 1969.)	First
Second	Carles, A. B. Sheep Production in the Tropics. Oxford and New York; Oxford University Press, 1983. 213p.	First
	Carter, G. R. Veterinarian's Guide to the Laboratory Diagnosis of Infectious Diseases. Lenexa, Kansas; Veterinary Medicine Pub. Co., 1986. 326p.	Second
	Carter, G. R., and M. M. Chengappa. Essentials of Veterinary Bacteriology and Mycology. 4th ed. Philadelphia; Lea & Febiger, 1991. 284p. (Earlier ed., by G. R. Carter. East Lansing;	Second

<table>
<tr><td>Developed
countries
ranking</td><td></td><td>Third
World
ranking</td></tr>
<tr><td></td><td>Michigan State University Press, 1976. 290p. Revision and enl. of earlier work: Outline of Veterinary Bacteriology and Mycology.)</td><td></td></tr>
<tr><td></td><td>Carter, G. R., and John R. Cole. Diagnostic Procedures in Veterinary Bacteriology and Mycology. 5th ed. San Diego; Academic Press, 1990. 620p. (1st ed. Springfield, Ill.; Thomas, 1967. 282p.) (Available in Spanish as Procedimientos de Diagnostico en Bacteriologia y Micologia Veterinarias. Zaragoza; Acribia, 1969.)</td><td>First</td></tr>
<tr><td></td><td>Carter, T. C., ed. Egg Quality: A Study of the Hen's Egg. Symposium organized by Scientific Advisory Committee of the British Egg Marketing Board, Harper Adams Agricultural College, Edgmond, Newport, Shropshire, September 1967. Edinburgh; Oliver & Boyd, 1968. 336p.</td><td>Third</td></tr>
<tr><td></td><td>Carter, T. C., and B. M. Freeman, eds. The Fertility and Hatchability of the Hen's Egg. Symposium of the British Egg Marketing Board Scientific Adivsory Committee, 5th, Harper Adams Agricultural College, September 1968. Edinburgh; Oliver & Boyd, 1969. 199p.</td><td>Third</td></tr>
<tr><td>Third</td><td>Casarett, Louis J., and John Doull, eds. Toxicology: The Basic Science of Poisons. New York; Macmillan, 1975. 768p.</td><td>Third</td></tr>
<tr><td></td><td>Castello, J. A. Diccionario Avicola-Ganadero Ingles-Espanol. Barcelona; Real Escuela Oficial y de Superior Avicultura, 1986. 135p.</td><td>Third</td></tr>
<tr><td>Third</td><td>Castle, Malcolm E., and Paul Watkins. Modern Milk Production: Its Principles and Applications for Students and Farmers. 2d ed. London and Boston; Faber & Faber, 1984. 310p. (1st ed., 1979. 308p.)</td><td>Second</td></tr>
<tr><td></td><td>Chakroff, Marilyn. Freshwater Fish Pond Culture and Management, edited by Laurel Druben. Washington, D.C.; ACTION, Peace Corps, 1976. 191p. (VITA Publications Manual Series no. 36E)</td><td>Third</td></tr>
<tr><td>Second</td><td>Chapman, A. B. General and Quantitative Genetics. Amsterdam and New York; Elsevier, 1985. 408p.</td><td></td></tr>
<tr><td>Second</td><td>Cheeke, Peter R. Rabbit Feeding and Nutrition. Orlando, Fla.; Academic Press, 1987. 376p.</td><td>Second</td></tr>
<tr><td>Second</td><td>Cheeke, Peter R., et al. Rabbit Production. 6th ed. Danville, Ill.; Interstate, 1987. 472p. (5th ed., 1982.)</td><td>Second</td></tr>
<tr><td>Third</td><td>Cheeke, Peter R., and Lee R. Shull. Natural Toxicants in Feeds and Poisonous Plants. Westport, Conn.; Avi Pub. Co., 1985. 492p.</td><td>Second</td></tr>
<tr><td></td><td>Chemineau, P., Y. Cognie, et al. Training Manual on Artificial Insemination in Sheep and Goats. Rome; Food and Agriculture Organization, 1991. 222p. (FAO Animal Production and Health Paper no. 83)</td><td>Third</td></tr>
</table>

Developed countries ranking		Third World ranking
	Chemineau, P., D. Gautier, and J. Thimonier, eds. Reproduction des Ruminants en Zone Tropicale = Reproduction of Ruminants in Tropical Areas; Reunion Internationale, Pointe-a-Pitre, Guadeloupe, June 1983. Paris; Institut National de la Recherche Agronomique, 1984. 519p. (Les Colloques de l'INRA no. 20)	Third
Third	Chen, Tung Pai. Aquaculture Practices in Taiwan. Farnham, U.K.; Fishing News Books, 1976. 162p.	Third
Second	Cheng, P. Livestock Breeds of China. Rome; Food and Agriculture Organization, 1984, 1985. 217p. (Rev. and expanded ed. of original, published in Chinese. Beijing, China; China Academic Publishers, 1980.)	
Second	Cheng, Thomas C. General Parasitology. 2d ed. Orlando, Fla.; Academic Press, 1986. 827p. (1st ed., New York; Academic Press, 1973. 965p.)	Third
Second	Cheville, Norman F. Cell Pathology. 2d ed. Ames; Iowa State University Press, 1983. 681p. (1st ed., 1976.)	Second
	Cheville, Norman F. Introduction to Veterinary Pathology. 1st ed. Ames; Iowa State University Press, 1988. 537p.	Second
Second	Child, R. Dennis, and E. K. Byington. Potential of the World's Forages for Ruminant Animal Production: Temperate Zone Cultivated Forages, Humid and Subhumid Tropical Rangelands, Tropical Zone Cultivated Forages, Arid and Semi-Arid Rangelands, Temperate and Tropical Forests. 2d ed. Morrilton, Ark.; Winrock International Livestock Research and Training Center, 1981. 111p. (1st ed., 1977. 91p.)	First
Second	Christie, William W. Lipid Metabolism in Ruminant Animals. 1st ed. Oxford and New York; Pergamon Press, 1981. 452p. (Supplement no. 1, 1981, to Progress in Lipid Research.)	Second
First	Church, David C. Livestock Feeds and Feeding. 3d ed. Englewood Cliffs, N.J.; Prentice-Hall, 1991. 549p. (2d ed., 1984. Corvallis, Oreg.; O & B Books. 549p.)	First
First	Church, David C., ed. The Ruminant Animal: Digestive Physiology and Nutrition. Englewood Cliffs, N.J.; Prentice-Hall, 1988. 564p. (Previously published as Digestive Physiology and Nutrition of Ruminants, 2d ed., vol. I, 1969, 1976, and vol. II, 1971, 1979, O & B Books.)	First
First	Church, David C., and W. G. Pond. Basic Animal Nutrition and Feeding. 3d ed. New York; J. Wiley, 1988. 472p.	Third
Second	Cioffi, L. A., W. P. T. James, and T. B. Van Itallie, eds. The Body Weight Regulatory System: Normal and Disturbed Mechanisms; Proceedings . . . 3d International Congress of Obesity, Rome, October 1980. New York; Raven Press, 1981. 380p.	
	Clark, Colin, and Margaret Haswell. 4th ed. The Economics of Subsistence Agriculture. London; Macmillan; New York; St.	Third

Developed countries ranking		Third World ranking
	Martin's Press, 1970. 267p. (1st ed., New York; St. Martin's Press, 1964. 218p.)	
Third	Clark, J. A., ed. Environmental Aspects of Housing for Animal Production; Based on the 31st Easter School in Agricultural Science. London and Boston; Butterworths, 1981. 511p.	
Third	Clark, J. A., K. Gregson, and R. A. Saffel, eds. Computer Applications in Agricultural Environments; Proceedings of the 42d Easter School in Agricultural Science. London and Boston; Butterworths, 1987. 304p.	Third
Third	Clarke, R. T. J., and T. Bauchop, eds. Microbial Ecology of the Gut. London and New York; Academic Press, 1977. 410p.	Third
	Clarkson, M. J., and W. B. Faull. Notes for the Sheep Clinician. 3d ed. Liverpool; Liverpool University Press, 1987. 175p. (1st ed., 1983. 115p.) (Available in Spanish as Notas para la Clinica Ovina. 1st ed. trans. by Pedro Ducar Maluenda. Zaragoza; Acribia, 1987.)	Second
Third	Clayton, G. A., et al. Turkey Production: Breeding and Husbandry. London; H.M.S.O., 1985. 123p.	Second
Second	Clutton-Brock, Juliet. A Natural History of Domesticated Animals. Cambridge; Cambridge University Press, 1987. 208p. (Originally published: London; Heineman, 1981.)	Second
	Coche, A. G. Soil and Freshwater Fish Culture. Rome; Food and Agriculture Organization, (UNIPUB), 1985. 174p. (FAO Training Series no. 6)	Third
	Cockrill, W. Ross. The Camelid: An All-Purpose Animal. Khartoum Workshop on Camels. Uppsala; Scandinavian Institute of African Studies, 1984–1985. 2 vols.	Second
Second	Cockrill, W. Ross. The Husbandry and Health of the Domestic Buffalo; A Project Sponsored by the Australian Freedom from Hunger Campaign. Rome; Food and Agriculture Organization, 1974. 993p.	First
First	Cole, D. J. A., and G. R. Foxcroft, eds. Control of Pig Reproduction; Proceedings of the 34th Easter School in Agricultural Science, University of Nottingham. London and Boston; Butterworths, 1982. 664p.	Second
Second	Cole, D. J. A., and William Haresign, eds. Recent Developments in Pig Nutrition: Nutrition Conference for Feed Manufacturers. London and Boston; Butterworths, 1985. 321p.	
Third	Cole, D. J. A., and William Haresign, eds. Recent Developments in Poultry Nutrition. London and Boston; Butterworths, 1989. 344p.	
First	Cole, Harold H., and W. N. Garrett. Animal Agriculture: The Biology, Husbandry, and Use of Domestic Animals. 2d ed. San Francisco; W. H. Freeman, 1980. 739p. (1st ed., by Cole and M. Ronning, 1974. 788p.)	First

Developed countries ranking		Third World ranking
	Cole, V. G. Helminth Parasites of Sheep and Cattle. Canberra; Australian Government Publishing Service, 1986. 255p.	Second
	Coles, Embert H. Veterinary Clinical Pathology. 4th ed. Philadelphia; Saunders, 1986. 486p. (1st ed., 1967. 455p.)	Second
Third	Colgan, Patrick W. Quantitative Ethology. New York; J. Wiley, 1978. 364p.	
Second	Collins, C. H., and John M. Grange. Isolation and Identification of Micro-Organisms of Medical and Veterinary Importance. London and Orlando, Fla.; Academic Press, 1985. 387p.	Third
	Collinson, Michael P. Farm Management in Peasant Agriculture. Rev. ed. Boulder, Colo.; Westview Press, 1983. 454p. (1st ed., Praegor, 1972. 444p.)	Third
Third	Commission of the European Communities. Scientific and Technical Information and Information Management, ed. Veterinrwissenschaft, Mehrsprachiger Thesaurus = Veterinary Multilingual Thesaurus = Thesaurus Multilingue v Ischen Gemeinschaften. New York; K. G. Saur, 1979. 5 vols. (The complete thesaurus consists of four monolingual volumes—German, English, French and Italian—and a quadrilingual index.)	Second
Third	Commonwealth Scientific and Industrial Research Organization (Australia). Nutritional Limits to Animal Production from Pastures: Proceedings of an International Symposium, St. Lucia, Queensland, Australia, August 1981. Farnham Royal, U.K.; Commonwealth Agricultural Bureaux, 1982. 536p.	
Second	Conant, Norman F., et al. Manual of Clinical Mycology. 3d ed. Philadelphia; Saunders, 1971. 755p. (1st ed., 1944. 348p.)	Third
Second	Conrad, H. Russell, Dean R. Zimmerman, and G. F. Combs, Jr. NFIA Literature Review on Iron in Animal and Poultry Nutrition. West Des Moines, Iowa; National Feed Ingredients Association, 1980. 118p.	
Second	Coop, I. E. Sheep and Goat Production. Amsterdam and New York; Elsevier, 1982. 492p.	
Third	Cooper, Malcolm M., and R. J. Thomas. Profitable Sheep Farming. 5th ed. Ipswich, U.K.; Farming Press, 1982. 192p. (Available in Spanish as Produccion del Cordero. 1st ed. Barcelona; Aedos, 1978.)	
	Cooper, Malcolm M., and Malcolm B. Willis. Profitable Beef Production. 4th ed. Ipswich, U.K.; Farming Press, 1984. 200p. (Available in Spanish as Produccion Rentable de Vacuno de Carne. Madrid; Mundi-Prensa, 1978.)	Second
Third	Cooper, Margaret E. An Introduction to Animal Law. London and San Diego; Academic Press, 1986. 213p.	
Third	Copland, J. W. Goat Production and Research in the Tropics: Proceedings of a Workshop, University of Queensland, Bris-	First

Developed countries ranking		Third World ranking
	bane, February 1984. Canberra; Australian Centre for International Agricultural Research, 1985. 118p.	
Third	Cornell Nutrition Conference for Feed Manufacturers, 1983, 1985–1986. Proceedings . . . Ithaca, N.Y.; Cornell University, 1983, 1985–1986. 128p.	
Second	Cornell Research Foundation, New York State College of Veterinary Medicine Pharmacy and Therapeutics Committee. Veterinary Drug Formulary. Baltimore; Williams & Wilkins, 1985. 168p.	Second
Third	Council for Agricultural Science and Technology. Animal Germplasm Preservation and Utilization in Agriculture. Ames, Iowa; Council for Agricultural Science and Technology, 1984. 35p. (Council for Agricultural Science and Technology Report no. 101)	Second
Third	Courot, M. The Male in Farm Animal Reproduction: A Seminar in the EEC Programme of Coordination of Research on Animal Production, Station de la Physiologie de la Reproduction. Boston; M. Nijhoff, 1984. 377p.	Third
First	Coutts, G. S. Poultry Diseases Under Modern Management. 3d ed. Alton, U.K.; Nimrod Press, 1987. 245p.	Second
Second	Cowey, C. B., A. M. Mackie, and J. G. Bell. Nutrition and Feeding in Fish. London and Orlando, Fla.; Academic Press, 1985. 489p.	Second
	Cox, C. Barry, and Peter D. Moore. Biogeography: An Ecological and Evolutionary Approach. 4th ed. Oxford and Boston; Blackwell Scientific, 1985. 244p. (1st ed., by C. B. Cox, Ian N. Healey and P. D. Moore, 1973. 179p.)	Third
	Cox, John E. Surgery of the Reproductive Tract in Large Animals. 3d ed., rev. Liverpool; Liverpool University Press, 1987. 194p. (Earlier ed., 1981? 212p.)	Second
Third	Craig, James V. Domestic Animal Behavior: Causes and Implications for Animal Care and Management. Englewood Cliffs, N.J.; Prentice-Hall, 1981. 364p.	
First	Crampton, Earle W., and L. E. Harris. Applied Animal Nutrition; The Use of Feedstuffs in the Formulation of Livestock Rations. 2d ed. San Francisco; W. H. Freeman, 1969. 753p. (1st ed., 1956. 458p.) (Available in Spanish as Nutricion Animal Aplicada. 3d ed. trans. by Pedro D. Maluenda. Zaragoza; Acribia, 1979.)	First
Second	Crawford, R. D., ed. Poultry Breeding and Genetics. Amsterdam and New York; Elsevier, 1990. 1123p.	Third
Second	Crighton, D. B., ed. Immunological Aspects of Reproduction in Mammals; Proceedings of the 38th Easter School in Agricultural Science. London and Boston; Butterworths, 1984. 529p.	

Developed countries ranking		Third World ranking
Second	Crighton, D. B., et al., eds. Control of Ovulation; Easter School in Agricultural Science. 1st ed. London and Boston; Butterworths, 1978. 492p.	Third
Second	Cross, H. Russell, and A. J. Overby. Meat Science, Milk Science, and Technology. Amsterdam and New York; Elsevier, 1988. 458p.	Second
Third	Croston, David, and Geoffrey Pollott. Planned Sheep Production. London and Dobbs Ferry, N.Y.; Collins & Sheridan House, 1985. 211p.	Second
	Crotty, Raymond D. Cattle, Economics and Development. Farnham Royal, U.K.; Commonwealth Agricultural Bureaux, 1980. 253p.	Second
Second	Crow, James F. Basic Concepts in Population, Quantitative, and Evolutionary Genetics. New York; W. H. Freeman, 1986. 273p.	Second
Third	Crowder, Loy V., and H. R. Chheda. Tropical Grassland Husbandry. London and New York; Longmans, 1982. 562p.	Third
First	Cullison, Arthur E., and Robert S. Lowrey. Feeds and Feeding. 4th ed. Englewood Cliffs, N.J.; Prentice-Hall, 1987. 645p. (1st ed., 1975. 486p.) (Available in Spanish as Alimentos y Alimentacion de Animales. 1st ed. trans. by Rene Ledesma. Mexico; Diana, 1983.)	First
First	Cunha, Tony J. Swine Feeding and Nutrition. Rev. ed. New York; Academic Press, 1977. 352p. (First published in 1957.)	
Second	Cunningham, E. P., ed. Modern Techniques in Animal Breeding. London; Butterworths, 1988. 288p.	First
	Cunningham, E. P., and O. Syrstad. Crossbreeding Bos Indicus and Bos Taurus for Milk Production in the Tropics. Rome; Food and Agriculture Organization, 1987. 90p. (FAO Animal Production and Health Paper no. 68)	First
Second	Cunningham, Frank E., and N. A. Cox. The Microbiology of Poultry Meat Products. Orlando, Fla.; Academic Press, 1987. 359p.	
First	Cupps, Perry T., ed. Reproduction in Domestic Animals. 4th ed. San Diego, Calif.; Academic Press, 1991. 670p. (1st ed., edited by Harold H. Cole and P. T. Cupps, published in New York, 1959.) (Available in Spanish as Reproduccion: Animales Domesticos. 1st ed. trans. by Luis Ariel Garica et al. Zaragoza; Acribia, 1984.)	First
First	Currie, W. Bruce. Structure and Function of Domestic Animals. Boston; Butterworths, 1988. 443p.	Second
First	Curtis, Stanley E. Environmental Management in Animal Agriculture. Ames; Iowa State University Press, 1983. 409p.	
Third	Czerkawski, J. W. An Introduction to Rumen Studies. 1st ed. Oxford and New York; Pergamon Press, 1986. 236p.	Third

Developed countries ranking		Third World ranking

D

Developed countries ranking	Entry	Third World ranking
Third	Dahl, Gudrun, and Anders Hjort. Having Herds: Pastoral Herd Growth and Household Economy. Stockholm; University of Stockholm, 1976. 335p. (Stockholm Studies in Social Anthropology no. 2)	Second
Second	Dalton, Clive. An Introduction to Practical Animal Breeding. 2d ed. London; Collins, 1985. 182p. (1st ed., 1980, Granada Publishing.) (Available in Spanish as Introduccion a la Genetica Animal Practica. Zaragoza; Acribia, 1982.)	Second
	Darling, F. Fraser. Wild Life in an African Territory; A Study Made for the Game and Tsetse Control Dept. of Northern Rhodesia. London and New York; Oxford University Press, 1960. 160p.	Third
	Dasmann, Raymond F., John P. Milton, and Peter H. Freeman. Ecological Principles for Economic Development. London and New York; J. Wiley, 1973. 252p.	Third
	Davies, William, and C. L. Skidmore, eds. Tropical Pastures. London; Faber & Faber, 1966. 215p.	Third
First	Davis, John W., Lars H. Karstad, and Daniel O. Trainer, eds. Infectious Diseases of Wild Mammals. 2d ed. Ames; Iowa State University Press, 1981. 446p. (1st ed., 1970. 421p.) (Available in Spanish as Enfermedades Infecciosas de los Mamiferos Salvajes. Zaragoza; Acribia, 1973.)	Second
Second	Davis, W. C., J. N. Shelton, and C. W. Weems, eds. Characterization of the Bovine Immune System and the Genes Regulating Expression of Immunity with Particular Reference to Their Role in Disease Resistance; Proceedings from a Symposium, East-West Center, Honolulu, May 1984. Pullman; Washington State University, 1985. 217p.	Third
Third	Dawkins, M. S. Animal Suffering: The Science of Animal Welfare. London; Chapman & Hall, 1980. 149p.	Third
Third	de Boer, H., and J. Martin, eds. Patterns of Growth and Development in Cattle: A Seminar in the EEC Programme of Coordination of Research on Beef Production, Ghent, October 1977. The Hague & Boston; M. Nijhoff, 1978. 767p.	
Second	De Lahunta, Alexander. Veterinary Neuroanatomy and Clinical Neurology. 2d ed. Philadelphia; Saunders, 1983. 471p. (1st ed., 1977.)	
	de Vos, Antoon. Deer Farming: Guidelines on Practical Aspects. Rome; Food and Agriculture Organization, 1982. 54p.	Third
	Dellmann, Horst D., and Esther M. Brown, eds. Textbook of Veterinary Histology. 3d ed. Philadelphia; Lea & Febiger, 1987. 468p. (1st ed., 1976. 513p.)	Second
Second	Demment, Montague W., and Peter J. Van Soest. Body Size, Digestive Capacity, and Feeding Strategies of Herbivores. Mor-	First

Developed countries ranking		Third World ranking
	rilton, Ark.; Winrock International Livestock Research & Training Center, 1983. 66p.	
Third	Dent, J. B., and J. R. Anderson. Systems Analysis in Agricultural Management. Sydney and New York; J. Wiley, 1971. 394p. (Available in Spanish.)	
	Dethier, V. G., and Eliot Stellar. Animal Behavior: Its Evolutionary and Neurological Basis. 2d ed. Englewood Cliffs, N.J.; Prentice-Hall, 1964. 118p. (1st ed., 1961. 118p.)	Second
Second	Devendra, C., and M. F. Fuller. Pig Production in the Tropics. Oxford; Oxford University Press, 1979. 172p.	First
First	Devendra, C., and Marca Burns, eds. Goat Production in the Tropics. 2d ed. Farnham Royal, U.K.; Commonwealth Agricultural Bureaux, 1983. 183p. (CAB Bureau of Animal Breeding & Genetics Technical Communication no. 19) (1st ed., 1970. 184p.)	First
First	Devendra, C., and R. I. Hutagalung, eds. Feedingstuffs for Livestock in South East Asia: Proceedings of a Symposium, Faculty of Medicine, National University of Malaysia, Kuala Lumpur, 1977. Serdang; Malaysian Society of Animal Production, 1978. 370p.	First
Third	Devendra, C., and G. B. McLeroy. Goat and Sheep Production in the Tropics. London; Longman, 1982. 271p. (Available in Spanish as Produccion de Cabras y Ovejas en los Tropicos. 1st ed. trans. by Luis Ocampo Camberos. Mexico; Manual Moderno, 1986.)	First
Second	Dickerson, G. E., and R. K. Johnson, eds. World Congress on Genetics Applied to Livestock Production, 3d, Lincoln, Nebraska, 1986. Lincoln; University of Nebraska, 1986. 4 vols.	Second
Second	Dietz, Olof, and Ekkehard Wiesner, eds. Diseases of the Horse: A Handbook for Science and Practice . . . trans. by A. S. Turner. Basel and New York; Karger, 1984. 3 vols. (Translation of Handbuch der Pferdekrankheiten.)	Third
Second	Diggins, Ronald V., Clarence E. Bundy, and V. W. Christensen. Beef Production. 4th ed. Englewood Cliffs, N.J.; Prentice-Hall, 1984. 256p. (1st ed., 1956.) (Available in Spanish as Produccion de Carne Bovina. Mexico; CECSA, 1985.)	Second
Second	Diggins, Ronald V., Clarence E. Bundy, and V. W. Christensen. Dairy Production. 5th ed. Englewood Cliffs, N.J.; Prentice-Hall, 1984. 326p. (1st ed., 1955. 342p.) (Available in Spanish as Vacas, Leche y. Sus Derivados. Mexico; CECSA, 1970.)	First
Second	Dmitriev, N. G., and L. K. Ernst, eds. Animal Genetic Resources of the USSR. Rome; Food and Agriculture Organization, 1989. 517p. (FAO Animal Production and Health Paper no. 65)	Second
Third	Dobie, J. Frank. The Longhorns. Tom Lea, illustrator. New	

Developed countries ranking		Third World ranking
	York; Bramnill House, 1941. 388p. (Reprinted, Austin and London; University of Texas Press, 1980.)	
Third	Dobson, A., and Marjorie J. Dobson, eds. Aspects of Digestive Physiology in Ruminants: Proceedings of a Satellite Symposium of the 30th International Congress of the International Union of Physiological Sciences, Cornell University, Ithaca, New York, July 1986. Ithaca, N.Y.; Comstock Pub. Associates, 1988. 311p.	Second
	Dolan, T. T., ed. Theileriosis in Eastern, Central and Southern Africa; Proceedings of a Workshop on East Coast Fever Immunization, Lilongwe, Malawi, 1988. Nairobi, Kenya; International Laboratory for Research on Animal Diseases, 1989. 191p.	Third
Second	Donald, A. D., W. H. Southcott, and J. K. Dineen, eds. The Epidemiology and Control of Gastrointestinal Parasites of Sheep in Australia. Melbourne; Commonwealth Scientific and Industrial Research Organization, Division of Animal Health, 1978. 153p.	Third
Third	Doolittle, Donald P. Population Genetics: Basic Principles. Berlin and New York; Springer-Verlag, 1987. 264p. (Advanced Series in Agricultural Sciences no. 16)	Third
Third	Doppler, Werner. The Economics of Pasture Improvement and Beef Production in Semi-Humid West Arica. Eschborn; Deutsche Gesellschaft fur Technische Zusammenarbeit (GTZ), 1980. 195p.	
	Dougherty, R. W. Experimental Surgery in Farm Animals. 1st ed. Ames; Iowa State University Press, 1981. 146p.	Third
Second	Dougherty, R. W., et al., eds. Physiology of Digestion in the Ruminant: Papers of International Symposium on the Physiology of Digestion in the Ruminant, 2d, 1964, Ames, Iowa. Washington, D.C.; Butterworths, 1965. 480p.	
	Douglas, S. W., M. E. Herrtage, and H. D. Williamson. Principles of Veterinary Radiography. 4th ed. London and Philadelphia; Bailliere Tindall, 1987. 371p. (Available in Spanish as Diagnostico Radiologico Veterinario. Zaragoza; Acribia, 1976.)	Second
Third	Downing, Elisabeth. Keeping Goats. 2d ed. London; Pelham Books, 1984. 128p. (1st ed., 1976. 128p.) (Available in Spanish as Usted Puede Criar Cabras. 2d ed. Buenos Aires; Ateneo, 1986.)	Second
Second	Doyle, Michael P. Foodborne Bacterial Pathogens. New York; M. Dekker, 1989. 796p.	Second
	Drochner, W. Aspects of Digestion in the Large Intestine of the Pig. Berlin; Paul Parey, 1987. 84p.	Second
Third	Drummond, Roger O., John E. George, and Sidney E. Kunz. Control of Arthropod Pests of Livestock: A Review of Technology. Boca Raton, Fla.; CRC Press, 1988. 245p.	Second

Developed countries ranking		Third World ranking
Third	Dubey, J. P., and Angela Towle. Toxoplasmosis in Sheep: A Review and Annotated Bibliography. Farnham Royal, U.K.; Commonwealth Agriculture Bureaux, 1986. 152p.	Third
	Dufty, J. H. Handbook of Bovine Obstetrics. Baltimore; Williams & Wilkins, 1980. 208p. (Available in Spanish.)	Third
Second	Duijn, C. van. Diseases of Fishes. 3d ed. London and Springfield, Ill.; Iliffe Books & Thomas, 1973. 372p. (1st ed., 1956.)	Third
First	Dukes, H. H., and Melvin J. Swenson, eds. Dukes' Physiology of Domestic Animals. 10th ed. Ithaca, N.Y.; Comstock Pub. Associates, 1984. 922p. (Available in Spanish as Fisiologia de los Animales Domesticos. 4th ed. Madrid; Aguilar, 1977.)	First
	Duncan, J. Robert, and Keith W. Prasse. Veterinary Laboratory Medicine: Clinical Pathology. 2d ed. Ames; Iowa State University Press, 1986. 285p. (1st ed., 1977. 243p.)	Second
	Dunn, Angus M. Veterinary Helminthology. 2d ed. London; W. Heinemann Medical, 1978. 323p. (Available in Spanish as Helmintologia Veterinaria . . . trans. by Alejandro R. Sanchez Rodriguez. Mexico; Manual Moderno, 1983.)	Second
First	Dunne, Howard W., and Allen D. Leman, eds. Diseases of Swine. 6th ed. Ames; Iowa State University Press, 1986. 930p. (1st ed., edited by H. W. Dunne, 1958. 716p.) (Available in Spanish as Enfermedades del Cerdo. Mexico City; UTEHA, 1988–1990.)	
Second	Duthil, J. Produccion de Forrajes (Forage Production). 3d ed., rev. Madrid; Ediciones Mundi-Prensa, 1989. 365p. (Earlier ed., 1980. 413p.)	Third
	Dvorak, Jaroslav, and M. Otcenasek. Mycological Diagnosis of Animal Dermatophytoses. Prague; Academia, 1969. 213p.	Third
	Dyce, K. M., W. O. Sack, and C. J. G. Wensing. Textbook of Veterinary Anatomy. Philadelphia; Saunders, 1987. 820p.	Second
	Dyer, Irwin A., and C. C. O'Mary. The Feedlot. 2d ed. Philadelphia; Lea & Febiger, 1977. 246p. (1st ed., 1977.) (Available in Spanish as Engorde a Corral. Buenos Aires; Hemisferio Sur, 1975.)	Second
	Dykstra, R. R. Animal Sanitation and Disease Control. 6th ed. Danville, Ill.; Interstate Printers & Publishers, 1961. 858p. (1st ed., 1942. 558p.) (Available in Spanish as Higiene Animal y Prevencion de Enfermedades. Spain; Labor, 1970.)	Second

E

Third	Eales, F. A., and J. Small. Practical Lambing: A Guide to Veterinary Care at Lambing. London and New York; Longman, 1986. 132p. (Available in Spanish as Parto de la Oveja: Con-	Third

Developed countries ranking		Third World ranking
	sejos Veterinarios e Instrucciones Practicas. Zaragoza; Acribia, 1986.)	
Third	Easmon, C. S. F., and C. Adlam, eds. Staphylococci and Staphylococcal Infections. London and New York; Academic Press, 1983. 2 vols.	Second
Second	Eckert, J., M. A. Gemmell, and E. J. L. Soulsby. Echinococcosis/Hydatidosis Surveillance, Prevention and Control: FAO/UNEP/WHO Guidelines. Rome; Food and Agriculture Organization, 1982. 147p.	Third
Second	Eckert, Roger, and David J. Randall. Animal Physiology: Mechanisms and Adaptations. 3d ed. New York; W. H. Freeman, 1988. 683p. (1st ed., San Francisco; W. H. Freeman, 1978. 558p.)	First
Third	Economides, Soterios. Intensive Sheep Production in the Near East. Rome; Food and Agriculture Organization, 1983. 67p. (FAO Animal Production and Health Paper no. 40)	Third
Second	Edqvist, Lars E., and Hans Kindahl, eds. Prostaglandins in Animal Reproduction; Proceedings from a Symposium, Swedish University of Agricultural Sciences, Uppsala, Sweden, May–June 1983. Amsterdam and New York; Elsevier, 1984. 304p. (Reprinted from Animal Reproduction Science, vol. 7, no. 1–3.)	Second
Third	Egerton, J. R., W. K. Yong, and G. G. Riffkin, eds. Footrot and Foot Abscess of Ruminants. Boca Raton, Fla.; CRC Press, 1989. 262p.	Second
Third	Eikelenboom, G. Stunning of Animals for Slaughter; Proceedings of a Seminar in the CEC Programme of Coordination of Research on Animal Welfare, Research Institute for Animal Production "Schoonoord," Zeist, Netherlands, October 1982. Boston; M. Nijhoff, 1983. 227p.	
Third	Eklund, Melvin W., and V. R. Dowell, eds. Avian Botulism: An International Perspective; Papers from a Conference Sponsored by the Toxic Micro-Organisms Panel of the Joint U.S.-Japan Cooperation on the Development and Utilization of Natural Resources Program. Springfield, Ill.; Thomas, 1987. 405p.	Third
Third	Ellendorf, F., M. Taverne, and D. Smidt, eds. Physiology and Control of Parturition of Domestic Animals; A Symposium, February 1979, Institute fur Tierzucht und Tierverhalten der Bundesforschungsanstalt fur Landwirtschaft Braunschweig-Volkenrode (FAL). Amsterdam and New York; Elsevier, 1979. 348p. (Developments in Animal and Veterinary Sciences no. 5)	Third
	Ellendorff, F., and F. Elsaesser, eds. Endocrine Causes of Seasonal and Lactational Anestrus in Farm Animals: A Seminar in the CEC Programme . . . at the Institute fur Tierzucht und Tierverhalten, Marienses, Bundesforschungsanstalt fur Land-	Second

Developed countries ranking		Third World ranking
	wirtschaft, October 1984, Sponsored by the Commission of the European Communities. Dordrecht and Boston; M. Nijhoff, 1985. 237p.	
Third	Ellis, Anthony E. Fish and Shellfish Pathology; Selected Papers of the International Conference of the EAFP, Plymouth Polytechnic, September 1983. U.S. ed. London and Orlando, Fla.; Academic Press, 1985. 412p.	Second
Third	Ellis, W. A., and T. W. A. Little. The Present State of Leptospirosis Diagnosis and Control: A Seminar in the CEC Programme of Coordination of Research on Animal Pathology, Veterinary Research Laboratories, Belfast, October 1984. Dordrecht; Boston and Hingham, Mass.; M. Nijhoff for the Commission of the European Communities Distributors for the U.S. and Canada, Kluwer Academic, 1986. 247p.	Second
Second	Elsden, R. P., and G. E. Seidel. Embryo Transfer Procedures for Cattle. Fort Collins; Colorado State University, 1982. 45p. (Colorado State University Experiment Station no. 1011)	
	English, Peter R., et al. The Growing and Finishing Pig: Improving Efficiency. Ipswich, Eng; Farming Press; Alexandria Bay, N.Y.; Distributed in North America by Diamond Farm Enterprises, 1988. 555p.	Third
First	Ensminger, M. Eugene. Animal Science. 8th ed. Danville, Ill.; Interstate Printers and Publishers, 1983. 1049p. (1st ed., 1950.) (Available in Spanish as Zootecnia General. 2d ed. Buenos Aires; El Ateneo, 1976.)	First
First	Ensminger, M. Eugene. Beef Cattle Science. 6th ed. Danville, Ill.; Interstate Printers & Publishers, 1987. 1030p. (First published as Beef Cattle Husbandry.) (Available in Spanish as Produccion Bovina para Carne. 3d ed. Buenos Aires; 1981.)	First
Second	Ensminger, M. Eugene. The Complete Encyclopedia of Horses. South Brunswick; A. S. Barnes, 1977. 487p.	
First	Ensminger, M. Eugene. Dairy Cattle Science. 2d ed. Danville, Ill.; Interstate Printers & Publishers, 1980. 625p. (1st ed., 1971. 524p.)	First
Second	Ensminger, M. Eugene. Poultry Science. 2d ed. Danville, Ill.; Interstate Printers & Publishers, 1980. 502p. (1st ed., 1971. 276p.) (Available in Spanish as Produccion Avicola. Mexico; Ateneo, 1979.)	First
Second	Ensminger, M. Eugene. The Stockman's Handbook. 7th ed. Danville, Ill.; Interstate Printers and Pub., 1992. 1029p. (1st ed., 1955. 598p.) (Available in Spanish as Manuel del Ganadero. Buenos Aires; Ateneo 1975.)	
First	Ensminger, M. Eugene, J. E. Oldfield, and W. W. Heinemann. Feeds and Nutrition. 2d ed. Clovis, Calif.; Ensminger Pub. Co., 1990. 1544p. 1st ed., 1978, by M. E. Ensminger and	First

Developed countries ranking		Third World ranking
	C. G. Olentine, Jr., as Feeds and Nutrition, Complete. 117p.) (Available in Spanish as Alimentos y Nutricion de los Animales. Buenos Aires; El Ateneo, 1983.)	
First	Ensminger, M. Eugene, and R. O. Parker. Sheep and Goat Science. 5th ed. Danville, Ill.; Interstate Printers & Publishers, 1986. 643p. (Rev. ed. of Sheep and Wool Science. 4th ed., 1970.) (Available in Spanish as Produccion Ovina. 2d ed. Buenos Aires; Ateneo, 1976.)	First
First	Ensminger, M. Eugene, and R. O. Parker. Swine Science. 5th ed. Danville, Ill.; Interstate Printers, 1984. 568p. (Available in Spanish as Produccion Porcina. 3d ed. Buenos Aires; Ateneo, 1980.)	Second
Second	Epstein, Hellmut, and I. L. Mason. The Origin of the Domestic Animals of Africa. New York; Africana Pub. Corp., 1971. 2 vols. (Also issued as a Leipzig ed., 1971.)	First
Third	Esmay, Merle L. Principles of Animal Environment. Textbook ed. Westport, Conn.; Avi Pub. Co., 1978. 358p. (1st ed., 1969. 325p.)	
Third	Esslemont, R. J., J. H. Bailie, and M. J. Cooper. Fertility Management in Dairy Cattle. London; Collins, 1985. 143p.	
Second	Etgen, W. M., ed. Dairy Cattle: Feeding and Management. 7th ed. New York; J. Wiley, 1987. 598p. (1st ed., 1917.) (Available in Spanish as Ganado Lechero: Alimentacion y Administracion. Mexico; Limusa-Noriega, 1989.)	Second
	Euroconsult. Agricultural Compendium for Rural Development in the Tropics and Subtropics. 3d rev. ed. Amsterdam and New York; Elsevier, 1989. 740p. (Prev. ed., 1981.)	Third
Second	European Association for Animal Production. Dictionary of Animal Production Terminology: English, French, Spanish, German, and Latin. Amsterdam and New York; Elsevier, 1985. 683p. (European Association for Animal Production Pub. no. 30) (Rev. ed. of Vocabulary of Animal Husbandry Terms, 1959.)	First
Third	European Grassland Federation. Quality of Herbage; Proceedings of the 5th General Meeting of the European Grassland Federation. Uppsala; Almqvist & Wiksell, 1974. 162p.	
Second	European Symposium on Poultry Nutrition, 6th, 1987, Konigslutter, Germany. Proceedings . . . Joint Conference with World's Poultry Science Association. Edited by H. Voot. Celle, Germany; Institut fur Kleintierzucht der FAL, 1987. 258p.	Second
Second	European Symposium on Poultry Nutrition, 7th, 1989, Lloret de Mar, Spain. Proceedings . . . Joint Conference with World's Poultry Science Association. Barcelona; World's Poultry Science Association, 1989. 309p.	Second
Third	European Symposium on Quality of Poultry Meat, 5th, 1981,	Third

Developed countries ranking		Third World ranking
	Apeldoorn, Netherlands. Quality of Poultry Meat; Proceedings . . . edited by R. W. A. W. Mulder, C. W. Scheele, C. H. Veerkamp. Beekbergen, Netherlands; Spelderholt Institute for Poultry Research, 1981. 488p.	
	Eusebio, J. A. Pig Production in the Tropics. London; Longman, 1980. 115p. (Intermediate Tropical Agriculture Series)	Second
Second	Evans, Gareth, W. M. C. Maxwell, and Steven Salamon. Salamon's Artificial Insemination of Sheep and Goats. Sydney and Boston; Butterworths, 1987. 194p. (Expansion of Artificial Insemination of Sheep, by Steven Salamon, 1976.)	Second

F

Developed countries ranking		Third World ranking
First	Falconer, D. S. Introduction to Quantitative Genetics. 3d ed. Burnt Mill, Harlow Essex, U.K.; Longman, Scientific & Technical; New York; Wiley, 1989. 438p. (1st ed., Edinburgh, 1960.) (Available in Spanish as Introduccion a la Genetica Cuantitativa. Mexico; CECSA, 1970.)	First
Third	Falconer, Ian R., ed. Lactation; Proceedings of an International Symposium, 17th Easter School in Agricultural Science, University of Nottingham, 1970. London; Butterworths, 1971. 467p.	
	Falloux, Francois, and Aleki Mukendi, eds. Desertification Control and Renewable Resource Management in the Sahelian and Sudanian Zones of West Africa; Proceedings of a Workshop . . . Oslo, 1986, sponsored by the Norwegian Ministry of Development Cooperation, the Canadian International Development Agency and the World Bank. Washington, D.C.; World Bank, 1988. 119p. (World Bank Technical Paper no. 70)	Third
	FAO/IAEA Joint Conference. Domestic Buffalo Production in Asia; Proceedings of the Final Research Coordination Meeting on the Use of Nuclear Techniques to Improve Domestic Buffalo Production in Asia, Phase II, Rockhampton, Australia, February 1989. Vienna; International Atomic Energy Agency, 1990. 225p.	Third
Third	Faull, W. B., J. W. Hughes, M. J. Clarkson, and G. S. Walton. Mastitis Notes for the Dairy Practitioner. 4th ed. Liverpool; Liverpool University Press, 1987. 82p.	Third
Third	Faure, Jean M., and Andrew D. Mills, eds. European Symposium on Poultry Welfare, 3d; Proceedings . . . sponsored by World's Poultry Science Association, France Branch. Tours, France; INRA, 1989. 284p.	
Third	Fell, Henry R. Intensive Sheep Management. 2d ed. Ipswich, Suffolk; Farming Press, 1985. 260p. (1st ed., 1979. 248p.)	Third
Third	Fenn, M. G., and I. Ozorai. Marketing Livestock and Meat. 2d ed. Rome; Food and Agriculture Organization, 1977. 198p. (1st	Second

<table>
<tr><td>Developed
countries
ranking</td><td></td><td>Third
World
ranking</td></tr>
<tr><td></td><td>ed., by R. F. Burdette and J. C. Abbott, 1960.) (Also available in Spanish.) (FAO Animal Production and Health Series no. 1)</td><td></td></tr>
<tr><td></td><td>Fenner, Frank, et al. Veterinary Virology. Orlando, Fla.; Academic Press, 1987. 660p.</td><td>Third</td></tr>
<tr><td>Second</td><td>Finney, David J. Statistical Method in Biological Assay. 3d ed. London; C. Griffin, 1978. 508p. (1st ed., 1952.)</td><td>Second</td></tr>
<tr><td>Second</td><td>Fisher, C., and K. N. Boorman, eds. Nutrient Requirements of Poultry and Nutritional Research; Proceedings of the 19th Poultry Science Symposium, Edinburgh, 1984. London and Boston; Butterworths, 1986. 224p. (Poultry Science Symposium no. 19)</td><td></td></tr>
<tr><td></td><td>Flora, Cornelia B., ed. Animals in the Farming System; Proceedings of Kansas State University's 1983 Farming Systems Research Symposium. Manhattan; Kansas State University, 1984. 924 numbered pages on 462p. (Farming Systems Research Paper no. 6)</td><td>Third</td></tr>
<tr><td></td><td>Flores Menendez, Jorge A. Bromatologia Animal. 3d ed. Mexico; Editorial Limusa, 1983. 1096p. (1st ed., 1977. 683p.)</td><td>Third</td></tr>
<tr><td>Third</td><td>Folsch, Detlef W., ed. The Ethology and Ethics of Farm Animal Production; Proceedings of the 28th Annual Meeting, Commission on Animal Management and Health, Brussels, 1977. Basel and Stuttgart; Birkhauser Verlag, 1978. 144p. (European Association for Animal Production Pub. no. 24)</td><td></td></tr>
<tr><td>Third</td><td>Folsch, Detlef W. Intensivhaltung von Nutztieren aus Ethischer, Rechtlicher und Ethologischer Sicht (Intensive Husbandry of Livestock from Ethical, Legal and Ethological Perspectives). Basel; Birkhauser, 1979. 228p. (In German with English, French, and Italian abstracts.)</td><td></td></tr>
<tr><td>First</td><td>Fonnesbeck, Paul V., Lorin E. Harris, and Leonard C. Kearl, eds. First International Symposium: Feed Composition, Animal Nutrient Requirements, and Computerization of Diets, Utah State University . . . Logan, Utah; International Feedstuffs Institute; Animal, Dairy, and Veterinary Sciences Dept., Utah Agricultural Experiment Station; Utah State University, 1977. 799p.</td><td>First</td></tr>
<tr><td>Third</td><td>Food and Agriculture Organization. Animal Energy in Agriculture in Africa and Asia: Technical Papers Presented at the FAO Expert Consultation, Rome, November 1982 = Energie Animale en Agriculture en Afrique et en Asie: Documents . . . Expert Consultation on the Appropriate Use of Animal Energy in Agriculture in Africa and Asia. Rome; Food and Agriculture Organization, 1984. 143p. (English and French.)</td><td>Second</td></tr>
<tr><td>Third</td><td>Food and Agriculture Organization. Animal Genetic Resources Data Banks. Rome; Food and Agriculture Organization, 1986. 3 vols. (FAO Animal Production and Health Paper no. 59)</td><td></td></tr>
<tr><td></td><td>Food and Agriculture Organization. Buffalo Reproduction and</td><td>Third</td></tr>
</table>

Developed countries ranking		Third World ranking
	Artificial Insemination, and National Dairy Research Institute, Karnal, India, December 1978; Proceedings of a Seminar . . . Rome; Food and Agriculture Organization, 1979. 363p. (FAO Animal Production and Health Paper no. 13)	
Second	Food and Agriculture Organization. Expert Consultation on Animal Disease Control in International Movement of Semen and Embryos: A Report. Rome; Food and Agriculture Organization, 1981. 101p.	First
	Food and Agriculture Organization. Expert Group Meeting on Livestock Programmes for Small Farmers and Agricultural Labourers in Asia and the Far East, 1976, Bangkok. Integration of Livestock with Crop Production at Small Farm Level. Bangkok; Food and Agriculture Organization, Regional Office for Asia and the Far East, 1976. 2 vols.	Second
Third	Food and Agriculture Organization. Integrating Crops and Livestock in West Africa. Rome; Food and Agriculture Organization, 1983. 112p.	Second
	Food and Agriculture Organization. International Expert Consultation. Dairy Cattle Breeding in the Humid Tropics, 2d, 1979, Hissar, India; Proceedings . . . Daya Singh Balaine, Chairman. Hissar, India; Haryana Agricultural University, 1980. 301p.	Second
Second	Food and Agriculture Organization/UNEP Technical Consultation. Animal Genetic Resources Conservation and Management: Proceedings of the . . . Consultation, 1980, Rome. Rome; Food and Agriculture Organization, 1981. 388p. (FAO Animal Production and Health Paper no. 24) (Papers in English, French or Spanish.)	First
	Food and Fertilizer Technology Center for the Asian and Pacific Region. Integrated Crop-Livestock-Fish Farming; Proceedings of a Symposium-Workshop . . . Philippine Council for Agriculture and Resources Research, Los Banos, 1979. Taipei, Taiwan; Food and Fertilizer Technology Center for the Asian and Pacific Region, 1980. 147p.	Third
Second	Forbes, J. M. The Voluntary Food Intake of Farm Animals. London and Boston; Butterworths, 1986. 206p.	Second
Second	Forrest, John C., et al. Principles of Meat Science. San Francisco; Freeman, 1975. 417p.	Second
	Forscey, Lance A., ed. Multi-Lingual Poultry Dictionary (English-French-German-Spanish). Bologna; European Federation of Branches of the World's Poultry Science Association, Edagricole, 1969. 356p. (Title also in French: Dictionnaire Multilingues de Volailles; German: Mehrsprachen-gefl.)	Second
Third	Fowler, Murray E. Restraint and Handling of Wild and Domes-	

<table>
<tr><td>Developed
countries
ranking</td><td></td><td>Third
World
ranking</td></tr>
<tr><td></td><td>tic Animals. 1st ed. Ames; Iowa State University Press, 1978.
332p.</td><td></td></tr>
<tr><td></td><td>Fowler, Murray E. Zoo and Wild Animal Medicine. 2d ed.
Philadelphia; Saunders, 1986. 1127p.</td><td>Second</td></tr>
<tr><td>Third</td><td>Fox, Michael W. Farm Animals: Husbandry, Behavior, and
Veterinary Practice: Viewpoints of a Critic. Baltimore; University Park Press, 1984. 285p.</td><td>Second</td></tr>
<tr><td>Third</td><td>Fox, P. F., ed. Developments in Dairy Chemistry. London and
New York; Applied Science; Elsevier sole distributor in the
U.S. and Canada, 1982–1986. 4 vols.</td><td></td></tr>
<tr><td>First</td><td>Frandson, R. D. Anatomy and Physiology of Farm Animals.
4th ed. Philadelphia; Lea & Febiger, 1986. 560p. (Available in
Spanish as Anotomia y Fisiologia de los Animales Domesticos.
2d ed. Mexico; Interamericana, 1983.)</td><td>First</td></tr>
<tr><td>Third</td><td>Franklin, Kenneth R., and H. Russell Cross, eds. Proceedings
. . . International Symposium—Meat Science and Technology,
1982, University of Nebraska. Chicago; National Livestock and
Meat Board, 1983. 398p.</td><td></td></tr>
<tr><td>Second</td><td>Fraser, Allan, and J. T. Stamp. Sheep Husbandry and Diseases.
6th ed., rev. by J. M. M. Cunningham and J. T. Stamp. London; Collins Professional and Technical, 1987. 344p. (3d rev.
ed., C. Lockwood, 1957. 444p.)</td><td>Second</td></tr>
<tr><td>First</td><td>Fraser, Andrew F. Animal Reproduction: Tabulated Data. Rev.
ed. London; Bailliere Tindall, 1971. 28p. (1st ed, 1968, as Tables of Data on Livestock Reproduction, Edinburgh University
Press.) (Available in Spanish as Reproduccion Animal: Datos
Tabulados. Montevideo, Uruguay; Mesiferio, Sur 1975.)</td><td></td></tr>
<tr><td>Third</td><td>Fraser, Andrew F. Ethology of Farm Animals: A Comprehensive Study of the Behavioural Features of the Common Farm
Animals. Amsterdam and New York; Elsevier Science Pub.,
1985. 500p.</td><td>First</td></tr>
<tr><td>Third</td><td>Fraser, Andrew F. Reproductive and Developmental Behaviour
in Sheep: An Anthology from Applied Animal Ethology. Amsterdam and New York; Elsevier, 1985. 439p. (Articles from
Applied Animal Ethology, December 1974–1984.)</td><td></td></tr>
<tr><td>First</td><td>Fraser, Andrew F., and D. M. Broom. Farm Animal Behaviour
and Welfare. 3d ed. London; Bailliere Tindall, 1990. 437p.
(Previous editions, 1974 and 1980 as Farm Animal Behaviour,
by A. F. Fraser.) (1980 ed. available in Spanish: Comportamiento de los Animales de Granja. Zaragoza; Acribia, 1982.)</td><td>First</td></tr>
<tr><td></td><td>Freeman, B. M., and P. E. Lake, eds. Egg Formation and Production. Edinburgh; British Poultry Science, 1972. 216p. (Poultry Science Symposium no. 8)</td><td>Third</td></tr>
<tr><td></td><td>French, M. H. Observations on the Goat. Rome; Food and Ag-</td><td>Second</td></tr>
</table>

Developed countries ranking		Third World ranking
	riculture Organization, 1970. 204p. (FAO Agricultural Studies no. 80) (Available in Spanish as *Observaciones sobre las Cabras*. Rome; FAO, 1970.)	
Second	French, M. H., and Ivar Johansson. *European Breeds of Cattle*. Rome; Food and Agriculture Organization, 1966. 2 vols.	
Third	Friedman, Mendel, ed. *Protein Nutritional Quality of Foods and Feeds; Proceedings of American Chemical Society Symposium on Chemical and Biological Methods for Protein Quality Evaluation, Atlantic City, N.J., 1974*. New York; M. Dekker, 1975. 2 vols.	Third
Third	Friend, John B. *Cattle of the World*. Poole, U.K.; Blandford Press, 1978. 198p.	Second
Second	Frimmer, Max. *Pharmakologie und Toxikologie; Bein Lehrbuch fur Veterinarmediziner und Naturwissenschaftler*. 3d ed. Stuttgart and New York; Schattauer, 1986. 432p. (1st ed., 1969. 331p.) (Available in Spanish as *Farmacologia y Toxicologia Veterinaria*. Zaragoza; Acribia, 1973.)	
Third	Frings, Hubert, and Mable Frings. *Animal Communication*. 2d ed., rev. and enlarged. Norman; University of Oklahoma Press, 1977. 207p.	
Third	Froystein, Terje, Erik Slinde, and Nils Standal, eds. *Porcine Stress and Meat Quality—Causes and Possible Solutions to the Problems; Proceedings of a Symposium . . . Refsnes Gods, Norway, November 1980*. As, Norway; Agricultural Food Research Society, 1981. 360p.	
Second	Fudenberg, H. Hugh, et al. *Basic Immunogenetics*. 2d ed. New York; Oxford University Press, 1978. 262p.	

G

Developed countries ranking		Third World ranking
Second	Gafaar, S. M., Walter E. Howard, and Rex E. Marsh. *Parasites, Pests, and Predators*. Amsterdam and New York; Elsevier, 1985. 575p.	Third
Second	Gall, C. *Goat Production*. London and New York; Academic Press, 1981. 619p.	Second
	Garner, Reuben J. *Veterinary Toxicology; formerly Lander's Veterinary Toxicology*. 3d ed., rev. by E. G. C. Clarke and M. L. Clarke. London and Baltimore; Bailliere Tindall & Cassell and Williams & Wilkins, 1967. 477p.	Third
First	Garnsworthy, Philip C. *Nutrition and Lactation in the Dairy Cow; Proceedings of the 46th Easter School in Agricultural Science*. London and Boston; Butterworths, 1988. 429p.	
	Garrett, Phillip D. *Guide to Ruminant Anatomy Based on the Dissection of the Goat*. 1st Iowa State University Press ed. Ames; Iowa State University Press, 1988. 102p.	Second

Developed countries ranking		Third World ranking
Third	Gatenby, Ruth M. Sheep Production in the Tropics and Sub-Tropics. London and New York; Longman, 1986. 351p.	First
	Gatenby, Ruth M., and J. C. Trail. Small Ruminant Breed Productivity in Africa; Proceedings of a Seminar . . . ILCA, Addis Ababa, Ethiopia, October 1982. Addis Ababa, Ethiopia; International Livestock Centre for Africa, 1982. 96p.	First
	Geering, W. A., and A. J. Forman. Exotic Diseases. Canberra, Australia; Australian Government Publishing Service, 1987. 260p.	Third
	Geerts, S., V. Kumar, and J. Brandt, eds. Helminth Zoonoses; Proceedings of the International Colloquium . . . Antwerp, December 1986. Dordrecht; Boston and Hingham, Mass.; Martinus Nijhoff; Distributors for the U.S. and Canada, Kluwer Academic Publishers, 1987. 240p.	Third
	Georgi, Jay R., Marion E. Georgi, and Vassilios J. Theodorides. Parasitology for Veterinarians. 5th ed. Philadelphia; Saunders, 1990. 412p. (4th ed., 1985. 344p.)	Second
Third	Georgievskii, V. I., B. N. Annenkov, and V. T. Samokhin. Mineral Nutrition of Animals. Translation of Mineral'noe Pitanie Zhivotnykh by Freund Publishing House; English translation verified by H. Brookes. London and Boston; Butterworths, 1982. 475p.	Second
	Gerhardt, Philipp, et al., eds. Manual of Methods for General Bacteriology. Washington, D.C.; American Society for Microbiology, 1981. 524p.	Third
	Ghoshal, Nani G., Tankred Koch, and Pete Popesko. The Venous Drainage of the Domestic Animals. Philadelphia; Saunders, 1981. 268p.	Third
Third	Giammattei, Victor M. Raising Small Meat Animals: Efficient Home Production of Cornish Game Hens, Chicken Broilers, Turkey Roasters, Fryer Rabbits, Squabs. Danville, Ill.; Interstate Printers & Publishers, 1976. 433p.	
	Gibson, T. E., ed. Weather and Parasitic Animal Disease. Geneva; Secretariat of the World Meterological Organization, 1978. 174p. (World Meterological Organization Technical Note no. 159)	Third
Third	Gil, J. Infante, and J. Costa Durao. A Colour Atlas of Meat Inspection. London; Wolfe Medical, 1990. 453p. (Translation of Manual de Inspeccao Sanitaria de Carnes. Lisbon; Fundacao Calouste Gulbenkian, 1985.)	Second
	Gilbert, Stephen G. Pictorial Anatomy of the Fetal Pig. 2d ed., rev. and enlarged. Seattle; University of Washington Press, 1966.	Third
Third	Gill, John L. Design and Analysis of Experiments in the Ani-	Third

Developed countries ranking		Third World ranking
	mal and Medical Sciences. 1st ed. Ames; Iowa State University Press, 1978. 3 vols.	
Third	Gillespie, James R. Modern Livestock and Poultry Production. 4th ed. Albany, N.Y.; Delmar Publishers, 1990. 964p. (1st ed., 1981. 662p.)	
	Gillies, R. R., and T. C. Dodds. Bacteriology Illustrated. 3d ed. Edinburgh; Churchill Livingstone; Baltimore; Williams & Wilkins, 1973. 244p.	Third
Third	Gilmore, Desmond, and Brian Cook, eds. Environmental Factors in Mammal Reproduction. Baltimore; University Park Press, 1981. 330p.	
Third	Gluzman, Yakov, ed. Eukaryotic Viral Vectors; Papers presented at a conference, Banbury Center, Dec. 1981. Cold Spring Harbor, N.Y.; Cold Spring Harbor Laboratory, 1982. 221p.	
Second	Gohl, Bo. Tropical Feeds: Feed Information Summaries and Nutritive Values. Updated ed. Rome; Food and Agriculture Organization, 1981. 529p. (FAO Animal Production and Health Series no. 12) (1st ed., 1975.) (This out-of-print book has been converted to an MS-DOS database with the same information and requiring 920 K disk space. It covers 500 tropical feeds and is available from FAO.)	First
Third	Goldstein, Lester, and David M. Prescott, eds. Cell Biology: A Comprehensive Treatise. New York; Academic Press, 1977. 4 vols.	
	Golub, Edward S. The Cellular Basis of the Immune Response: An Approach to Immunobiology. 2d ed. Sunderland, Mass.; Sinauer Associates, 1981. 330p. (1st ed., 1977. 278p.) (Available in Spanish as Base Celular de la Respuesta Immunologica. 1st ed. trans. by Jorge Barbe Garcia. Barcelona; Reverte, 1987.)	Second
Third	Gomez, Kwanchai A., and Arturo A. Gomez. Statistical Procedures for Agricultural Research. 2d ed. New York; J. Wiley, 1984. 680p.	Third
Third	Goodall, Daphne M. Horses of the World: An Illustrated Survey . . . of Breeds of Horses and Ponies. 3d ed., rev. Newton Abbot, U.K.; David & Charles, 1973. 272p. (Earlier ed., New York; Macmillan, 1965.)	Second
	Goodwin, Derek H. Pig Management and Production: A Practical Guide for Farmers and Students. London; Hutchinson Educational, 1973. 203p. (Available in Spanish as Produccion y Manejo del Cerdo. 2d ed. Zaragoza; Acribia, 1986.)	Second
	Goodwin, Derek H. Pigeons and Doves of the World. 3d ed. London; British Museum (Natural History); Ithaca, N.Y.; Com-	Third

Developed countries ranking		Third World ranking
	stock Pub. Associates, 1983. 363p. (1st ed., London; British Museum, 1967. 446p.)	
Third	Goodwin, Derek H. Sheep Management and Production. 2d ed. Brookfield, Vermont; Brookfield Publishing, 1982. 224p. (1st ed., 1971, as The Production and Management of Sheep.) (Available in Spanish as Produccion y Manejo del Ganado Ovino. Zaragoza; Acribia, 1975.)	Second
Second	Gordon, Ian R. Controlled Breeding in Farm Animals. 1st ed. Oxford and New York; Pergamon Press, 1983. 436p.	Third
Second	Gordon, Malcolm S., in collaboration with George A. Bartholomew et al. Animal Physiology: Principles and Adaptations. 4th ed. New York and London; Macmillan and Collier Macmillan, 1982. 635p. (1st ed. as Animal Function: Principles and Adaptations, 1968. 560p.) (Available in Spanish as Fisiologia Animal. Mexico; CECSA, 1979.)	Third
Second	Gordon, R. F., and F. T. W. Jordan, eds. Poultry Diseases. 2d ed. London; Bailliere Tindall, 1982. 401p. (1st ed., edited by R. F. Gordon, 1977. 352p.) (Available in Spanish, 1980.)	Second
Second	Goss, Richard J. The Physiology of Growth. New York; Academic Press, 1978. 441p.	Third
Third	Gould, Sylvester E., ed. Trichinosis in Man and Animals. Springfield, Ill.; Thomas, 1970. 540p.	
	Graber, M., and C. Perrotin. Helminthes et Helminthoses des Ruminants Domestiques d'Afrique Tropicale. Maisons-Alfort; Editions du Point Veterinaire, 1983. 378p.	Third
Second	Gracey, J. F., and Horace Thornton. Meat Hygiene. 8th ed. London and Philadelphia; Bailliere Tindall, 1986. 517p. (First published, 1949, as Textbook of Meat Inspection by H. Thornton. 4th ed., 1981, as Thornton's Meat Hygiene by J. F. Gracey.) (Available in Spanish as Higiene de la Carne. 8th ed. Madrid; McGraw-Hill/Interamericana, 1988.)	
Second	Graffis, Don W., E. M. Juergenson, and Malcolm H. McVickar. 4th ed. Danville, Ill.; Interstate Printers & Publishers, 1985. 356p. (Rev. ed. of 3d ed. by M. H. McVickar, 1974.)	Third
Second	Graham, Horace D., ed. The Safety of Foods. 2d ed. Westport, Conn.; Avi Pub. Co., 1980. 774p. (1st ed., edited by J. C. Ayres, H. D. Graham et al., 1968. 367p.)	Third
Third	Gravert, Hans Otto. Dairy-Cattle Production. Amsterdam and New York; Elsevier Science Publishers, 1987. 309p.	Second
Third	Gray, Annie P. Mammalian Hybrids; A Check-List with Bibliography. 2d ed., rev. Farnham Royal, U.K.; Commonwealth Agricultural Bureaux, 1972. 262p.	
Third	Great Britain. Agricultural Development and Advisory Service. Dairy Herd Fertility. London; H.M.S.O., 1984. 80p.	Third

Developed countries ranking		Third World ranking
Third	Great Britain. Meteorological Office. Tables of Temperature, Relative Humidity and Precipitation, and Sunshine for the World. London; H.M.S.O., 1972. 6 vols. (Published, 1958, as Tables of Temperature, Relative Humidity, and Precipitation for the World.)	Second
Second	Great Britain. Ministry of Agriculture, Fisheries and Food. Energy Allowances and Feeding Systems for Ruminants. 2d ed. London; H.M.S.O., 1984. 85p. (1st ed., 1975. 79p.)	Second
First	Great Britain. Ministry of Agriculture, Fisheries and Food. Feed Composition: UK Tables of Feed Composition and Nutritive Value for Ruminants. Rev. of 1986 ed., with corrections. Berks, U.K.; Chalcombe Publications, 1987. 69p.	First
	Great Britain. Ministry of Agriculture, Fisheries and Food. Manual of Veterinary Investigation Laboratory Techniques. 3d ed. London; H.M.S.O., 1984. 2 vols.	Second
	Greenland, D. J., and R. Lal, eds. Soil Conservation and Management in the Humid Tropics. Papers from the Conference Sponsored by the International Institute of Tropical Agriculture and the Agricultural Research Council of Nigeria. Chichester, U.K. and New York; Wiley, 1977. 283p.	Second
Third	Greenough, Paul R., Finlay J. MacCallum, and A. David Weaver. Lameness in Cattle. 2d ed., edited by A. David Weaver. Philadelphia; Lippincott, 1981. 471p. (1st ed., 1972. 478p.)	Second
Third	Griffiths, John F. Climates of Africa. Amsterdam and New York; Elsevier Pub. Co., 1972. 604p.	
	Grigg, David B. The Agricultural Systems of the World: An Evolutionary Approach. London and New York; Cambridge University Press, 1974. 358p.	Third
	Gross, F., ed. Iron Metabolism; An International Symposium, Sponsored by CIBA, Aix-en-Provence, July 1963. Berlin; Springer, 1964. 629p.	Third
	Gual, Carlos, and F. J. G. Ebling, eds. Progress in Endocrinology; Proceedings of the Third International Congress of Endocrinology, Mexico, June-July 1968. Amsterdam; Excerpta Medica Foundation, 1969. 1276p.	Third
Third	Gulland, J. A. Manual of Methods for Fish Stock Assessment. Rome; Food and Agriculture Organization, 1969–1976. 5 vols. (FAO Manuals in Fisheries Science no. 4)	Third
Third	Gurtler, Herbert. Lehrbuch der Physiologie der Haustiere . . . edited by Erich Kolb. 2d ed. Jena; G. Fischer, 1967. 989p. (1st ed., 1962. 942p.) (Available in Spanish as Fisologia Veterinaria. 2d ed. Zaragoza; Acribia, 1975.)	
Second	Guss, Samuel B. Management and Diseases of Dairy Goats. Scottsdale, Ariz.; Dairy Goat Journal, 1977. 222p.	

<table>
<tr><td>Developed
countries
ranking</td><td></td><td>Third
World
ranking</td></tr>
<tr><td>Second</td><td>Gyles, C. L., and Charles O. Thoen. Pathogenesis of Bacterial Infections in Animals. 1st ed. Ames; Iowa State University Press, 1986. 227p.</td><td>Third</td></tr>
<tr><td></td><td style="text-align:center">H</td><td></td></tr>
<tr><td></td><td>Hann, Cornelis de, and Nico J. Nissen. Animal Health Services in Sub-Saharan Africa: Alternative Approaches. Washington, D.C.; World Bank, 1985. 83p. (World Bank Technical Paper no. 44)</td><td>Third</td></tr>
<tr><td></td><td>Habel, Robert E. Guide to the Dissection of Domestic Ruminants. 4th ed. Ithaca, N.Y.; R. E. Habel, 1989. 233p. (3d ed., 1983. 165p.) (Available in Spanish as Anatomia y Manual de Diseccion de los Ruminantes Domesticos. Zaragoza; Acribia, 1968.)</td><td>Second</td></tr>
<tr><td>First</td><td>Hacker, J. B., ed. Nutritional Limits to Animal Production from Pastures; Proceedings of an International Symposium, St. Lucia, Queensland, Australia, August 1981. Farnham Royal, U.K.; Commonwealth Agricultural Bureaux, 1982. 536p.</td><td>First</td></tr>
<tr><td>First</td><td>Hacker, J. B., and J. H. Ternouth. The Nutrition of Herbivores; Proceedings . . . 2d International Symposium, University of Queensland, July, 1987. Sydney and Orlando, Fla.; Academic Press, 1987. 552p.</td><td>First</td></tr>
<tr><td>First</td><td>Hafez, E. S. E. The Behaviour of Domestic Animals. 3d ed. London; Bailliere Tindall, 1975. 532p. (1st ed., Baltimore; Williams & Wilkins, 1962. 619p.)</td><td>First</td></tr>
<tr><td>Second</td><td>Hafez, E. S. E., ed. The Mammalian Fetus: Comparative Biology and Methodology; Mammalian Fetus Symposium, Wayne State University, 1973. Springfield, Ill.; Thomas, 1975. 352p.</td><td></td></tr>
<tr><td>First</td><td>Hafez, E. S. E., ed. Reproduction in Farm Animals. 5th ed. Philadelphia; Lea & Febiger, 1987. 649p. (1st ed., 1962.) (Available in Spanish as Reproduccion e Insemination Artificial en Animales. 5th ed. Madrid; Interamericana, 1990.)</td><td>First</td></tr>
<tr><td></td><td>Hafez, E. S. E., and I. A. Dyer, eds. Animal Growth and Nutrition. Philadelphia; Lea & Febiger, 1969. 402p. (Available in Spanish as Desarrollo y Nutricion Animal. Zaragoza; Acribia, 1973.)</td><td>Third</td></tr>
<tr><td>First</td><td>Hagan, William A., Dorsey W. Bruner, and John F. Timoney. Microbiology and Infectious Diseases of Domestic Animals. 8th ed. Ithaca, N.Y.; Comstock Pub. Associates, 1988. 951p. (Rev. ed. of Hagan and Bruner's Infectious Diseases of Domestic Animals. 7th ed., 1981. 1st ed., 1943, by Hagan and Bruner.) (3d English ed. trans. to 2d Spanish ed. as Enfermedades Infecciosas de los Animales Domesticos. Mexico; Prensa Medica, 1984.)</td><td>Second</td></tr>
<tr><td>First</td><td>Hall, Harold T. B. Diseases and Parasites of Livestock in the</td><td>Second</td></tr>
</table>

Developed countries ranking		Third World ranking
	Tropics. 2d ed. London and New York; Longman, 1985. 328p. (1st ed., 1977. 288p.)	
	Hall, J. M., and R. Sansoucy. Open Yard Housing for Young Cattle. Rome; Food and Agriculture Organization, 1981. 133p.	Third
	Halliwell, Richard E. W., and Neil T. Gorman. Veterinary Clinical Immunology. Philadelphia; Saunders, 1989. 548p.	Third
Second	Halnan, Clive R. E., ed. Cytogenetics of Animals. Wallingford, Oxon, U.K.; CAB International, 1989. 519p.	Third
Third	Halpin, Brendan. Patterns of Animal Disease. London; Bailliere Tindall, 1975. 184p.	Third
Second	Halver, John E. Fish Nutrition. 2d ed. San Diego; Academic Press, 1989. 798p. (1st ed., New York; 1972. 713p.)	
First	Hammond, John, ed. Progress in the Physiology of Farm Animals. London; Butterworths Scientific Pub., 1954–1957. 3 vols.	First
Third	Hamori, Dezso. Constitutional Disorders and Hereditary Diseases in Domestic Animals . . . trans. by Ilona Koch of Haziallatok Oroklodo Alkati Hibai es Betegsegei. Amsterdam and New York; Elsevier Scientific Pub. Co., 1983. 727p. (Developments in Animal and Veterinary Sciences no. 11)	
Second	Handbook of Physiology: A Critical, Comprehensive Presentation of Physiological Knowledge and Concepts. Edited by S. R. Geiger. Rev. ed. Bethesda & Baltimore; American Physiological Society, 1977 to the present, and under constant revision. Currently in 23 vols. divided into 6 sections. (Supersedes original ed., 1959–1976, 39 vols.)	
Second	Handbook on Animal Diseases in the Tropics . . . edited by M. M. H. Sewell and D. W. Brocklesby. 4th ed. London and Philadelphia; Bailliere Tindall, 1990. 385p. (1st ed., London; British Veterinary Assoc., 1968. 3d ed. edited by Alexander Robertson.)	First
Second	Hanrahan, J. P. Beta-Agonists and Their Effects on Animal Growth and Carcass Quality; A Seminar in the EEC Programme of Coordination of Research in Animal Husbandry, Brussels, May, 1987. London and New York; Elsevier Applied Science, 1987. 201p. (Sponsored by the Commission of the European Communities, Directorate-General for Agriculture, Division for the Coordination of Agricultural Research.)	
Third	Hansel, W., and Barbara J. Weir, eds. Genetic Engineering of Animals; Proceedings . . . 2d Symposium, Cornell University, Ithaca, N.Y., June 1989. Dorset, U.K.; Journal of Reproduction & Fertility, 1990. (Journal of Reproduction & Fertility, Supplement no. 41)	
	Hansen, Jorgen, and Brian Perry. The Epidemiology, Diagnoses and Control of Gastro-Intestinal Parasites of Ruminants in	Third

<table>
<tr><td valign="top">

Developed
countries
ranking

</td><td></td><td valign="top" align="right">

Third
World
ranking

</td></tr>
<tr><td></td><td>

Africa. Nairobi, Kenya; International Laboratory for Research on Animal Diseases, 1990. 121p.

</td><td></td></tr>
<tr><td></td><td>

Hansen, Richard M., Benson M. Woie, and R. Dennis Child, eds. Range Development and Research in Kenya; Proceedings of a conference, Agricultural Resources Centre, Egerton College, Njoro, Kenya, April 1986, cosponsored by Kiboko Range Research Expansion Project and Winrock International. Morrilton, Ark.; Winrock International Institute for Agricultural Development, 1986. 474p.

</td><td align="right">Third</td></tr>
<tr><td valign="top">Third</td><td>

Hanson, Robert P., and Martha G. Hanson. Animal Disease Control: Regional Programs. 1st ed. Ames; Iowa State University Press, 1983. 331p.

</td><td></td></tr>
<tr><td valign="top">Third</td><td>

Harden Jones, F. R. Fish Migration. London; Edward Arnold, 1968. 325p.

</td><td align="right" valign="top">Third</td></tr>
<tr><td></td><td>

Hardy, James D., Adolf P. Gagge, and Jan A. J. Stolwijk, eds. Physiological and Behavioral Temperature Regulation. Springfield, Ill.; Thomas, 1970. 944p. (Revised papers of the International Symposium on Temperature Regulation, Aug. 1970, New Haven, Conn.)

</td><td align="right" valign="top">Third</td></tr>
<tr><td valign="top">Third</td><td>

Hardy, Ron, and Sam Meadowcroft. Indoor Beef Production. Ipswich, U.K.; Farming Press, 1986. 159p.

</td><td></td></tr>
<tr><td></td><td>

Haresign, William, ed. Sheep Production; Proceedings of the 35th Easter School in Agricultural Science. London and Boston; Butterworths, 1983. 576p.

</td><td align="right" valign="top">Second</td></tr>
<tr><td valign="top">First</td><td>

Haresign, William, and D. J. A. Cole, eds. Recent Advances in Animal Nutrition, 1991. London; Butterworth-Heinemann, 1991. 255p. (W. Haresign and Dyfed Lewis, 1964–1984.)

</td><td align="right" valign="top">First</td></tr>
<tr><td valign="top">Second</td><td>

Haresign, William, and D. J. A. Cole. Recent Developments in Ruminant Nutrition 2. London and Boston; Butterworths, 1988. 387p. (1st ed., 1981. 367p.)

</td><td align="right" valign="top">Second</td></tr>
<tr><td valign="top">Second</td><td>

Haresign, William, Henry Swan, and Dyfed Lewis, eds. Nutrition and the Climatic Environment; Papers of Nutrition Conference for Feed Manufacturers. London and Boston; Butterworths, 1977. 200p.

</td><td></td></tr>
<tr><td valign="top">Second</td><td>

Harkness, John E., and Joseph E. Wagner. The Biology and Medicine of Rabbits and Rodents. 3d ed. Philadelphia; Lea & Febiger, 1989. 230p. (1st ed., 1977.) (Available in Spanish as Biologia y Clinica de Conejos y Roedores. Zaragoza; Acribia, 1980.)

</td><td align="right" valign="top">Second</td></tr>
<tr><td valign="top">First</td><td>

Harris, Lorin E., compiler and ed. Chemical and Biological Methods for Feed Analysis. Gainesville, Fla.; Center for Tropical Agriculture, Feed Composition Project, Livestock Pavilion, University of Florida, 1970. 142p. (Available in Spanish as Metodos para el Analisis Quimico y la Evaluacion Biologica de Alimentos para Animales, 1970.)

</td><td align="right" valign="top">Third</td></tr>
</table>

Developed countries ranking		Third World ranking
Second	Harris, Lorin E. Nutrition Research Techniques for Domestic and Wild Animals; Vol. I: An International Record System and Procedures for Analyzing Samples. Logan, Utah; The author, 1970. 1 vol. (Various paging.)	
	Harris, Marvin. Cows, Pigs, Wars, and Witches: The Riddles of Culture. Rev. ed. New York; Vintage Books, 1978. 238p. (1st ed. New York; Random House, 1974. 276p.)	Third
Third	Harris, Marvin. Good to Eat: Riddles of Food and Culture. New York; Simon and Schuster, 1985. 289p.	Third
	Harrison, Greg J., and Linda Harrison. Clinical Avian Medicine and Surgery, Including Aviculture. Philadelphia; Saunders, 1986. 717p.	Third
Third	Hart, Benjamin L. The Behavior of Domestic Animals. New York; Freeman, 1985. 390p.	Third
Third	Hartl, D. L. Principles of Population Genetics. 2d ed. Sutherland, Mass.; Sinauer Associates, 1989. 682p. (1st ed., 1980. 488p.)	Second
Third	Harwood, Robert F. Entomology in Human and Animal Health. 7th ed. New York; Macmillan, 1979. 548p. (1st–5th ed. by W. B. Herms as Medical Entomology. 6th ed., 1969, by M. T. James as Herms' Medical Entomology.) (Available in Spanish.)	Third
Third	Hathcock, John N., and Julius Coon, eds. Nutrition and Drug Interrelations; Proceedings of a Symposium . . . Iowa State University, 1976. New York; Academic Press, 1978. 927p.	
	Hawkey, C. M., T. B. Dennett, and M. A. Peirce. Color Atlas of Comparative Veterinary Hematology. 1st ed. Ames; Iowa State University Press, 1989. 192p.	Third
	Hay, John B. Animal Models of Immunological Processes. London and New York; Academic Press, 1982. 295p.	Third
Second	Hayami, Y., and Vernon W. Ruttan. Agricultural Development: An International Perspective. Rev. and expanded. Baltimore; Johns Hopkins University Press, 1985. 506p. (1st ed., 1971.)	Second
Third	Hazlett, Brian A. Quantitative Methods in the Study of Animal Behavior. Papers from a Symposium, University of Illinois at Chicago Circle, 1976. New York; Academic Press, 1977. 222p.	
Third	Heady, Earl O., and Shashanka Bhide. Livestock Response Functions. 1st ed. Ames; Iowa State University Press, 1984. 331p.	Third
	Heady, Harold F., and Eleanor B. Heady. Range and Wildlife Management in the Tropics. London and New York; Longman, 1982. 140p.	Third
	Heath, Everett, and Segun Olusanya, eds. Anatomy and Physiology of Tropical Livestock. London and New York; Longman, 1985. 138p.	Third
Second	Heath, Maurice E., Robert F. Barnes, and Darrel S. Metcalfe,	Third

Developed countries ranking		Third World ranking
	eds. Forages: The Science of Grassland Agriculture. 4th ed. Ames; Iowa State University Press, 1985. 643p. (1st ed. by Harold D. Hughes, 1951. 724p.) (Available in Spanish as Forrajes: La Ciencia de la Agricultura Basada en la Produccion de Pastos . . . trans. by Jose Luis de la Loma. Mexico; CECSA, 1974.)	
Third	Heathcote, John G., and J. R. Hibbert. Aflatoxins: Chemical and Biological Aspects. Amsterdam and New York; Elsevier Scientific Pub. Co.; Distributors for the U.S. and Canada, Elsevier North-Holland, 1978. 212p.	Third
Second	Herman, Harry A. Improving Cattle by the Millions: NAAB and the Development and Worldwide Application of Artificial Insemination. Columbia; University of Missouri Press, 1981. 377p.	Third
First	Herman, Harry A., and F. W. Madden. The Artificial Insemination and Embryo Transfer of Dairy and Beef Cattle, Including Techniques for Goats, Sheep, Horses, and Swine: A Handbook and Laboratory Manual for Students, Herd Operators, and Workers in the AI Field. 7th ed. Danville, Ill.; Interstate Printers & Publishers, 1987. 279p. (5th ed., Columbia, Mo.; Lucas Brothers, 1974. 234p.)	First
	Herschodoerfer, S. M., ed. Quality Control in the Food Industry. 2d ed. London and Orlando, Fla.; Academic Press, 1984–1988. 4 vols. (1st ed., London and New York; Academic Press, 1967–1972. 3 vols.)	Second
Third	Hetherington, Lois. All About Goats. 4th ed., rev. Ipswich, U.K.; Farming Press, 1992. 196p. (1st ed., 1977.) (Available in Spanish as Cabras: Manejo, Produccion Patologia Barcelona; Aedos, 1980. 236p.)	
Third	Hickling, Charles F. Fish Culture. Rev. ed. London; Faber & Faber, 1971. 317p. (1st ed., 1962. 295p.)	Third
	Hickman, John, and Robert G. Walker. An Atlas of Veterinary Surgery. 2d ed. Bristol, U.K.; John Wright & Sons, 1980. 244p. (1st ed. Philadelphia; Lippincott, 1973.) (Available in Spanish as Atlas de Cirugia Veterinaria. Mexico; CECSA, 1976.)	Third
	Higgins, A. J., ed. The Camel in Health and Disease. London; Bailliere Tindall, 1986. 168p.	Third
Third	Hill, Desmond H. Cattle and Buffalo Meat Production in the Tropics. Harlow, U.K.; Longman, 1988. 210p.	Second
Second	Hill, William G. and Trudy F. C. Mackay, eds. Evolution and Animal Breeding: Review on Molecular and Quantitative Genetic Approaches in Honour of Alan Robertson. Wallingford, U.K.; CAB International, 1989. 313p.	Third
Third	Hillyer, G. M., et al., eds. Computers in Animal Production;	Second

Developed countries ranking		Third World ranking
	Proceedings of a Symposium Organized by the British Society of Animal Production, Harrogate, Nov. 1980. Thames Ditton, Surrey, U.K.; British Society of Animal Production, 1981. 155p. (BSAP Occasional Publication no. 5)	
Third	Hinks, John. Breeding Dairy Cattle. Ipswich, U.K.; Farming Press, 1983. 106p. (Available in Spanish as Cria del Ganado Lechero. 1st ed. trans. by Ingrid Adam. Buenos Aires; Ateneo, 1987.)	Second
Third	Hoar, William Stewart, D. J. Randall, and Frank P. Conte. Fish Physiology. New York; Academic Press, 1969+. (Vols. 8–10 edited by W. S. Hoar et al.)	Third
First	Hobson, P. N. The Rumen Microbial Ecosystem. London and New York; Elsevier Applied Science, 1988. 527p.	Second
Third	Hodges, John, ed. Animal Genetic Resources: Strategies for Improved Use and Conservation. Proceedings . . . 2d Meeting of the FAO/UNEP Expert Panel, Warsaw, Poland, June 1986, with Proceedings of the EAAP/PSAS Symposium on Small Populations of Domestic Animals. Rome; Food and Agriculture Organization, 1987. 316p. (FAO Animal Production and Health Paper no. 66)	Second
Third	Hodges, Robert D. The Histology of the Fowl. London and New York; Academic Press, 1974. 648p.	Third
Second	Hoekstra, W. G., et al., eds. Trace Element Metabolism in Animals; Proceedings of the 2d International Symposium . . . Madison, June, 1973. Sponsored jointly by the Steenbock Symposium Fund; Dept. of Biochemistry, University of Wisconsin, Madison; and the U.S. Dept. of Agriculture. Baltimore; University Park Press, 1974. 775p.	Third
	Hoff, Gerald L., Fredric L. Frye, and Elliott R. Jacobson. Diseases of Amphibians and Reptiles. New York; Plenum Press, 1984. 784p.	Third
Third	Holechek, Jerry L., Rex D. Pieper, and Carlton H. Herbel. Range Management: Principles and Practices. Englewood Cliffs, N.J.; Prentice-Hall, 1989. 501p. (Earlier ed., by Arthur W. Sampson. New York; Wiley, 1952. 570p.)	Third
Third	Hoobler, Icie G. Macy. The Composition of Milks; A Compilation of the Comparative Composition and Properties of Human, Cow, and Goat Milk, Colostrum, and Transitional Milk . . . prepared by Icie G. Macy, Harriet J. Kelly and Ralph E. Sloan for the Food and Nutrition Board, with the Consultation of the Committee of Maternal and Child Feeding. Washington, D.C.; National Academy of Sciences, National Research Council, 1953. 70p. (1950 ed., 54p.)	
Third	Hood, D. E., and P. V. Tarrant. The Problem of Dark-Cutting in Beef: A Seminar in the EEC Programme of Coordination of	

Developed countries ranking		Third World ranking

Research on Animal Welfare, Brussels, October 1980. The Hague; Boston and Hingham, Mass.; M. Nijhoff for the Commission of the European Communities, 1981. 504p.

Hormones in Animal Production: Selected Papers Presented to the Joint FAO/WHO Expert Committee on Food Additives, Geneva, March–April 1981 Rome; Food and Agriculture Organization, 1982. 53p. (FAO Animal Production and Health Paper no. 31) — *Third World: Second*

Horton-Smith, Clifford, and Emmanuel C. Amoroso, eds. Physiology of the Domestic Fowl. Proceedings of a Symposium of the Scientific Advisory Committee of the British Egg Marketing Board. Edinburgh and London; Oliver & Boyd, 1966. 329p. — *Third World: Second*

Le Houerou, H. N., ed. Browse in Africa: The Current State of Knowledge. Papers presented at an International Symposium . . . Addis Ababa, April 1980. Addis Ababa, Ethiopia; International Livestock Centre for Africa, 1980. 491p. — *Third World: Second*

Developed: Second — Houpt, Katherine A., and Thomas R. Wolski. Domestic Animal Behavior for Veterinarians and Animal Scientists. 1st ed. Ames; Iowa State University Press, 1982. 356p. — *Third World: Second*

Developed: Second — Howard, Dexter H., and Lois F. Howard, eds. Fungi Pathogenic for Humans and Animals. New York; M. Dekker, 1983. 2 pts. — *Third World: Third*

Developed: Third — Howard, Jimmy L., ed. Current Veterinary Therapy: Food Animal Practice 2. Philadelphia; W. B. Saunders, 1986. 1008p. (1st ed. as Current Veterinary Therapy, 1981.) — *Third World: Second*

Developed: Second — Hubbert, William T., William F. McCulloch, Paul R. Schnurrenberger, and Thomas G. Hull, eds. Diseases Transmitted from Animals to Man. 6th ed. Springfield, Ill.; C. C. Thomas, 1975. 1206p. (Previous editions edited by T. G. Hull.) — *Third World: Second*

Developed: Third — Hudlicka, Olga. Muscle Blood Flow; Its Relation to Muscle Metabolism and Function. Amsterdam; Swets & Zeitlinger, 1973. 219p.

Developed: Third — Huet, Marcel. Textbook of Fish Culture: Breeding and Cultivation of Fish. 2d ed. trans. by Henry Kahn from the 4th French ed. Farnham, U.K.; Fishing News Books, 1986. 438p. (1st ed., 1973.) (Available in Spanish as Tratado de Piscicultura. 3d ed. Madrid; Mundi-Prensa, 1983.) — *Third World: Second*

Developed: Second — Hughes, P. E., and M. A. Varley. Reproduction in the Pig. London; Butterworth, 1980. 241p. (Available in Spanish as Reproduccion del Cerdo. 1st ed. trans. by Mariano Illero Martin. Zaragoza; Acribia, 1984.) — *Third World: Second*

Developed: Third — Humphreys, D. J. Veterinary Toxicology. 3d ed. London and Philadelphia; Bailliere Tindall, 1988. 356p. (2d ed., by M. L. Clark, D. G. Harvey and D. J. Humphreys, 1981.) — *Third World: Second*

Developed countries ranking		Third World ranking
Second	Humphreys, L. R. Tropical Pastures and Fodder Crops. 2d ed. London and New York; Longman Scientific & Technical; Wiley, 1987. 155p. (1st ed., 1978. 135p.)	First
Second	Hungate, Robert E. The Rumen and Its Microbes. New York; Academic Press, 1966. 533p.	
Second	Hungerford, Thomas Gordon. Diseases of Livestock. 8th ed. Sydney; McGraw-Hill, 1975. 1318p. (4th ed., 1959. 623p.)	Second
Second	Hunter, R. H. F. Physiology and Technology of Reproduction in Female Domestic Animals. London and New York; Academic Press, 1980. 393p. (Available in Spanish as Fisiologica y Tecnologia de la Reproduccion de la Hembra de los Animales Domesticos. Zaragoza; Acribia, 1982.)	Second
Third	Hurnik, J. F., A. B. Webster, and P. B. Siegel. Dictionary of Farm Animal Behaviour. Guelph, Ontario, Canada; University of Guelph, 1985. 176p.	Second
Third	Hutt, Frederick B. Genetic Resistance to Disease in Domestic Animals. Ithaca, N.Y.; Comstock Pub. Associates, 1958. 198p.	Second
Second	Hutt, Frederick B., and Benjamin A. Rasmusen. Animal Genetics. 2d ed. New York; Wiley, 1982. 582p. (1st ed., 1964. 546p.)	First
	Hyams, Edward. Animals in the Service of Man. Philadelphia; Lippincott, 1972. 209p.	Third

I

Developed countries ranking		Third World ranking
	IDRC/ILCA Workshop, 1983, Addis Ababa. Pastoral Systems Research in Sub-Saharan Africa; Proceedings. . . . Addis Ababa, Ethiopia; International Livestock Centre for Africa, 1983. 480p.	Third
Second	Ingram, D. G., W. R. Mitchell, and S. Wayne Martin, eds. Animal Disease Monitoring: Proceedings of an International Symposium, University of Guelph, July 1974. Springfield, Ill.; Thomas, 1975. 215p.	Third
	Innis, George S., ed. Grassland Simulation Model. New York; Springer-Verlag, 1978. 295p. (Ecological Studies no. 26)	Third
Second	Institute of Laboratory Animal Resources (U.S.). Committee on Care and Use of Laboratory Animals, and National Institutes of Health (U.S.) Division of Research Resources. Guide for the Care and Use of Laboratory Animals. Rev. ed. Bethesda, Md.; Dept. of Health and Human Services, Public Health Service, National Institutes of Health, 1985. 83p. (NIH Publication no. 85-23)	Third
Third	Interactions of Mycotoxins in Animal Production. Proceedings of Symposium, July 1978, Michigan State University; Jointly Sponsored by American Society of Animal Sience, American	Second

Developed countries ranking		Third World ranking
	Dairy Science Association, Committee on Animal Nutrition, National Research Council. Washington, D.C.; National Academy of Sciences, 1979. 197p.	
Third	International Association of Biological Standardization. International Symposium on Brucellosis, IIIrd: Proceedings of a Symposium . . . Institut Scientifique et Technique des Sports, Algiers, Algeria, April 1983. Basel and New York; S. Karger, 1984. 779p. (English and French.)	Second
Third	International Association of Biological Standardization. Symposium on Reduction of Animal Usage in the Development and Control of Biological Products: Proceedings . . . Basel and New York; S. Karger, 1986. 324p. (English and French.)	
	International Conference of Institutions of Tropical Veterinary Medicine, 2d, Berlin, 1976. Results of the Conference. Eschborn, Germany; Deutsche Gesellschaft fur Technische Zusammenarbeit, 1978. 503p.	Third
Third	International Conference on Cattle Diseases, 6th, 1970, Philadelphia. Proceedings of the VI International Conference on Cattle Diseases; edited by the Congress of Publication Committee, Richard A. McFeely, Guy E. Morse and Eric I. Williams. Stillwater, Okla.; Published by the American Association of Bovine Practitioners at Heritage Press, 1971. 456p.	
Second	International Conference on Forage Quality Evaluation and Utilization, 1969. Proceedings . . . edited by R. F. Barnes et al. Lincoln; Nebraska Center for Continuing Education, 1970. 356p.	
Third	International Conference on Goat Breeding, 2d, 1971, Tours, France. Proceedings . . . Institut Technique de l'Elevage Ovin et Caprin, 1971. 381p. (In English, German and French.)	Third
	International Conference on Goat Production and Disease, 3d, 1982, Tucson. Proceedings . . . Scottsdale, Ariz.; Dairy Goat Journal, 1982. 604p.	Second
	International Conference on Goats, 4th, 1987, Brasilia. Proceedings . . . Brasilia; Embrapa, Departamento de Difusao de Tecnologia, 1987. 2 vols.	Second
Second	International Conference on Production Disease in Farm Animals, 4th, 1980, Munich. Metabolic Disorders in Farm Animals; Proceedings . . . edited by D. Giesecke, G. Dirksen nad M. Stangassinger. Munchen, Germany; Institut fur Physiologie, Physiologische Chemie und Ernahrungsphsiologie, Tierarztliche Fakultat der Universitat Munchen; Distributed by Fotodruch Frank, 1981. 291p.	Third
Second	International Conference on Production Disease in Farm Animals, 6th, 1986, Belfast, Northern Ireland. Proceedings . . . Belfast; Veterinary Research Laboratories, 1987. 340p.	Second

Developed countries ranking		Third World ranking
Third	International Conference on Proteins of Iron Metabolism, 7th, 1985, Villeneuve-d'Ascq, France. Proteins of Iron Storage and Transport; Proceedings . . . edited by G. Spik et al. Amsterdam and New York; Elsevier Science Publishers, 1985. 380p.	Third
Second	International Congress on Animal Reproduction and Artificial Insemination, 8th, 1976, Krakow. Proceedings . . . Krakow; Wrocawska Druckarnia Naukowa, 1976. 5 vols.	
Third	International Congress on Animal Reproduction and Artificial Insemination, 9th, 1980, Madrid. IX Congreso Internacional de Reproduccion Animal e Inseminacion Artificial. Proceedings . . . Madrid, Spain; Editorial Garsi, 1980. 3 vols.	
Second	International Congress on Animal Reproduction and Artifical Insemination, 10th, 1984, University of Illinois. Congress Proceedings . . . Urbana-Champaign, Ill.; University of Illinois, 1984. 4 vols.	
Second	International Congress on Animal Reproduction and Artificial Insemination, 11th, 1988, Dublin. Proceedings . . . Belfast; The Congress, 1988. 5 vols.	
Third	International Congress on Diseases of Cattle, 11th, 1980, Tel-Aviv. Reports and Summaries = Congres International sur les Maladies du Betail: Rapports et resumes. Scientific editor, E. Mayer. Haifa, Israel; Israel Association for Buiatrics, 1980. 2 vols. (1559 p.) (In English, French, German or Spanish.)	Third
Second	International Dairy Federation. Dairying Throughout the World. Brussels, Belgium; International Dairy Federation, 1986. 129p.	Second
Second	International Dairy Federation. Dictionary of Dairy Terminology: In English, French, German, and Spanish. Amsterdam and New York; Elsevier Scientific Pub. Co., 1983. 328p.	Second
Second	International Grassland Congress, 13th, 1977, Leipzig, Germany. Congress Proceedings . . . edited by E. Wojahn and H. Thons. Berlin; Akademie-Verlag, 1980. 2 vols.	
Second	International Grassland Congress, 14th, 1981, Lexington. Proceedings . . . edited by J. Allan Smith and Virgil W. Hays. Boulder, Colo.; Westview Press, 1983. 878p.	
Third	International Grassland Congress, 16th, 1989, Nice, France. Proceedings . . . Congres International des Herbages. Nice, France; Association Francaise pour la Production Fourragere (The French Grassland Society), 1989. 3 vols.	Third
Third	International Livestock Centre for Africa. Livestock Production in the Subhumid Zone of West Africa; A Regional Review. Addis Ababa, Ethiopia; International Livestock Centre for Africa, 1979. 184p. (ILCA Systems Study no. 2)	Second
	International Livestock Centre for Africa. Livestock Systems Research Manual. Addis Ababa, Ethiopia; ILCA, 1990. 2 vols. (ILCA Working Paper no. 1) (Second volume concerned with on-farm trials.)	Third

Developed countries ranking		Third World ranking
Third	International Livestock Centre for Africa. Small Ruminant Production in the Humid Tropics. Addis Ababa, Ethiopia; International Livestock Centre for Africa, 1979. 122p. (ILCA Systems Study no. 3)	First
Third	International Minerals Conference, 3d, 1980, Orlando, Florida. Proceedings . . . Mundelein, Ill.; International Minerals & Chemical Corporation, 1980. 90p.	
Second	International Rangeland Congress, 2d, 1984, Adelaide, S. Australia. Rangelands: A Resource Under Siege; Proceedings . . . edited by P. J. Joss, P. W. Lynch, and O. B. Williams. Cambridge & New York; Cambridge University Press, 1986. 634p.	
Third	International Reindeer and Caribou Symposium, 1st, 1972, University of Alaska. Proceedings . . . edited by Jack R. Luick et al. Fairbanks; University of Alaska, 1975. 551p. (Biological Papers of the University of Alaska. Special Report no. 1)	
Second	International Silage Research Conference, 1st, 1971, Washington, D.C. Technological Papers Presented . . . Sponsored by the National Silo Association, Inc., Dec. 1971. Cedar Falls, Iowa; The Association, 1972. 322p.	
	International Symposium on Animal Production in the Tropics, 1973, University of Ibadan. Proceedings . . . Ibadan; Published for the Dept. of Animal Science, University of Ibadan, Nigeria, by Heinemann Educational Books, 1974.	Second
Third	International Symposium on Avian Endocrinology, 2d, 1980, Benalmadena, Spain. Proceedings . . . edited by August Epple and Milton H. Stetson. New York; Academic Press, 1980. 577p.	Third
Second	International Symposium on Avian Endocrinology, 3d. Environmental and Ecological Perspectives . . . edited by Shin-ichi Mikami, Kazutaka Homma and Masaru Wada. Tokyo; Japan Scientific Societies Press; Berlin and New York; Springer-Verlag, 1983. 334p.	Third
	International Symposium on Genetics and Horse-Breeding, 1975, Dublin. Proceedings . . . Dublin, Irish Republic; Royal Dublin Society, 1976. 96p.	Third
Third	International Symposium on Livestock Wastes, 3d, 1975, University of Illinois. Managing Livestock Wastes; Proceedings . . . St. Joseph, Mich.; American Society of Agricultural Engineers, 1975. 631p.	
Third	International Symposium on Livestock Wastes, 4th, 1980, Amarillo, Texas. Livestock Waste; A Renewable Resource; Proceedings . . . St. Joseph, Mich.; American Society of Agricultural Engineers, 1981. 430p.	Second
	International Symposium on Proteases: Protential Role in Health and Disease, 1982, Wurzburg, Germany. Proceedings . . . edited by Walter H. Horl and August Heidland. New York;	Third

Developed countries ranking		Third World ranking
	Plenum Press, 1984. 591p. (Advances in Experimental Medicine and Biology no. 167)	
	International Symposium on Protein Metabolism and Nutrition, 1st, 1974, Nottingham, England. Proceedings . . . edited by D. J. A. Cole et al. London and Boston; Butterworth, 1976. 515p. (European Association for Animal Production Publication no. 16)	Second
Second	International Symposium on Protein Metabolism and Nutrition, 3d, 1980, Braunschweig, Germany. Proceedings . . . edited by H. J. Oslage and K. Rohr. Braunschweig; Infromation Centre of Bundesforschungsanstalt fur Landwirtschaft, 1980. 3 vols. (European Association for Animal Production Publication no. 27)	Third
	International Symposium on Protein Metabolism and Nutrition, 6th, 1973, Hohenheim, Germany. Energy Metabolism on Farm Animals; Proceedings . . . edited by K. H. Menke, H. J. Lantzsch and J. R. Reichl. Honhenheim; Universitat Hohenheim Dokumentstionsstelle, 1974. 308p. (European Association for Animal Production. Pub. no. 14)	Third
First	International Symposium on Ruminant Physiology, 4th, 1974, Sydney. Digestion and Metabolism in the Ruminant: Proceedings . . . edited by I. W. McDonald and A. C. I. Warner. Armidale, Australia; University of New England Pub. Unit, 1975. 602p.	
First	International Symposium on Ruminant Physiology, 5th, 1979, Clermont-Ferrand, France. Digestive Physiology and Metabolism in Ruminants; Proceedings . . . edited by Y. Ruckebusch and P. Thivend. Lancaster, U.K.; MTP Press, 1980. 854p.	First
Second	International Symposium on Ruminant Physiology, 7th, 1989, Sendai, Japan. Physiological Aspects of Digestion and Metabolism in Ruminants; Proceedings . . . edited by T. Tsuda, Y. Sasaki and R. Kawashima. San Diego, Calif.; Academic Press, 1991. 779p.	Third
Second	International Symposium on Selenium in Biology and Medicine, 3d, 1984, Peking. Selenium in Biology and Medicine; Proceedings . . . edited by Gerald F. Combs, Jr.; Sponsored by the International Selenium Symposium Organizing Committee in Cooperation with the Chinese Academy of Medical Sciences. New York; Van Nostrand Reinhold, 1987. 2 vols.	Second
Second	International Symposium on Selenium in Biology and Medicine, 4th, 1988, Tubingen, Germany. Proceedings . . . edited by A. Wendel. Berlin and New York; Springer-Verlag, 1989. 330p.	Second
Third	International Symposium on Trace Element Metabolism in Man and Animals, 3d, 1977, Freising, Germany. Proceedings . . .	Third

<table>
<tr><td>Developed
countries
ranking</td><td></td><td>Third
World
ranking</td></tr>
<tr><td></td><td>edited by M. Kirchgessner et al. Freising, Germany; Arbeits-
kreis fur Tierernahrungsforschung Weihenstephan, 1978. 684p.</td><td></td></tr>
<tr><td>First</td><td>International Symposium on Trace Element Metabolism in Man
and Animals, 4th, 1982, Perth. Proceedings . . . edited by J.
M. Gawthorne, J. McC. Howell, and C. L. White. Berlin and
New York; Springer-Verlag, 1982. 715p.</td><td>Second</td></tr>
<tr><td>Third</td><td>International Symposium on Trace Elements in Man and Ani-
mals, 6th, 1987, Pacific Grove, California. Proceedings . . .
edited by L. S. Hurley, G. L. Keen, B. Lonnerdal, and R.
Rucker. New York; Plenum Press, 1988. 724p.</td><td>Second</td></tr>
<tr><td>Second</td><td>International Symposium on Veterinary Epidemiology and Eco-
nomics, 2d, 1979, Canberra. Proceedings . . . edited by W. A.
Geering, R. T. Roe and L. A. Chapman; Sponsored by the
Australian Bureau of Animal Health. Canberra; Australian Gov-
ernment Publishing Service, 1980. 661p.</td><td></td></tr>
<tr><td></td><td>International Symposium on Veterinary Epidemiology and Eco-
nomics, 3d, 1982, Arlington, Virginia. Proceedings . . . Spon-
sored by the Association of Teachers of Veterinary Public
Health and Preventive Medicine under the auspices of the Inter-
national Society for Veterinary Epidemiology and Economics.
Edwardsville, Kans.; Veterinary Medicine Pub. Co., 1983.
682p.</td><td>Third</td></tr>
<tr><td>Third</td><td>Isaac, Erich. Geography of Domestication. Englewood Cliffs,
N.J.; Prentice-Hall, 1970. 132p.</td><td>Third</td></tr>
</table>

J

<table>
<tr><td>Second</td><td>Jackson, George, Robert Herman, and Ira Singer, eds. Immu-
nity to Parasitic Animals. New York; Appleton-Century-Crofts,
1969–1970. 2 vols.</td><td></td></tr>
<tr><td>Second</td><td>Jackson, I. J. Climate, Water, and Agriculture in the Tropics.
2d ed. Essex, U.K.; New York; Longman Scientific & Techni-
cal; Copublished in the U.S. with Wiley, 1989. 377p.</td><td>Second</td></tr>
<tr><td>Third</td><td>Jackson, M. G. Treating Straw for Animal Feeding: An As-
sessement of Its Technical and Economic Feasibility. Rome;
Food and Agriculture Organization, 1978. 81p. (FAO Animal
Production and Health Paper no. 10)</td><td>Second</td></tr>
<tr><td>Third</td><td>Jagiello, Georgiana, and Henry J. Vogel, eds. Bioregulators of
Reproduction. New York; Academic Press, 1981. 584p.</td><td></td></tr>
<tr><td>Second</td><td>Jahnke, Hans E. Livestock Productions Systems and Livestock
Development in Tropical Africa. Kiel; Kieler Wissen-
schaftsverlag Vauk, 1982. 253p.</td><td>First</td></tr>
<tr><td>Third</td><td>Jahnke, Hans E. Tsetse Flies and Livestock Development in
East Africa: A Study in Environmental Economics. Munich;
Weltforum Verlag, 1976. 180p.</td><td>Second</td></tr>
</table>

136   Wallace C. Olsen

<table>
<tr><td>Developed
countries
ranking</td><td></td><td>Third
World
ranking</td></tr>
<tr><td>Second</td><td>Jainudeen, M. R., and A. R. Omar, eds. Animal Production and Health in the Tropics; Proceedings . . . 1st Asian-Australian Animal Science Congress, Serdang, Sept., 1980. Serdang, Selangor; Universiti Pertanian Malaysia, 1980. 482p.</td><td>First</td></tr>
<tr><td></td><td>Janssen, W. M. M. A., et al. Feeding Values for Poultry. 2d ed. Beekbergen, Netherlands; Spelderholt Institute for Poultry Research, 1979. 59p.</td><td>Third</td></tr>
<tr><td>Third</td><td>Jarrige, Robert. Alimentation des Bovins, Ovins et Caprins. (Feeding of Cattle, Sheep, and Goats). Paris; Institute Nationale de la Recherche Agronomique, 1988. 471p.</td><td>Second</td></tr>
<tr><td>Second</td><td>Jarrige, Robert. Principes de la Nutrition et de l'Alimentation des Ruminants: Besoins Alimentaires des Animaux, Valeur Nutritive des Aliments. Paris; Institut National de la Recherche Agronomique, 1978. 597p. (Available in Spanish as Alimentacion de los Rumiantes. Madrid; Mundi-Prensa, 1981.)</td><td>Second</td></tr>
<tr><td>Second</td><td>Jarrige, Robert, ed. Ruminant Nutrition: Recommended Allowances and Feed Tables. Versailles, France; INRA Editions, 1989. 389p.</td><td>First</td></tr>
<tr><td></td><td>Jasiorowski, H., and J. Rudzka, eds. Optimum Methods of Cattle Breeding for Increasing Meat and Dairy Production; Proceedings of a Symposium . . . Warsaw Agricultural University, May–June, 1978. Warsaw, Poland; Warsaw Agricultural University, 1979. 255p.</td><td>Third</td></tr>
<tr><td></td><td>Jennings, Paul B. The Practice of Large Animal Surgery. Philadelphia; Saunders, 1984–1985. 2 vols. 1233p.</td><td>Third</td></tr>
<tr><td>Third</td><td>Jensen, P., Bo Algers, and Ingvar Ekesbo. Methods of Sampling and Analysis of Data in Farm Animal Ethology. Basel; Birkhauser, 1986. 86p.</td><td></td></tr>
<tr><td>First</td><td>Jensen, Rue, Brinton L. Swift, and Cleon V. Kimberling. Jensen and Swift's Diseases of Sheep. 3d ed., by Cleon V. Kimberling. Philadelphia; Lea & Febiger, 1988. 394p. (2d ed., by R. Jensen and B. L. Swift, as Diseases of Sheep, 1982. 394p. 1st ed., by R. Jensen, 1974. 389p.)</td><td>Second</td></tr>
<tr><td>Second</td><td>Jensen, Rue, and Donald R. Mackey. Diseases of Feedlot Cattle. 3d ed. Philadelphia; Lea & Febiger, 1979. 300p. (Available in Spanish as Enfermedades de los Bovinos en los Corrales de Engorda. 2d ed. Mexico; UTEHA, 1973.)</td><td>Second</td></tr>
<tr><td>Second</td><td>Johansson, Ivar, and Jan Rendel. Genetics and Animal Breeding. San Francisco; W. H. Freeman, 1968. 498p. (Translation, by Michael Taylor, of Arftlighet och Husdjursforadling.) (Available in Spanish as Genetica y Mejora Animal. Zaragoza; Acribia, 1971.)</td><td>Third</td></tr>
<tr><td></td><td>Johnson, A. D., W. R. Gomes, and N. L. Vandemark, eds. The Testis. New York; Academic Press, 1970–1977. 4 vols.</td><td>Second</td></tr>
<tr><td>Second</td><td>Johnson, Harold D. Bioclimatology and the Adaptation of Live-</td><td>First</td></tr>
</table>

Developed countries ranking		Third World ranking
	stock. Amsterdam and New York; Elsevier, 1987. 279p. (Earlier eds. as Progress in Animal Biometeorology.)	
	Johnson, Russell C., ed. The Biology of Parasitic Spirochetes. New York; Academic Press, 1976. 402p.	Third
Third	Johnston, R. G. Introduction to Sheep Farming. London and New York; Granada, 1983. 266p.	
Third	Joint ESACT/IABS Meeting on the Diagnostics and Vaccines for Parasitic Diseases, Royal Academy of Science, Stockholm, Sweden, February 1985; Proceedings . . . Basel and New York; S. Karger, 1985. 158p. (Developments in Biological Standardization no. 62)	Third
	Joint FAO/IAEA Div. of Nuclear Techniques in Food and Agriculture. Livestock Reproduction in Latin America; Proceedings of the Final Research Coordinating Meeting of the FAO/IAEA/ARCAL III Regional Network for Improving the Reproductive Management of Meat- and Milk-Producing Livestock in Latin Amercia with the Aid of Radioimmunoassay . . . held at Bogota, Sept. 1988. Vienna, International Atomic Energy Agency, 1990. 446p.	Third
	Joint FAO/WHO Expert Committee on Brucellosis. Sixth Report. Geneva; World Health Organization, 1986. 132p. (World Health Organization, Technical Paper Series no. 740)	Third
	Jones, J. G. W., ed. The Biological Efficiency of Protein Production; Proceedings of a Symposium . . . University of Reading, September 1971. Cambridge; University Press, 1973. 385p.	Third
Third	Jones, Richard W. Principles of Biological Regulation: An Introduction to Feedback Systems. New York; Academic Press, 1973. 359p.	Second
	Jones, Thomas C., Ronald D. Hunt, and Hilton A. Smith. Veterinary Pathology. 5th ed. Philadelphia; Lea & Febiger, 1983. 1792p. (1st ed., 1957, by Smith and Jones.) (Available in Spanish as Patologia Veterinaria. 1st ed. trans. by C. H. Lightowler. Buenos Aires; Hemisferio Sur, 1984–1988.)	Second
Second	Jones, William E. Genetics and Horse Breeding. Rev. ed. Philadelphia; Lea & Febiger, 1982. 660p. (1st ed., by W. E. Jones and Ralph Bogert, as Genetics of the Horse. Fort Collins, Colo.; Caballus Pub., 1971. 356p.)	Second
Second	Jordan, Anthony M. Trypanosomiasis Control and African Rural Development. London and New York; Longman, 1986. 357p.	
	Joshi, N. R. Types and Breeds of African Cattle. Rome; Food and Agriculture Organization, 1957. 297p. (Also available in Spanish.)	Second
First	Jubb, K. V. F., Peter C. Kennedy, and Nigel Palmer. Pathol-	Second

Developed countries ranking		Third World ranking
	ogy of Domestic Animals. 3d ed. Orlando Fla.; Academic Press, 1985. 3 vols. (1st ed., 1963–1965.)	
Third	Juergenson, Elwood M. Approved Practices in Beef Cattle Production. 5th ed. Danville, Ill.; Interstate Printers & Publishers, 1980. 467p. (1st ed., 1958.) (Available in Spanish as Metodos Aprobados en la Produccion de Ganado Para Carne. Mexico; Trillas, 1979.)	Second
Third	Juergenson, Elwood M. Approved Practices in Sheep Production. 4th ed. Danville, Ill.; Interstate Printers & Publishers, 1981. 455p. (Available in Spanish as Practicas Aprobadas en la Explotacion de Ganado Lanar. 2d ed. Mexico; CECSA, 1975.)	Second
Third	Juergenson, Elwood M. Handbook of Livestock Equipment. 2d ed. Danville, Ill.; Interstate Printers & Publishers, 1979. 371p. (1st ed., 1971. 266p.)	Second
Third	Juergenson, Elwood M., and W. P. Mortenson. Approved Practices in Dairying. 4th ed. Danville, Ill.; Interstate Printers & Publishers, 1977. 353p. (Available in Spanish as Practicas Aprobadas en la Produccion de Leche. Mexico; CECSA, 1977.)	Second
Third	Jurgens, Marshall H. Animal Feeding and Nutrition. 6th ed. Dubuque, Iowa; Kendall-Hunt Publishing Co., 1988. 626p. (1973 rev. ed. as Applied Animal Feeding and Nutrition: An Outline. 171p.)	Second

K

Developed countries ranking		Third World ranking
	Kabata, Z. Parasites and Diseases of Fish Cultured in the Tropics. London and Philadelphia; Taylor & Francis, 1985. 318p. (Spine title: Diseases and Parasites of Fish Cultured in the Tropics.)	Third
First	Kahrs, Robert F. Viral Diseases of Cattle. 1st ed. Ames; Iowa State University Press, 1981. 299p. (Available in Spanish as Enfermedades Viricas del Ganado Vacuno. 1st ed. trans. by Manuel Ramis Verges. Zaragoza; Acribia, 1985.)	Second
Third	Kamil, Alan C., and Theodore D. Sargent, eds. Foraging Behavior: Ecological, Ethological, and Psychological Approaches; Papers from a Symposium . . . held as Part of the Animal Behavior Society Meetings, Seattle, 1978. New York; Garland STPM Press, 1981. 534p.	
Third	Kaneko, Jiro J., ed. Clinical Biochemistry of Domestic Animals. 4th ed. San Diego; Academic Press, 1989. 932p. (1st ed., 1963, edited by C. E. Cornelius and J. J. Kaneko.)	Second
Second	Kaplan, Martin M., and Hilary Koprowski, eds. Laboratory Techniques in Rabies. 3d ed. Geneva; World Health Organization, 1973. 367p. (1st ed., 1954. 150p.)	Second
	Karasszon, Denes. A Concise History of Veterinary Medicine	Third

<table>
<tr><td>Developed
countries
ranking</td><td></td><td>Third
World
ranking</td></tr>
<tr><td></td><td>. . . trans. by E. Farkas; translation rev. by Iringo K. Kecskes. Budapest; Akademiai Kiado; Boca Raton, Fla.; H. Stillman, 1988. 458p.</td><td></td></tr>
<tr><td>Third</td><td>Karg, H., and E. Schallenberger. Factors Influencing Fertility in the Postpartum Cow: A Seminar in the CEC Programme of Coordination of Research on Beef Production, Freising, 1981. The Hague, Boston and Hingham, Mass.; M. Nijhoff for The Commission of the European Communities, 1982. 585p.</td><td></td></tr>
<tr><td></td><td>Kearl, Leonard C. Nutrient Requirements of Ruminants in Developing Countries. Logan; International Feedstuffs Institute, Utah Agricultural Experiment Station, Utah State University, 1982. 381p.</td><td>Third</td></tr>
<tr><td>Third</td><td>Keeler, Richard F., Kent R. Van Kampen, and Lynn F. James, eds. Effects of Poisonous Plants on Livestock; Proceedings of a Joint U.S.-Australian Symposium . . . Utah State University, Logan, June 1977. New York; Academic Press, 1978. 600p.</td><td>Third</td></tr>
<tr><td>Third</td><td>Kellerman, T. S., J. A. W. Coetzer, and T. W. Naude. Plant Poisonings and Mycotoxicoses of Livestock in Southern Africa. Cape Town; Oxford University Press, 1988. 243p.</td><td>Third</td></tr>
<tr><td>Third</td><td>Kempster, Tony, Alastair Cuthbertson, and Geoffrey Harrington. Carcass Evaluation in Livestock Breeding, Production, and Marketing. London and New York; Granada, 1982. 306p.</td><td>Second</td></tr>
<tr><td>Second</td><td>Kenneth, John H., and G. R. Ritchie. Gestation Periods: A Table and Bibliography. 3d ed. Farnham Royal, U.K.; Commonwealth Agricultural Bureaux, 1953. 39p. (1st ed., Edinburgh and London; Oliver & Boyd, 1943. 23p.)</td><td></td></tr>
<tr><td></td><td>Kerr, Morag G. Veterinary Laboratory Medicine: Clinical Biochemistry and Haematology. Oxford and Boston; Blackwell Scientific Publications, 1989. 270p.</td><td>Second</td></tr>
<tr><td></td><td>Kersjes, A. W., and L. J. E. Rutgers. Atlas of Large Animal Surgery. Baltimore; Williams & Wilkins, 1985. 143p.</td><td>Second</td></tr>
<tr><td>Third</td><td>Kerslake, D. Mc. The Stress of Hot Environments. Cambridge, U.K.; University Press, 1972. 316p.</td><td>Second</td></tr>
<tr><td>Second</td><td>Kettle, D. S. Medical and Veterinary Entomology. London; Croom Helm, 1984. 658p.</td><td>Second</td></tr>
<tr><td>Second</td><td>Kidder, D. E., and M. J. Manners. Digestion in the Pig. Bristol, U.K.; Scientechnica, 1978. 201p.</td><td>Third</td></tr>
<tr><td></td><td>Kiley-Worthington, M. Behavioural Problems of Farm Animals. Stocksfield, U.K.; Boston; Oriel Press, 1977. 134p.</td><td>Third</td></tr>
<tr><td>Third</td><td>Kilgour, Ronald, and Clive Dalton. Livestock Behavior: A Practical Guide. St. Albans, U.K.; Granada, 1983. 256p.</td><td>Third</td></tr>
<tr><td></td><td>Kilian, M., W. Frederiksen, and E. L. Biberstein, eds. Haemophilus, Pasteurella and Actinobacillus; Proceedings of an International Symposium, Copenhagen, August 1980. London and New York; Academic Press, 1981. 294p.</td><td>Third</td></tr>
</table>

Developed countries ranking		Third World ranking
	Kim, Ke Chung, and Richard W. Merritt. Black Flies: Ecology, Population Management, and Annotated World List. University Park; Pennsylvania State University Press, 1987. 528p.	Third
	King, A. S., J. McLelland, and A. S. King. Birds; Their Structure and Function. 2d ed. London and Philadelphia; Bailliere Tindall, 1984. 334p. (First published, 1975, as Outlines of Avian Anatomy.)	Second
Third	King, J. W. B., and F. Nissier. Muscle Hypertrophy of Genetic Origin and Its Use to Improve Beef Production: A Seminar in the CEC Programme of Coordination of Research on Beef Production, Toulouse, June 1980. The Hague, Boston and Hingham, Mass.; M. Nijhoff for the Commission of the European Communities, 1982. 658p.	Third
Third	King, John M., et al. An Atlas of General Pathology: With Special Reference to Swine Diseases. Taipei; Joint Commission on Rural Reconstruction, 1976. 300p. (Vol. II, by J. M. King and R. C. T. Lee. Taipei; Council for Agricultural Planning and Development, Executive Yuan and the Pig Research Institute of Taiwan; Ithaca, N.Y.; Cornell University, 1983. 376p.)	Third
Second	Kingsbury, John M. Poisonous Plants of the United States and Canada. Englewood Cliffs, N.J.; Prentice-Hall, 1964. 626p.	
Third	Kinney, Terry B. A Summary of Reported Estimates of Heritabilities and of Genetic and Phenotypic Correlations for Traits of Chickens. Washington, D.C.; U.S. Agricultural Research Service, 1969. 49p. (USDA Agriculture Handbook no. 363)	
Third	Kinsman, Donald M., ed. International Meat Science Dictionary: English-French-German-Spanish-Russian-Chinese-Danish-Italian-Japanese. Boston; American Press, 1991. 282p. (1st ed. Storrs, Conn.; Kinsman, 1978. 282p.)	Third
	Kirk, Robert W. Handbook of Veterinary Procedures and Emergency Treatment. 5th ed. Philadelphia; Saunders, 1990. 1016p. (1st ed., 1969, by Kirk and Bistner. 474p.) (Available in Spanish as Manual de Urgencias en Veterinaria. 3d ed., rev. Barcelona; Salvat, 1989.)	Second
Second	Kirkbride, Clyde A. Control of Livestock Diseases. Springfield, Ill.; Thomas, 1986. 152p.	Second
First	Kleiber, Max. The Fire of Life; An Introduction to Animal Energetics. Rev. ed. Huntington, N.Y.; R. E. Krieger Pub. Co., 1975. 453p. (1st ed., Wiley, 1961. 454p.) (Available in Spanish as Bioenergetica Animal. Zaragoza; Acribia, 1973.)	First
Second	Klein, Jan. Natural History of the Major Histocompatibility Complex. New York; Wiley, 1986. 775p.	Third
Second	Kleinbaum, David G., and Lawrence L. Kupper. Epidemiologic Research: Principles and Quantitative Methods. Belmont, Calif.; Lifetime Learning Publications, 1982. 529p.	Second

Developed countries ranking		Third World ranking
	Knecht, Charles D. Fundamental Techniques in Veterinary Surgery. 3d ed. Philadelphia; W. B. Saunders, 1987. 349p. (1st ed., 1975.) (Available in Spanish as Tecnicas Fundamentales de Cirugia Veterinaria. Zaragoza; Acribia, 1977.)	Second
Second	Koch, Tankred. Anatomy of the Chicken and Domestic Birds. Edited and trans. by Bernard H. Skold and Louis De Vries. 1st ed. Ames; Iowa State University Press, 1973. 170p. Translation of Bau und Funktion des Geflugelkorpers. (Reprinted by UMI, 1978.)	Second
Second	Koeman, J. H., F. Balk, and W. Takken. The Environmental Impact of Tsetse Control Operation: A Report on Present Knowledge. Rome; Food and Agriculture Organization, 1980. 71p.	Third
	Koger, Marvin, Tony J. Cunha, and Alvin C. Warnick. Crossbreeding Beef Cattle: Series 2. Gainesville; University of Florida Press, 1973. 459p. (Selection of papers presented at the 20th Annual Beef Cattle Short Course, University of Florida, May 1971.)	Second
Third	Kon, S. K., and A. T. Cowie, eds. Milk: The Mammary Gland and Its Secretion. New York; Academic Press, 1961. 2 vols.	First
	Konczacki, Zbigniew A. The Economics of Pastoralism: A Case Study of Sub-Saharan Africa. London and Totowa, N.J.; F. Cass, 1978. 185p.	Second
Third	Korver, S., and J. A. M. van Arendonk, eds. Modelling of Livestock Production Systems: A Seminar in the European Community Programme for the Coordination of Agricultural Research, Brussels, April 1987. Dordrecht and Boston; Kluwer Academic Publishers for the Commission of the European Communities, 1988. 215p. (Current Topics in Veterinary Medicine and Animal Science no. 46)	
	Kowal, Jan M., and A. H. Kassam. Agricultural Ecology of Savanna: A Study of West Africa. Oxford and New York; Clarendon Press, Oxford University Press, 1978. 403p.	Third
	Kreier, Julius P., and John R. Baker. Parasitic Protozoa. Boston; Allen & Unwin, 1987. 241p.	Third
Second	Krider, J. L., J. H. Conrad, and W. E. Carroll. Swine Production. 5d ed. New York; McGraw-Hill, 1982. 679p. (1st ed., by W. E. Carroll and J. L. Krider, 1950. 498p.)	Second
Second	Krol, B., P. S. van Roon, and J. H. Houben, eds. Trends in Modern Meat Technology 2; Proceedings of the International Symposium, Den Dolder, Netherlands, Nov. 1987. Wageningen; Pudoc, 1988. 150p.	

Developed countries ranking		Third World ranking

L

	Ladds, P. W. A Colour Atlas of Lymph Node Pathology in Cattle. Ames; Iowa State University Press, 1986. 80p.	Third
	Laing, J. A. Vibrio Fetus Infection of Cattle. Rev. ed. Rome; Food and Agriculture Organization, 1960. 62p.	Third
Second	Laing, J. A., W. J. Brinley Morgan, and W. C. Wagner. Fertility and Infertility in Veterinary Practice. 4th ed. London and Philadelphia; Bailliere Tindall, 1988. 280p. (2d ed. as Fertility and Infertility in Domestic Animals . . . Baltimore; Williams & Wilkins, 1970.)	First
	Laird, Marshall, and James W. Miles. Integrated Mosquito Control Methodologies. London and New York; Academic Press, 1983. 2 vols.	Third
Second	Lamond, D. R. Control of Reproductive Functions in Domestic Animals. The Hague, Boston and Hingham, Mass.; M. Nijhoff, 1980. 248p.	Second
Third	Lampert, Lincoln M. Modern Dairy Products; Composition, Food Value, Processing, Chemistry, Bacteriology, Testing, Imitation Dairy Products. 3d ed. New York; Chemical Pub. Co., 1975. 437p. (First published, 1947, as Milk and Dairy Products.)	
Third	Lancaster, J. L., and M. V. Meisch. Arthropods in Livestock and Poultry Production. Chichester, U.K.; E. Horwood; New York; Halsted Press, 1986. 402p.	Second
Second	Land, R. B., and D. W. Robinson, eds. Genetics of Reproduction in Sheep. London and Boston; Butterworths, 1985. 427p.	Second
Third	Landauer, Walter. The Hatchability of Chicken Eggs as Influenced by Environment and Heredity. Rev. ed. Storrs, Conn.; Storrs Agricultural Experiment Station, The University of Connecticut, 1967. 315p. (Connecticut, Agricultural Experiment Station, Storrs, Monograph no. 1 Rev. ed) (Originally published as Conn. AES Bulletins 216, 236 and 262.)	
Second	Lapage, Geoffrey. Veterinary Parasitology. Edinburgh; Oliver & Boyd, 1956. 964p. (Available in Spanish as Paratistologia Veterinaria. Mexico City; CECSA, 1983.)	Third
First	Larson, Bruce L., and Vearl R. Smith, eds. Lactation: A Comprehensive Treatise. New York; Academic Press, 1974–1978. 4 vols. (Earlier ed., 1974. 3 vols.)	First
Third	Lasley, John F. Beef Cattle Production. Englewood Cliffs, N.J.; Prentice-Hall, 1981. 468p.	Second
Second	Lasley, John F. Genetics of Livestock Improvement. 4th ed. Englewood Cliffs, N.J.; Prentice-Hall, 1987. 477p. (1st ed., 1963. 342p.) (Available in Spanish as Genetica del Mejoramiento del Ganado . . . trans. by Gustavo Reta. Mexico; UTEHA, 1970.)	First

Developed countries ranking		Third World ranking
	Latin American Symposium on Mineral Nutrition Research with Grazing Ruminants, 1976, Belo Horizonte, Brazil. Proceedings of the Conference . . . edited by Joe H. Conrad and Lee R. McDowell. Gainesville; University of Florida, 1978. 200p.	Second
	Latshaw, William K. Veterinary Developmental Anatomy: A Clinically Oriented Approach. Toronto, Philadelphia, Saint Louis; B. C. Decker; U.S. distribution, C. V. Mosby Co., 1987. 283p.	Third
	Laver, W. Graeme, and Gillian M. Air, eds. Immune Recognition of Protein Antigens. Cold Spring Harbor, N.Y.; Cold Spring Harbor Laboratory, 1985. 197p. (Reports from a Conference held in March 1985 at Cold Spring Harbor Laboratory.)	Third
Second	Lawrence, Carl A., Seymour S. Block, and George F. Reddish. Disinfection, Sterilization, and Preservation. Philadelphia; Lea & Febiger, 1968. 808p. (Successor to Antiseptics, Disinfectants, Fungicides, and Chemical and Physical Sterilization, edited by G. Reddish and published in 1954 and 1957.)	Second
First	Lawrence, T. L. J. Growth in Animals. London and Boston; Butterworths, 1980. 308p.	First
First	Lawrie, Ralston A., ed. Developments in Meat Science. London; Elsevier Applied Science Publishers, 1980–1988. 4 vols.	First
Second	Lawrie, Ralston A. Meat Science. 5th ed. Oxford and New York; Pergamon Press, 1991. 300p. (1st ed., 1966. 368p.) (Available in Spanish as Ciencia de la Carne. 2d ed. Zaragoza; Acribia, 1977.)	First
Third	Lean, Ian. Nutrition of Dairy Cattle. Sydney; University of Sydney Post-Graduate Foundation in Veterinary Science, 1987. 485p.	Second
Second	Leaver, J. D. Herbage Intake Handbook. Hurley, Berkshire, U.K.; British Grassland Society, 1982. 143p.	
Third	Leaver, J. D. Milk Production: Science and Practice. London and New York; Longman, 1983. 173p.	
Third	Lebas, F. The Rabbit: Husbandry, Health and Production. Rome; Food and Agriculture Organization, 1986. 235p. (FAO Animal Production and Health Series no. 21)	Second
	Leech, Frederick B., and Kenneth C. Sellers. Statistical Epidemiology in Veterinary Science. London; C. Griffin, 1979. 158p.	Second
	Lefevre, P. C. Peste des Petits Ruminants et Infection Bovipestique des Ovins et Caprins. 2d ed. Maison-Alfort, France; Institut d'Elevage et de Medecine Veterinaire des Pays Tropicaux, 1987. (Etudes et Syntheses de l'IEMVT no. 5)	Third
First	Legates, J. Edward, and Everett J. Warwick. Breeding and Improvement of Farm Animals. 8th ed. New York; McGraw-Hill, 1990. 624p. (1st–6th ed. by V. A. Rice et al.; 7th ed., War-	First

Developed countries ranking		Third World ranking
	wick's name appears first.) (Available in Spanish as Cria y Mejoramiento del Ganado. 3d ed. Mexico; McGraw-Hill, 1984.)	
	Lehninger, Albert L. Biochemistry: The Molecular Basis of Cell Structure and Function. 2d ed. New York; Worth Publishers, 1975. 1104p. (1st ed., 1970.) (Available in Spanish as Bioquimica. 2d ed. Barcelona; Omega.)	Third
First	Leman, Allen D., et al., eds. Diseases of Swine. 6th ed. Ames; Iowa State University Press, 1986. 930p. (1st–4th eds. edited by Howard W. Dunne.)	First
Third	Lenkeit, Walter, Knut Breirem, and Edgar Crasemann, eds. Handbuch der Tierernahrung. Hamburg, Berlin; Parey, 1969–1972. 2 vols. (Text partly in English.)	
	Lennette, Edwin H., et al. Manual of Clinical Microbiology. 4th ed. Washington, D.C.; American Society for Microbiology, 1985. 1149p. (1st ed., 1970. 727p.)	Second
Third	Lerner, I. Michael. The Genetic Basis of Selection. New York; Wiley, 1958. 208p.	Third
Third	Leuthold, Walter. African Ungulates; A Comparative Review of Their Ethology and Behavioral Ecology. Berlin and New York; Springer-Verlag, 1977. 307p.	Third
	Levandowsky, Michael, S. H. Hutner, and Andre Lwoff. Biochemistry and Physiology of Protozoa. 2d ed. New York; Academic Press, 1979–1980. 3 vols. (First ed., 1951–1964, by A. Lwoff.)	Third
Third	Levi, W. M. The Pigeon. Sumter, S.C.; Levi Publishing, 1974. 667p. (Reprinted, 1981.)	Third
Third	Levie, Albert. Meat Handbook. 4th ed. Westport, Conn.; Avi Pub. Co., 1979. 338p. (3d ed., 1970.)	Third
	Levine, Norman D. Veterinary Protozoology. 1st ed. Ames; Iowa State University Press, 1985. 414p. (Based on Protozoan Parasites of Domestic Animals and of Man.) (Available in Spanish as Tratado de Parasitologia Veterinaria. Zaragoza; Acribia, 1983.)	Second
Second	Levine, Norman D., and Virginia Ivens. The Coccidian Parasites (Protozoa, Apicomplexa) of Artiodactyla. Urbana; University of Illinois Press, 1986. 265p. (Illinois Biological Monographs no. 55)	Third
	Lewis, Benjamin P., and Leon O. Wilken. Veterinary Drug Index. Philadelphia; Saunders, 1982. 327p.	Second
Second	Liener, Irvin E., ed. Toxic Constituents of Plant Foodstuffs. 2d ed. New York; Academic Press, 1980. 502p. (1st ed., 1969. 500p.)	Second
Third	Lillie's Development of the Chick: An Introduction to Embryology. 3d ed., rev. by Howard L. Hamilton. New York; Henry Holt, 1952. 624p. (1st ed., 1908. 463p.)	

Developed countries ranking		Third World ranking
Second	Lindsay, D. R., and D. T. Pearce. Reproduction in Sheep. Cambridge and New York; Cambridge University Press, 1984. 403p.	Second
Third	Lister, D., ed. In Vivo Measurement of Body Composition in Meat Animals; Proceedings of a Workshop at Langford, Bristol, Nov.–Dec. 1983; Sponsored by the Commission of the European Communities, Coordination of Agricultural Research. London and New York; Elsevier Applied Science, 1984. 241p.	
Second	Lister, D., ed. Meat Animals: Growth and Productivity; Proceedings of a Symposium . . . 1974, Prestbury, England. New York; Plenum Press, 1976. 541p. (NATO Advanced Study Institutes Series: Series A, Life Sciences no. 8)	
	Lloyd, D. H., and Kenneth C. Sellers. Dermatophilus Infection in Animals and Man: Proceedings of a Symposium, University of Ibadan, Nigeria, and Sponsored by the Agricultural Research Council of Nigeria. London and New York; Academic Press, 1976. 322p. (Summaries in French.)	Second
	Lodge, G. A., and G. E. Lamming, eds. Growth and Development of Mammals; Proceedings of 14th Easter School in Agricultural Science, University of Nottingham, 1967. New York; Plenum Press, 1968. 527p.	Third
	Loosli, John K., Victor A. Oyenuga, and Gabriel M. Babatunde, eds. Animal Production in the Tropics; Proceedings of an International Symposium . . . Ibadan; Published for the Dept. of Animal Science, University of Ibadan, Nigeria by Heinemann Educational Books (Nigeria), 1974. 402p.	First
Third	Losos, George J. Infectious Tropical Diseases of Domestic Animals. Essex; Longman; New York; Churchill Livingstone, Inc., 1986. 938p.	Second
Second	Lovell, Tom. Nutrition and Feeding of Fish. New York; Van Nostrand Reinhold, 1989. 260p.	Second
Third	Low, A. G., and I. G. Partridge, eds. Current Concepts of Digestion and Absorption in Pigs; Proceedings of a Seminar, National Institute for Research in Dairying, July 1979. Reading, U.K.; National Institute for Research in Dairying; Ayr, Scotland; Hannah Research Institute, 1980. 222p. (National Institute for Research in Dairying Technical Bulletin no. 3)	
	Lu, Frank C., and Jan Rendel, eds. Anabolic Agents in Animal Production: FAO/WHO Symposium, Rome, March 1975. Stuttgart; Thieme, 1976. 277p.	Third
Third	Lucas, Alfred M. Atlas of Avian Hematology . . . illustrated by Casimir Jamroz. Washington, D.C.; U.S. Dept. of Agriculture, 1961. 271p. (USDA Agriculture Monograph no. 25)	Third
Third	Lucas, Alfred M., and Peter R. Stettenheim. Avian Anatomy: Integument. Washington, D.C.; U.S. Agricultural Research	

Developed countries ranking		Third World ranking
	Service; U.S. Government Printing Office, 1972. 2 vols. (Prepared as part of the Avian Anatomy Project conducted by U.S. Agricultural Research Service, and Michigan State University, Dept. of Poultry Science.)	
First	Lush, Jay L. Animal Breeding Plans. 3d ed. Ames; Iowa State University Press, 1945. 443p. Reprinted, 1969. (1st ed., 1937. 350p.) (Available in Spanish as Bases para la Seleccion Animal. 1st ed. Buenos Aires; Ediciones Agropecuarias Peri, 1969.)	
Second	Lush, Jay L. Proceedings of the Animal Breeding and Genetics Symposium in Honor of Dr. Jay L. Lush, July 1972, Virginia Polytechnic Institute and State University, Blacksburg, Virginia. Champaign, Ill.; American Society of Animal Science, 1973. 104p.	Second
Third	Luttmann, Rick, and Gail Luttmann. Chickens in Your Backyard: A Beginner's Guide. Emmaus, Pa.; Rodale Press, 1976. 157p.	

M

Developed countries ranking		Third World ranking
	Maar, A., M. A. E. Mortimer, and I. Van der Lingen. Fish Culture in Central East Africa. Rome; Food and Agriculture Organization, 1966. 158p.	Third
Second	Mack, Roy. Dictionary for Veterinary Science and Biosciences: German-English/English-German: With Trilingual Appendix, Latin Terms = Waterbuck for Medizin und Biowissenschaften: Deutsch-Englisch/Englisch-Deutsch: Mit Einem Dreisprachigen Anhang, Lateinische Begriffe. Berlin; Paul Parey, 1988. 321p.	Third
Third	Mack, Roy. Russian-English Veterinary Dictionary = Russko-Angli. Farnham Royal, U.K.; Commonwealth Agricultural Bureaux, 1972. 104p.	Third
Second	Mackenzie, David, and Jean Laing. Goat Husbandry. 4th ed., rev. and edited by J. Laing. London and Boston; Faber & Faber, 1980. 375p. (1st ed., 1957. 349p.)	First
	MacMillan, Susan, ed. Wildlife/Livestock Interfaces on Rangelands; Proceedings of a Conference, Taita Hills Lodge, Kenya, April 1985. Nairobi, Kenya; Inter-African Bureau for Animal Resources, 1986. 212p.	Third
First	Mahadevan, P. Breeding for Milk Production in Tropical Cattle. Farnham Royal, U.K.; Commonwealth Agricultural Bureaux, 1966. 154p. (CAB Technical Communication no. 17)	
	Malluche, H. H., and M. C. Faugere. Atlas of Mineralized Bone Histology. Basel and New York; Karger, 1986. 136p.	Third
Second	Mannetje, L. 't, ed. Measurement of Grassland Vegetation and Animal Production. Farnham Royal, U.K.; Commonwealth Ag-	First

Developed countries ranking		Third World ranking
	ricultural Bureaux, 1978. 260p. (Commonwealth Bureau of Pastures and Field Crops Bulletin no. 52)	
Second	Manning, Aubrey. An Introduction to Animal Behaviour. 3d ed. Reading, Mass.; Addison-Wesley, 1979. 329p. (1st ed. London; Edward Arnold, 1967. 208p.) (Available in Spanish as Introduccion a la Conducta Animal. Madrid; Alianza.)	
	Manning, Margaret J., and Mary F. Tatner, eds. Fish Immunology; Proceedings of a Conference . . . by the Fisheries Society of the British Isles, Plymouth, July 1983. London and Orlando, Fla.; Academic Press, 1985. 374p.	Third
	Manual of Tropical Veterinary Parasitology . . . trans. by Mira Shah-Fischer and R. Ralph Say. Wallingford, Oxon, U.K.; CAB International, 1989. 473p. (From French ed., 1981. Paris, Ministere de la Cooperation et du Developpment.)	Second
Third	Marai, I. Fayez M., and John B. Owen. New Techniques in Sheep Production. London and Boston; Butterworths, 1987. 292p.	Second
Second	Marasas, W. F. O., and Paul E. Nelson. Mycotoxicology: Introduction to the Mycology, Plant Pathology, Chemistry, Toxicology, and Pathology of Naturally Occurring Mycotoxicoses in Animals and Man. University Park; Pennsylvania State University Press, 1987. 102p.	Third
	Marcenac, Louis-Noel, and H. Aublet. Encyclopedie du Cheval. 3d ed., rev. by P. D'Autheville. Paris; Maloine, 1974. 1252p. (1st ed., 1964.)	Third
First	Marshall's Physiology of Reproduction. 4th ed., edited by G. E. Lamming. Edinburgh and New York; Churchill Livingstone, 1984–1990. 3 vols. (1st ed., Longman, Green Pub., 1922.)	First
Second	Marshall, Adrian G. The Ecology of Ectoparasitic Insects. London and New York; Academic Press, 1981. 459p.	Third
Third	Martin, S. Wayne, Alan H. Meek, and Preben Willeberg. Veterinary Epidemiology: Principles and Methods. 1st ed. Ames; Iowa State University Press, 1987. 343p.	Second
First	Martin, W. B. Diseases of Sheep. Oxford and Boston; Blackwell Scientific, 1983. 282p. (Available in Spanish as Enfermedades de la Oveja. 1st ed. trans. by J. L. Muzquiz M. Zaragoza; Acribia, 1987.)	Second
Third	Martin, W. B. Respiratory Diseases in Cattle: A Seminar in the EEC Programme of Coordination of Research on Beef Production, Edinburgh, 1977. The Hague and Boston; M. Nijhoff for the Commission of the European Communities, 1978. 562p.	
	Mason, I. L. The Classification of West African Livestock. Farnham Royal, U.K.; Commonwealth Agricultural Bureaux, 1951. 39p. (Commonwealth Bureau of Animal Breeding and Genetics, Technical Communication no. 7)	First

Developed countries ranking		Third World ranking
Second	Mason, I. L. Evolution of Domesticated Animals. London and New York; Longman, 1984. 452p.	Second
Third	Mason, I. L. Prolific Tropical Sheep. Rome; Food and Agriculture Organization, 1980. 124p. (FAO Animal Production and Health Paper no. 17)	First
Third	Mason, I. L. Sheep Breeds of the Mediterranean. Farnham Royal, U.K.; Published by arrangement with the Food and Agriculture Organization by the Commonwealth Agricultural Bureaux, 1967. 215p.	Third
First	Mason, I. L. A World Dictionary of Livestock Breeds, Types and Varieties. 3d ed. Wallingford, Oxon, U.K.; CAB International, 1988. 348p. (1st ed., 1951. 272p.)	First
Second	Mason, I. L., and V. Buvanendran. Breeding Plans for Ruminant Livestock in the Tropics. Rome; Food and Agriculture Organization, 1982. 89p. (FAO Animal Production and Health Paper no. 34)	First
Third	Mason, I. L., and W. Pabst, eds. Crossbreeding Experiments and Strategy of Beef Utilization to Increase Beef Production. Luxembourg; Commission of the European Communities, 1976. 490p.	
Third	Mason, Jim, and Peter Singer. Animal Factories. 1st ed. New York; Crown Publishers, 1980. 174p.	Third
Third	Matches, Arthur G., ed. Anti-Quality Components of Forages; A Symposium sponsored by the Crop Science Society of America, Miami Beach, Fla., 1972. Madison, Wis.; Crop Science Society of America, 1973. 140p. (CSSA Special Publication no. 4)	
Third	Maton, A., J. Daelemans, and J. Lambrecht. Housing of Animals: Construction and Equipment of Animal Houses. Amsterdam and New York; Elsevier; Distributors for the U.S. and Canada, Elsevier Science, 1985. 458p. (Translation of De Huisvesting van Dieren.) (Available in Spanish as Construcciones Para el Ganado. Madrid; Mundi-Prensa, 1975.)	
	Matyas, Z. Salmonellosis Control: The Role of Animal and Product Hygiene; Report of a WHO Expert Committee. Geneva; World Health Organization, 1988. 83p. (WHO Technical Report Series no. 774)	Second
Third	Maule, J. P. The Cattle of the Tropics. Edinburgh; University of Edinburgh Centre for Tropical Veterinary Medicine, 1990. 225p.	Second
	May, Cheryl. Cattle Management. Reston, Va.; Reston Pub. Co., 1981. 333p.	Second
Third	May, Neil D. The Anatomy of the Sheep; A Dissection Manual. 3d ed. St. Lucia, Australia; University of Queensland Press,	

<table>
<tr><td>Developed
countries
ranking</td><td></td><td>Third
World
ranking</td></tr>
<tr><td></td><td>1970. 369p. (Distributed in the U.S. by International Scholarly Book Services.)</td><td></td></tr>
<tr><td>First</td><td>Maynard, Leonard A., et al. Animal Nutrition. 7th ed. New York; McGraw-Hill, 1979. 602p. (1st ed., 1937. 483p. 4th–6th eds. by L. A. Maynard and J. K. Loosli.) (Available in Spanish as Nutricion Animal. 4th ed. Mexico; McGraw-Hill, 1981.)</td><td>First</td></tr>
<tr><td>Third</td><td>Mayr, A., G. Eissner, and B. Mayr-Bibrack. Handbuch der Schutzimpfungen in der Tiermedizin. Berlin; Paul Parey, 1984. 1006p.</td><td></td></tr>
<tr><td>Third</td><td>McCullough, Marshall E., ed. NFIA Literature Review on Fermentation on Silage: A Review. West Des Moines, Iowa; Grants-In-Aid Committee, National Feed Ingredients Association, 1978. 332p.</td><td>Third</td></tr>
<tr><td>Third</td><td>McCullough, Marshall E. Optimum Feeding of Dairy Animals: For Meat and Milk. 2d ed. Athens; University of Georgia Press, 1973. 200p. (1st ed., 1969. 180p.) (Available in Spanish as Alimentacion Practica de la Vaca Lechera. 2d ed. Barcelona; Aedos, 1976.)</td><td></td></tr>
<tr><td>First</td><td>McDonald, L. E., and M. H. Pineda, eds. Veterinary Endocrinology and Reproduction. 4th ed. Philadelphia; Lea & Febiger, 1989. 571p. (1st ed., by L. E. McDonald, 1969. 460p.)</td><td>First</td></tr>
<tr><td>Second</td><td>McDonald, Peter, R. A. Edwards, and J. F. D. Greenhalgh. Animal Nutrition. 4th ed. Harlow, Essex, U.K.; Longman; New York; Copublished in the U.S. with J. Wiley, 1988. 543p. (1st ed., 1966, by Oliver & Boyd. 407p.) (Available in Spanish as Nutricion Animal. 3d ed. Zaragoza; Acribia, 1985.)</td><td>First</td></tr>
<tr><td>Third</td><td>McDonald, Peter, Nancy Henderson, and Shirley Heron. The Biochemistry of Silage. Bucks, U.K.; Chalcombe Publications, 1991. 340p. (Earlier ed., by P. McDonald. Chichester and New York; Wiley, 1981. 226p.)</td><td></td></tr>
<tr><td>First</td><td>McDowell, Lee R. Nutrition of Grazing Ruminants in Warm Climates. Orlando, Fla.; Academic Press, 1985. 443p.</td><td>First</td></tr>
<tr><td>Second</td><td>McDowell, Lee R. Vitamins in Animal Nutrition: Comparative Aspects to Human Nutrition. San Diego; Academic Press, 1989. 486p.</td><td>First</td></tr>
<tr><td></td><td>McDowell, Lee R., J. E. Conrad, J. E. Thomas, and L. E. Harris. Latin American Tables of Feed Composition. 2d ed. Gainesville; University of Florida, Dept. of Animal Science, 1974. 509p. (Available in Spanish as Tabelas de Composicao de Alimentos de America Latina.)</td><td>First</td></tr>
<tr><td>Second</td><td>McDowell, R. E. Feasibility of Commercial Dairying with Cattle Indigenous to the Tropics. Ithaca; New York State College of Agriculture, Cornell University, 1971. 22p. (Cornell Inst. Agric. Devel. Bulletin no. 21)</td><td>First</td></tr>
</table>

Developed countries ranking		Third World ranking
First	McDowell, R. E. Improvement of Livestock Production in Warm Climates. San Francisco; W. H. Freeman, 1972. 711p. (Available in Spanish as Bases Biologicas de la Produccion Animal en Zonas Tropicales . . . trans. by Pedro Ducar Malvenda. Zaragoza; Acribia, 1975.)	First
	McDowell, R. E., and P. E. Hildebrand, eds. Integrated Crop and Animal Production: Making the Most of Resources Available to Small Farms in Developing Countries; a Bellagio Conference, October 1978. New York; Rockefeller Foundation, 1980. 78p.	Third
Second	McFerran, J. B., and M. S. McNulty. Acute Virus Infections of Poultry: A Seminar in the CEC Agricultural Research Programme, Brussels, June 1985. Dordrecht, Boston and Hingham, Mass.; M. Nijhoff for the Commission of the European Communities, 1986. 242p.	Third
	McIlory, Robert J. An Introduction to Tropical Grassland Husbandry. 2d ed. London and New York; Oxford University Press, 1972. 160p. (1st ed., 1964. 128p.) (Available in Spanish as Introduccion al Cultivo de los Pastos Tropicales . . . trans. by Agustin Contin. Mexico; Limusa, 1976.)	Third
	McLoughlin, Peter F. M., ed. African Food Production Sytems; Case and Theory. Baltimore; Johns Hopkins Press, 1970. 318p.	Third
Third	McNitt, J. I. Livestock Husbandry Techniques. London and New York; Granada, 1983. 280p.	Second
Third	Mead, G. C., and B. M. Freeman, eds. Meat Quality in Poultry and Game Birds; Proceedings of the Joint 15th Poultry Science Symposium, and 4th European Symposium on Poultry Meat Quality, September 1979. Edinburgh; British Poultry Science, 1980.	
Third	Mead, Roger, and R. N. Curnow. Statistical Methods in Agriculture and Experimental Biology. London and New York; Chapman & Hall, 1983. 335p.	
Second	Mehlhorn, Heinz, and D. Bunnag. Parasitology in Focus: Facts and Trends. Berlin and New York; Springer-Verlag, 1988. 924p.	Third
Second	Melby, Edward C., and Norman H. Altman, eds. CRC Handbook of Laboratory Animal Science. Cleveland, Ohio; CRC Press, 1974–1976. 3 vols.	
Second	Menke, K. H., H. J. Lantzsch, and J. R. Reichl, eds. Energy Metabolism of Farm Animals; Proceedings of the 6th Symposium, Hohenheim, Germany, Sept. 1973. Stuttgart; Universitaet Hohenheim Kodkumentationsstelle, 1974. 308p. (European Association for Animal Production no. 14)	
First	Mepham, T. B., ed. Biochemistry of Lactation. Amsterdam and	Third

Developed countries ranking		Third World ranking
	New York; Elsevier; Distributors for the U.S. and Canada, Elsevier, 1983. 500p.	
Third	Mertz, Walter, and W. E. Cornatzer, eds. New Trace Elements in Nutrition; Proceedings of an International Symposium . . . Grand Forks, N.Dak., 1970. New York; Dekker, 1971. 438p.	
First	Mertz, Walter, ed. Trace Elements in Human and Animal Nutrition. 5th ed. Orlando, Fla.; Academic Press, 1986–1987. 2 vols. (1st ed., by E. J. Underwood. New York; Academic Press, 1956. 430p.)	
Second	Midwest Plan Service. Sheep Handbook: Housing and Equipment. 3d ed. Ames, Iowa; Midwest Plan Service, 1982. 115p. (1st ed., 1960.)	
Second	Midwest Plan Service. Structures and Environment Handbook. 11th ed. Ames, Iowa; Midwest Plan Service, 1983. 1 vol. (Various pagings.) (7th ed., 1975. 412p.)	
First	Midwest Plan Service. Swine Housing and Equipment Handbook. 4th ed. Ames, Iowa; Midwest Plan Service, 1983. 112p. (Earlier rev. ed., 1968. 74p.)	
	Miert, A. S. J. van, J. Frens, and F. W. Van der Kreek. Trends in Veterinary Pharmacology and Toxicology: Proceedings of the First European Congress on Veterinary Pharmacology and Toxicology, September 1979, Zeist, Netherlands. Amsterdam and New York; Elsevier Scientific Pub. Co., 1980. 363p.	Third
Third	Miller, E. L., I. H. Pike, and A. J. H. van Es, eds. Protein Contribution of Feedstuffs for Ruminants: Application to Feed Formulation. London and Boston; Butterworth Scientific, 1982. 160p.	Second
Second	Miller, W. J. Dairy Cattle Feeding and Nutrition. New York; Academic Press, 1979. 411p.	Second
Third	de Milliano, W. A. J., R. A. Frederiksen, and G. D. Bengston, eds. Sorghum and Millets Diseases: A Second World Review. Patancheru, India; International Crops Research Institute for the Semi-Arid Tropics, 1992. 370p.	Third
First	Milligan, L. P., W. L. Grovum, and A. Dobson. Control of Digestion and Metabolism in Ruminants; Proceedings of the 6th International Symposium on Ruminant Physiology, Banff, Canada, September 1984. Englewood Cliffs, N.J.; Prentice-Hall, 1986. 567p.	Second
Third	Mills, Colin F., ed. Trace Element Metabolism in Animals; Proceedings of WAAP/IBP International Symposium, Aberdeen, Scotland, July 1969. Edinburgh; Livingstone, 1970. 549p.	Second
	Mims, Cedric A. The Pathogenesis of Infectious Disease. 3d ed. London and Orlando, Fla.; Academic Press, 1987. 342p.	Second

Developed countries ranking		Third World ranking
	(1st ed., London; Academic Press; New York; Grune & Stratton, 1976. 246p.)	
Second	Minish, Gary L., and Danny G. Fox. Beef Production and Management. 2d ed. Reston, Va.; Reston Pub. Co., 1982. 470p. (1st ed., 1979. 416p.)	Second
Third	Minvielle, Francis. Principes d'Amelioration Genetique des Animaux Domestiques. Paris; INRA, 1990. 211p.	
Third	Mitchell, Harold H. Comparative Nutrition of Man and Domestic Animals. New York; Academic Press, 1963–1964. 2 vols.	
	Mitchell, J. R. Guide to Meat Inspection in the Tropics. 2d ed. Farnham Royal, U.K.; Commonwealth Agricultural Bureaux, 1980. 95p.	Second
Third	Mloszewski, Mark J. The Behavior and Ecology of the African Buffalo. Cambridge and New York; Cambridge University Press, 1983. 256p.	Third
Third	Moberg, Gary P., ed. Animal Stress. Papers Delivered at a Symposium, July 1983, Sponsored by the College of Agriculture and Environmental Sciences at the University of California, Davis. Bethesda and Baltimore; American Physiological Society, Distributed by Williams & Wilkins, 1985. 324p.	Second
Third	Mocsy, Janos. Lehrbuch der Klinischen Diagnostik der Inneren Krankheiten der Haustiere. 6th ed. Jena; G. Fischer, 1960. 659p. (Earlier ed., by Josef Marek, 1912. 957p.) (Available in Spanish as Tratado de Diagnostico Clinico de las Enfermedades Internas de los Animales Domesticos. 4th ed. Barcelona; Labor, 1973.)	
	Molyneux, D. H., and R. W. Ashford. The Biology of Trypanosoma and Leishmania; Parasites of Man and Domestic Animals. New York; International Publications Service, 1983. 294p.	Third
Third	Monod, Theodore, èd. Pastoralism in Tropical Africa. Les Societies Pastorales en Afrique Tropicale: Studies Presented and Discussed . . . = International African Seminar on Pastoralism in Tropical Africa, 13th, Niamey, December 1972. London; Published for the International African Institute by Oxford University Press, 1975. 502p. (English and/or French with summaries in French.)	Third
Third	Monteith, John L., and Lawrence E. Mount, eds. Heat Loss from Animals and Man: Assessment and Control; Proceedings of the 20th Easter School in Agricultural Science, University of Nottingham, 1973. London; Butterworths, 1974. 457p.	Third
	Moore-Landecker, Elizabeth. Fundamentals of the Fungi. 2d ed. Englewood Cliffs, N.J.; Prentice-Hall, 1982. 578p. (1st ed., 1972. 482p.)	Second

Developed countries ranking		Third World ranking
Third	Moreng, Robert E., and John S. Avens. Poultry Science and Production. Reston, Va.; Reston Pub. Co., 1985. 438p.	Third
	Morgan, Joe P., and Sam Silverman. Techniques of Veterinary Radiography. 4th ed. Davis, Calif.; Veterinary Radiology Associates, 1984. 334p. (1st ed., 1975. 388p.)	Third
First	Morley, Frederick H. W. Grazing Animals. Amsterdam and New York; Elsevier Scientific Pub. Co., 1981. 411p. (World Animal Science. B, Disciplinary Approach no. 1)	First
Third	Morris, Bede, and Masayuki Miyasaka, eds. Immunology of the Sheep; International Symposium on the Immune Responses in Foetal and Adult Sheep, Basel Institute for Immunology, 1984. Basel; Editiones Roche, 1985. 520p.	
First	Morrison, Frank B. Feeds and Feeding; A Handbook for the Student and Stockman. 22d ed., unabridged. Ithaca, N.Y.; Morrison Pub. Co., 1956. 1165p. (1st–9th eds. edited by W. A. Henry; 10th-14th eds. by W. A. Henry assisted by F. B. Morrison; 15th-21st eds. revised and rewritten by F. B. Morrison.) (Available in Spanish as Alimentos y Alimentacion del Ganado. Mexico City; UTEHA, 1980.)	Third
Second	Morrison, W. Ivan, ed. The Ruminant Immune System in Health and Disease. Cambridge and New York; Cambridge University Press, 1986. 570p.	Second
	Morrow, David A. Current Therapy in Theriogenology. 2d ed. Philadelphia; Saunders, 1986. 1143p.	Second
Third	Moss, R. The Laying Hen and its Environment: A Seminar in the EEC Programme of Coordination of Research on Animal Welfare, Luxembourg, March 1980. The Hague and Boston; M. Nijhoff for the Commission of the European Communities, 1980. 333p.	
Second	Moss, R. Transport of Animals Intended for Breeding, Production, and Slaughter: A Seminar in the CEC Programme of Coordination of Research on Animal Welfare, Brussels, July 1981. The Hague, Boston and Hingham, Mass.; M. Nijhoff for the Commission of the European Communities, 1982. 236p.	
Second	Mount, L. E. Adaptation to Thermal Environment: Man and His Productive Animals. Baltimore; University Park Press, 1979. 333p.	Second
Second	Mount, L. E. The Climatic Physiology of the Pig. London; Edward Arnold, 1968. 271p. (Physiological Society Monographs no. 18)	
Third	Mountney, George J. Poultry Products Technology. 2d ed. Westport, Conn.; Avi Pub. Co., 1976. 369p. (1st ed., 1966. 264p.)	
	Mouwen, J. M. V., E. C. B. de Groot, and J. E. van Dijk.	Third

Developed countries ranking		Third World ranking
	Atlas of Veterinary Pathology. Philadelphia; W. B. Saunders, 1982. 160p. (Available in Spanish as Atlas de Patalogia Veterinaria. Barcelona; Salvat, 1984.)	
Second	Mugero, G. M., O. Bwongomi, and J. G. Wondera. Diseases of Cattle in Tropical Africa. Nairobi; Kenya Literature Bureau, 1979.	Second
Third	Muir, J. F., and Ronald J. Roberts. Recent Advances in Aquaculture. London; Croom Helm; Boulder, Colo.; Westview Press, 1982. 2 vols.	Third
	Mukasa-Mugerwa, E. The Camel (Camelus Dromedarius): A Bibliographical Review. Addis Ababa, Ethiopia; International Livestock Centre for Africa, 1981. 147p.	Second
Third	Muller, Z. O. Feed from Animal Wastes: Feeding Manual. Rome; Food and Agriculture Organization, 1982. 214p. (Continuation of Feed from Animal Wastes: State of Knowledge.)	Second
	Mulligan, Hugh, and W. H. Potts, eds. The African Trypanosomiases. New York; Wiley-Interscience, 1970. 950p.	Third
Third	Munro, Hamish N., and J. B. Allison, eds. Mammalian Protein Metabolism. New York; Academic Press, 1964–1970. 4 vols.	Third
Second	Murty, A. S. Toxicity of Pesticides to Fish. Boca Raton, Fla.; CRC Press, 1986. 2 vols.	Third

N

Second	Nalbandov, Andrew V. Reproductive Physiology of Mammals and Birds: The Comparative Physiology of Domestic and Laboratory Animals and Man. 3d ed. San Francisco; W. H. Freeman, 1976. 334p. (Previously published as Reproductive Physiology.) (Available in Spanish as Fisiologia de la Reproduccion. Zaragoza; Acribia, 1969.)	Second
Third	Nansen, Peter J., and E. J. L. Soulsby. Epidemiology and Control of Nematodiasis in Cattle: An Animal Pathology in the CEC Programme of Coordination of Agricultural Research, Royal Veterinary and Agricultural University, Copenhagen, Denmark, February 1980. The Hague, Boston and Hingham, Mass.; M. Nijhoff for the Commission of the European Communities, 1981. 606p.	Third
Third	National Academy of Sciences (U.S.). Body Composition in Animals and Man; Proceedings of a Symposium, May 1967, University of Missouri, Columbia. Washington, D.C.; National Academy of Sciences, 1968. 521p. (National Academy of Sciences, Washington, D.C. Publication no. 1598)	
Third	National Academy of Sciences (U.S.). The Use of Drugs in Animal Feeds; Proceedings of a Symposium. Washington,	

Developed countries ranking		Third World ranking
	D.C.; National Academy of Sciences, 1969. 407p. (National Academy of Sciences Publication no. 1679)	
Second	National Mastitis Council. Microbiological Procedures for Use in the Diagnosis of Bovine Mastitis. 2d ed. Washington, D.C.; National Mastitis Council, 1981. 35p. (1st ed., 1969. 27p.)	Second
Second	National Research Council (U.S.). Effect of Environment on Nutrient Requirements of Domestic Animals; compiled by Subcommittee on Environmental Stress, Committee on Animal Nutrition, Board on Agricultural and Renewable Resources and Commission on Natural Resources of the National Research Council. Washington, D.C.; National Academy Press, 1981. 152p.	
Second	National Research Council (U.S.). Board on Agriculture and Renewable Resources. Urea and Other Nonprotein Nitrogen Compounds in Animal Nutrition, Board on Agriculture and Renewable Resources, Commission on Natural Resources. Washington, D.C.; National Academy of Sciences, 1976. 120p.	Second
	National Research Council (U.S.). Board on Science and Technology for International Development. The Improvement of Tropical and Subtropical Rangelands. Washington, D.C.; National Academy Press, 1990. 379p.	Third
First	National Research Council (U.S.). Committee on Animal Nutrition. Alternative Sources of Protein for Animal Production; Proceedings of a Symposium. Washington, D.C.; National Academy of Sciences, 1973. 183p.	First
First	National Research Council (U.S.). Committee on Animal Nutrition and Subcommittee on Biological Energy. Nutritional Energetics of Domestic Animals & Glossary of Energy Terms. 2d ed., rev. Washington, D.C.; National Academy Press, 1981. 45p. (1966 ed. as Biological Energy Interrelationships and Glossary of Energy Terms.)	First
Second	National Research Council (U.S.). Committee on Physiological Effects of Environmental Factors on Animals. A Guide to Environmental Research on Animals. Washington, D.C.; National Academy of Sciences, 1971. 374p.	
First	National Research Council (U.S.). Subcommittee on Beef Cattle Nutrition. Nutrient Requirements of Beef Cattle. 6th ed., rev. Washington, D.C.; National Academy Press, 1984. 90p. (5th ed., 1976. 56p.) (Available in Spanish as Necesidades Nutritivas del Ganado Vacuno de Carne. 2d ed. Buenos Aires; Hemisferio Sur, 1980.)	First
First	National Research Council (U.S.). Subcommittee on Coldwater Fish Nutrition. Nutrient Requirements of Coldwater Fishes. Washington, D.C.; National Academy Press, 1981. 63p.	Second
First	National Research Council (U.S.). Subcommittee on Dairy Cat-	First

156   Wallace C. Olsen

<table>
<tr><td>Developed
countries
ranking</td><td></td><td>Third
World
ranking</td></tr>
<tr><td></td><td>tle Nutrition. Nutrient Requirements of Dairy Cattle. 6th ed., rev. Washington, D.C.; National Academy of Sciences, 1988. 157p. (1st ed., 1958.) (Available in Spanish as Necesidades Nutritivas del Ganado Lechero. Buenos Aires; Hemisferio Sur, 1982.)</td><td></td></tr>
<tr><td>Second</td><td>National Research Council (U.S.). Subcommittee on Feed Composition. Atlas of Nutritional Data on United States and Canadian Feeds, by the Subcommittee on Feed Composition . . . and the Committee on Feed Composition, Research Branch, Dept. of Agriculture, Canada. Washington, D.C.; National Academy of Sciences, 1972. 772p.</td><td>Second</td></tr>
<tr><td>First</td><td>National Research Council (U.S.). Subcommittee on Feed Composition. United States-Canadian Tables of Feed Composition; Nutritional Data for United States and Canadian Feeds. Washington, D.C.; National Academy of Sciences, 1982. 92p. (2d rev. of the Joint U.S.-Canadian Tables of Feed Composition prepared in 1959 and 1964 by the Committee on Animal Nutrition, National Research Council, Washington and the National Committee on Animal Nutrition, Canada.)</td><td>Third</td></tr>
<tr><td>First</td><td>National Research Council (U.S.). Subcommittee on Furbearer Nutrition. Nutrient Requirements of Mink and Foxes. Rev. ed. Washington, D.C.; National Academy of Sciences, 1982. (Nutrient Requirements of Domestic Animals no. 7) (1953 ed. as National Academy of Sciences-National Research Council Publication 296.)</td><td>Second</td></tr>
<tr><td>First</td><td>National Research Council (U.S.). Subcommittee on Genetic Variance in Animal Nutrition. The Effect of Genetic Variance on Nutritional Requirements of Animals: Proceedings of a Symposium, University of Maryland, 1974. Washington, D.C.; National Academy of Sciences, 1975. 123p.</td><td></td></tr>
<tr><td>First</td><td>National Research Council (U.S.). Subcommittee on Goat Nutrition. Nutrient Requirements of Goats: Angora, Dairy, and Meat Goats in Temperate and Tropical Countries. Washington, D.C.; National Academy Press, 1981. 91p.</td><td>First</td></tr>
<tr><td>First</td><td>National Research Council (U.S.). Subcommittee on Horse Nutrition. Nutrient Requirements of Horses. 5th ed. Washington, D.C.; National Academy of Sciences, 1989. (Earlier eds. as National Academy of Sciences, National Research Council Publication no. 912, 1401.) (Available in Spanish as Necesidades Nutritivas de los Caballos. Buenos Aires; Hemisferio Sur, 1975.)</td><td>First</td></tr>
<tr><td>First</td><td>National Research Council (U.S.). Subcommittee on Laboratory Animal Nutrition. Nutrient Requirements of Laboratory Animals: Rat, Mouse, Gerbil, Guinea Pig, Hamster, Vole, Fish. 3d</td><td>First</td></tr>
</table>

Developed countries ranking		Third World ranking
	ed., rev. Washington, D.C.; National Academy of Sciences, 1978. 96p.	
First	National Research Council (U.S.). Subcommittee on Mineral Toxicity in Animals. Mineral Tolerance of Domestic Animals. Washington, D.C.; National Academy of Sciences, 1980. 577p.	First
First	National Research Council (U.S.). Subcommittee on Poultry Nutrition. Nutrient Requirements of Poultry. 8th ed. Washington, D.C.; National Academy of Sciences, 1984. 71p. (Editions for 1954, 1960, and 1966 as National Academy of Sciences-National Research Council Publications no. 301, 827 & 1345.) (Available in Spanish as Necesidades Nutritivas de las Aves de Corral. Buenos Aires; Hemisferio Sur, 1975.)	First
First	National Research Council (U.S.). Subcommittee on Rabbit Nutrition. Nutrient Requirements of Rabbits. 2d ed., rev. Washington, D.C.; National Academy of Sciences, 1977. 30p. (Available in Spanish as Necesidades Nutritivas del Conejo. Buenos Aires; Hemisferio Sur, 1979.)	First
First	National Research Council (U.S.). Subcommittee on Sheep Nutrition. Nutrient Requirements of Sheep. 6th ed., rev. Washington, D.C.; National Academy of Sciences, 1985. 72p. (Available in Spanish as Necesidades Nutritivas de los Ovinos. Buenos Aires; Hemisferio Sur, 1979.)	First
Second	National Research Council (U.S.). Subcommittee on Standard Methods for Veterinary Microbiology. Manual of Standardized Methods for Veterinary Microbiology. Committee on Animal Health, Board on Agriculture and Renewable Resources, National Academy of Sciences-National Research Council, Washington; edited by George E. Cottral. Ithaca, N.Y.; Comstock Pub. Associates, 1978. 731p. (Available in Spanish, 1986.)	Third
First	National Research Council (U.S.). Subcommittee on Swine Nutrition. Nutrient Requirements of Swine. 9th ed., rev. Washington, D.C.; National Academy of Sciences, 1988. 93p. (Title varies slightly. 1st ed., 1953.) (Available in Spanish as Necesidades Nutritivas del Cerdo. Buenos Aires; Hemisferio Sur, 1980.)	First
Second	National Research Council (U.S.). Subcommittee on Underutilized Resources as Animal Feedstuffs. Underutilized Resources as Animal Feedstuffs. Washington, D.C.; National Academy Press, 1983. 253p.	
First	National Research Council (U.S.). Subcommittee on Warmwater Fish Nutrition. Nutrient Requirements of Warmwater Fishes and Shellfishes. Rev. ed. Washington, D.C.; National Academy Press, 1983. 102p. (Rev. ed. of Nutrient Requirements of Warmwater Fishes, 1977.)	Second

Developed countries ranking		Third World ranking
	Navarro Pruneda, G. Diccionario Tecnologico de Ciencias Veterinarias y Zootecnica: Ingles-Espanol. Havana; Editorial Cientifico-Tecnica, 1982. 167p.	Third
Third	Nehring, K. Lehrbuch der Tierernahrung und Futtermittelkunde. 6th ed. Radebeul; Neumann, 1972. 460p. (3d ed., 1953. 415p.)	
	Nelson, Michael. The Development of Tropical Lands: Policy Issues in Latin America. Baltimore; Published for Resources for the Future by Johns Hopkins University Press, 1973. 306p. (Available in Spanish as Aprovechamiento de las Tierras Tropicales en America Latina. 1st ed. Mexico; Siglo XXI, 1977.)	Third
Third	Nestel, Barry L. Development of Animal Production Systems. Amsterdam and New York; Elsevier, 1984. 435p.	Second
Second	Neumann, A. L., and Keith S. Lusby. Beef Cattle. 8th ed. New York; Wiley, 1986. 326p. (1st–4th ed. by R. R. Snapp; 5th ed. by R. R. Snapp and A. L. Neumann.)	Second
Second	Neundorf, Rudolf, and Heinrich Seidel, eds. Schweinekrankheiten; Aetiologie, Pathogenese, Klinik, Therapie, Prophylaxe. Jena; Fischer, 1972. 719p. (Available in Spanish as Enfermeda del Cerdo; Etiologia, Patogenia, Sintomas Clinicos, Tratamiento, Profilaxis. Zaragoza; Acribia, 1974. 758p.)	Third
Third	Neville, Margaret C., and Charles W. Daniel, eds. The Mammary Gland: Development, Regulation, and Function. New York; Plenum Press, 1987. 625p.	Second
	New Zealand Dairy Research Institute. Jubilee Conference on Dairy Science and Technology, 1977, Palmerston North. Proceedings of Jubilee Conference . . . Palmerston North; New Zealand Dairy Research Institute, 1977. 196p.	Third
	Nicholas, F. W. Veterinary Genetics. Oxford and New York; Clarendon Press, Oxford University Press, 1987. 580p.	Second
Third	Nickel, R., A. Schummer, and E. Seiferle. Anatomy of the Domestic Birds . . . trans. by W. G. Siller and P. A. L. Wright. Berlin; Parey; New York; Springer-Verlag, 1977. 202p. (Translation of Lehrbuch der Anatomie der Haustiere (Textbook of the Anatomy of the Domestic Animals), Vol. V: Anatomie der Hausvogel.)	Second
	Nicolet, J. Compendio de Bacteriologia Medica Veterinaria. Zaragoza, Spain; Acribia, 1985. 275p.	Third
	Nicoletti, Paul. Diagnosis and Vaccination for the Control of Brucellosis in the Near East. Rome; Food and Agriculture Organization, 1982. 42p.	Third
	Nieuwolt, S. Tropical Climatology: An Introduction to the Climates of the Low Latitudes. London and New York; Wiley, 1977. 207p.	Third
Third	Nilsson, Stefan, and Susanne Holmgren, eds. Fish Physiology:	Third

Developed countries ranking		Third World ranking
	Recent Advances. London and Dover, N.H.; Croom Helm, 1986. 198p.	
Second	Nixey, C., and T. C. Grey, eds. Recent Advances in Turkey Science. Papers from the 21st Poultry Science Symposium, Harper Adams Agricultural College, Shropshire, Sept. 1987; Organized by the U.K. Branch of the World's Poultry Science Association. London and Boston; Butterworths, 1989. 373p. (Poultry Science Symposium no. 21)	Second
	Noakes, David E. Fertility and Obstetrics in Cattle. Oxford and Boston; Blackwell Scientific Publications, 1986. 139p.	Second
	Noden, Drew M., and Alexander DeLahunta. The Embryology of Domestic Animals: Developmental Mechanisms and Malformations. Baltimore; Williams & Wilkins, 1985. 367p.	Second
	Norris, David O. Vertebrate Endocrinology. 2d ed. Philadelphia; Lea & Febiger, 1985. 505p. (1st ed., 1980.)	Second
Second	North, Mack O., and Donald D. Bell. Commercial Chicken Production Manual. 4th ed. New York; Van Nostrand Reinhold, 1990. 913p. (1st ed., Avi, 1972.)	
Third	Novin, Donald, Wanda Wyrwicka, and George A. Bray, eds. Hunger: Basic Mechanisms and Clinical Implications. New York; Raven Press, 1976. 494p.	
	Nunez, J. L., and H. L. Moltedo. Sarna Psoroptica en Ovinos y Bovinos. Buenos Aires; Editorial Hemisferio Sur, 1985. 145p.	Third
Third	Nunez, J. L., M. E. Munoz-Cobenas, and H. L. Moltedo. Boophilus Microplus: The Common Cattle Tick . . . trans. by Harry Bailie, Constanza Michelsohn and Cecilia Paris. Berlin and New York; Springer-Verlag, 1985. 204p. (Original ed., Buenos Aries, Editorial Hemisferio Sur, 1982 and later ed., 1987.)	
Second	Nutrition Conference for Feed Manufacturers, 9th, University of Nottingham, 1975. Feed Energy Sources for Livestock; Papers . . . edited by Henry Swan and Dyfed Lewis. London and Boston; Butterworths, 1976. 158p.	Third
	Nutting, William B. Mammalian Diseases and Arachnids. Boca Raton, Fla.; CRC Press, 1984. 2 vols.	Third

O

Developed countries ranking		Third World ranking
Second	O'Dell, Boyd, Elwyn R. Miller, and William J. Miller. NFIA Literature Review on Copper and Zinc in Poultry, Swine and Ruminant Nutrition. West Des Moines, Iowa; Literature Review Committee, National Feed Ingredients Association, 1979. 279p.	Second
	O'Keefe, Philip, and Benjamin Wisner. Land Use and Development. London; Published by the International African Institute	Third

Developed countries ranking		Third World ranking
	in association with the Environment Training Programme, UNEP-IDEP-SIDA, 1977. 232p. (Papers in English or French.)	
Second	O'Mary, Clayton C., and Irwin A. Dyer, eds. Commerical Beef Cattle Production. 2d ed. Philaelphia; Lea & Febiger, 1978. 414p. (1st ed., 1972. 393p.)	Second
Third	Odend'hal, S. The Geographical Distribution of Animal Viral Diseases. New York; Academic Press, 1983. 493p.	
	Oehme, Frederick W. Textbook of Large Animal Surgery. 2d ed. Baltimore; Williams & Wilkins, 1988. 714p.	Second
Third	Ogbourne, Colin P. Bovine Dictyocauliasis: A Review and Annotated Bibliography. Farnham Royal, Slough, U.K.; Published on behalf of Commonwealth Institute of Parasitology by the Commonwealth Agricultural Bureaux, 1985. 104p.	Third
Second	Okerman, Lieve. Diseases of Domestic Rabbits. Boston and Oxford; Blackwell Scientific Publications, 1988. 120p.	Second
	Olds, R. J. A Colour Atlas of Microbiology. London; Wolfe Medical, 1975. 288p.	Third
	Oliver, John E., B. F. Hoerlein, and Ian G. Mayhew. Veterinary Neurology. Philadelphia; Saunders, 1987. 554p.	Second
	Oliver, John E., and Michael D. Lorenz. Handbook of Veterinary Neurologic Diagnosis. Philadelphia; Saunders, 1983. 371p.	Second
Third	Oluyemi, J. A., and F. A. Roberts. Poultry Production in Warm Wet Climates. London; Macmillan, 1979. 197p.	Second
Third	Onions, W. J. Wool; An Introduction to its Properties, Varieties, Uses and Production. New York; Interscience Publishers, 1962. 278p.	Third
	Organization of African Unity. Animal Genetic Resources in Africa: High Potential and Endangered Livestock; Proceedings of the 2d OAU Expert Committee Meeting on Animal Genetic Resources in Africa, Bulawayo, Zimbabwe, Nov. 1983. Nairobi; OAU/STRC/IBAR, 1985. 155p.	Third
First	Orskov, E. R. Protein Nutrition in Ruminants. London and New York; Academic Press, 1982. 160p.	First
First	Orskov, E. R., and M. Ryle. Energy Nutrition in Ruminants. London and New York; Elsevier Science Publishers, 1990.	First
Second	Orskov, E. R., ed. Feed Science. Amsterdam; Elsevier Science Publishers, 1988. 336p.	Second
Third	Ortavant, Robert, Jean Pelletier, and Jean-Paul Ravault, eds. Photoperiodism and Reproduction in Vertebrates: International Colloquim = Photoperiodisme et Reproduction chez les Vertebries: Colloque International, Nouzilly, France, September 1981. Paris; Institut National de la Recherche Agronomique, 1981. 337p. (Les Colloques de l'INRA no. 6)	Third
Third	Osbourn, D. F., D. E. Beever, and D. J. Thomson, eds. Rumi-	

Developed countries ranking		Third World ranking
	nant Digestion and Feed Evaluation; A Seminar held under the auspices of the Agricultural Research Council, Grassland Research Institute, Hurley, January 1978. London; Publication arranged by Agricultural Research Council, 1978. 1 vol.	
Second	Osweiler, Gary D., et al. Clinical and Diagnostic Veterinary Toxicology. 3d ed. Dubuque, Iowa; Kendall/Hunt Pub. Co., 1985. 494p. (Earlier eds. by W. B. Buck, G. Osweiler, and G. A. Van Gelder.)	Third
	Ott, Randall S., and Mushtaq A. Memon. Sheep and Goat Manual. Hastings, Nebr.; Society for Theriogenology, 1980. 50p. (Society for Theriogenology. "Volume X.")	Third
	Outteridge, P. M. Veterinary Immunology. London and Orlando; Academic Press, 1985. 280p.	Third
	Owen, Den. Animal Ecology in Tropical Africa. San Francisco; W. H. Freeman, 1966.	Third
Second	Owen, John B. Cattle Feeding. Ipswich, Suffolk; Farming Press, 1983. 170p. (Available in Spanish as Alimentacion del Ganado Vacuno. 1st ed. trans. by Mariana Bosenberg. Buenos Aires; Ateneo, 1987.)	Second
Third	Owen, John B. Complete Diets for Cattle and Sheep. Ipswich, U.K.; Farming Press, 1979. 159p. (Available in Spanish as Sistemas de Alimentacion Integral para Vacuno y Ovino. Madrid; Mundi-Prensa, 1981.)	Second
Second	Owen, John B. Sheep Production. London; Balliere Tindall, 1976. 436p.	
First	Owens, F. N., ed. Protein Requirements for Cattle: Proceedings of an International Symposium at Oklahoma State University, November 1980. Stillwater, Okla.; Division of Agriculture, Oklahoma State University, 1982. 363p. (MP-109.) (Running title: 1980 Protein Symposium.)	Second
	Oyenuga, Victor A. Nigeria's Foods and Feeding-Stuffs; Their Chemistry and Nutritive Value. 3d ed., rev. Ibadan; Ibadan University Press, 1968. 99p. (1st ed., 1955, as Nigerian Feedstuffs.)	Second

P

Developed countries ranking		Third World ranking
	Pagot, Jean. Animal Production in the Tropics. Macmillan, 1991. 480p. (Translation of L'Elevage en Pays Tropicaux. Paris; Editions G.-P. Maisonneuve & Larose; Agence de Cooperation Culturelle et Technique, 1985. 526p. Techniques Agricoles et Productions Tropicales, Serie Elevage no. 34, 1)	First
	Paling, R. W. A Contribution to the Understanding of the Epidemiology and Control of Livestock Diseases in Africa. Utrecht, Netherlands; Rijksuniversiteitsbibliotheek, 1990. 223p.	Third

Developed countries ranking		Third World ranking
	Palmer, Dan F., et al. Serodiagnosis of Mycotic Diseases. Springfield, Ill.; C. C. Thomas, 1977. 191p.	Third
	Pandey, R., ed. Biotechnology and Comparative Medicine. Basel and New York; Karger, 1987. 266p. (Progress in Veterinary Microbiology and Immunology no. 3)	Second
Second	Pandey, R., ed. Infection and Immunity in Farm Animals. Basel and New York; Karger, 1985. (Progress in Veterinary Microbiology and Immunology no. 1)	Second
Third	Parker, Ronald B. The Sheep Book: A Handbook for the Modern Shepherd. New York; Scribner, 1983. 344p.	Third
Second	Parker, W. H. Health and Disease in Farm Animals: An Introduction to Farm Animal Medicine. 3d ed. Oxford and New York; Pergamon Press, 1980. 307p. (Available in Spanish as Manejo de los Animales: Salud y Enfermedad. 2d ed. Barcelona; Aedos, 1978.)	Second
Third	Parks, John R. A Theory of Feeding and Growth of Animals. Berlin and New York; Springer-Verlag, 1982. 322p.	
Second	Parry, H. B., and D. R. Oppenheimer. Scrapie Disease in Sheep: Historical, Clinical, Epidemiological, Pathological, and Practical Aspects of the Natural Disease. London and New York; Academic Press, 1983. 192p.	Third
	Pasquini, Chris J. Atlas of Bovine Anatomy. Eureka, Calif.; Sudz, 1982. 335p.	Third
	Passmore, R. Handbook on Human Nutritional Requirements. Geneva; World Health Organization, 1974. 66p. (Also issued by Food and Agriculture Organization, 1974.)	Third
Third	Patrick, Homer, and Philip J. Schaible. Poultry, Feeds and Nutrition. 2d ed. Westport, Conn.; Avi Pub. Co., 1980. 668p. (1st ed., by Schaible, 1970.)	
First	Paul, William E., ed. Fundamental Immunology. 2d ed. New York; Raven Press, 1989. 1123p. (1st ed., 1984. 809p.)	Second
	Pavaux, Claude. A Color Atlas of Bovine Visceral Anatomy. Translation of Atlas en Couleurs d'Anatomie des Bovins, Splanchnologie. London; Wolfe Medical Publications, 1983. 167p.	Third
Second	Payne, Jack M. Metabolic and Nutritional Diseases of Cattle. Oxford; Blackwell Scientific, 1989. 176p.	Second
Third	Payne, Jack M. Metabolic Diseases in Farm Animals. London; W. Heinemann Medical Books, 1977. 206p. (Available in Spanish as Enfermedades Metabolicas, Animales Zootecnicos. Zaragoza; Acribia, 1981.)	Second
Third	Payne, Jack M., and S. Payne. The Metabolic Profile Test. Oxford and New York; Oxford University Press, 1987. 179p.	Second
Third	Payne, W. J. A. Cattle Production in the Tropics. London; Longman, 1970. 2 vols.	First
Second	Payne, W. J. A. An Introduction to Animal Husbandry in the	First

Developed countries ranking		Third World ranking
	Tropics. 4th ed. Harlow, U.K.; Longman; New York; Wiley, 881p. (1st–3d eds. by Grahame Williamson and W. Payne. 1st ed., 1959.)	
Third	Pearson, Albert M., and T. R. Dutson, eds. Edible Meat By-Products. London and New York; Elsevier Applied Science, 1988. 439p. (Advances in Meat Research no. 5)	Third
Third	Pearson, Albert M., and T. R. Dutson, eds. Electrical Stimulation. Westport, Conn; Avi Pub. Co., 1985. 327p. (Advances in Meat Research no. 1)	
Second	Pearson, Albert M., and F. W. Tauber. Processed Meats. 2d ed. Westport, Conn.; Avi Pub. Co., 1984. 427p. (Revision of Processed Meats, by W. E. Kramlich, A. M. Pearson, F. W. Tauber, 1973.)	
	Pearson, Mark L., and Henry F. Epstein, eds. Muscle Development—Molecular and Cellular Control. Cold Spring Harbor, N.Y.; Cold Spring Harbor Laboratory, 1982. 581p.	Third
Second	Peel, L., and D. E. Tribe. Domestication, Conservation, and Use of Animal Resources. Amsterdam and New York; Elsevier; Distributors for the U.S. and Canada, Elsevier Science Pub. Co., 1983. 357p. (World Animal Science. A. Basic Information no. 1)	Second
	Penning De Vries, F. W. T., and M. A. Djiteye, eds. La Productivite des Paturages Saheliens: Une Etude des Sols, des Vegetations et de l'Exploitation de Cette Ressource Naturelle. Wageningen; Centre for Agricultural Publishing and Documentation, 1982. 525p.	Third
Third	Perry, Tilden W. Animal Life-Cycle Feeding and Nutrition. Orlando, Fla.; Academic Press, 1984. 319p.	Third
Second	Perry, Tilden W. Beef Cattle Feeding and Nutrition. New York; Academic Press, 1980. 383p.	
	Perspectives in World Agriculture. Farnham Royal, U.K.; Commonwealth Agriculutral Bureaux, 1980. 532p.	Third
First	Phillipson, A. T., et al., eds. Physiology of Digestion and Metabolism in the Ruminant; Proceedings of the Third International Symposium, Cambridge, England, 1969. Newcastle upon Tyne; Oriel, 1970. 636p.	Second
	Phillipson, A. T., Leslie W. Hall, and W. R. Pritchard. Scientific Foundations of Veterinary Medicine. London; William Heinemann Medical Books, 1980. 438p.	Second
	Phillis, J. W., and Norman F. Clinch. Veterinary Physiology. Philadelphia; Saunders, 1976. 882p.	Third
	Pigden, W. J., C. C. Balch, and Michael Graham. Standardization of Analytical Methodology for Feeds: Proceedings of a Workshop, Ottawa, Canada, March 1979. Ottawa; International Development Research Centre, 1980. 128p.	Second
	Pillay, T. V. R., and William A. Dill, eds. Advances in Aqua-	Third

Developed countries ranking		Third World ranking
	culture: Papers Presented at FAO Technical Conference on Aquaculture, Kyoto, May–June 1976. Farnham, U.K.; Fishing News Books, 1979. 653p. (Published by arrangement with the Food and Agriculture Organization.)	
Third	Pimentel, David, and Marcia Pimentel. Food, Energy, and Society. New York; Wiley; London; E. Arnold, 1979. 165p.	
Second	Pirchner, Franz. Population Genetics in Animal Breeding = Populationsgenetik in der Tierzucht. 2d ed. New York; Plenum Press, 1983. 414p. (Translated from German with the assistance of D. L. Frape. 1st ed., San Francisco; W. H. Freeman, 1969. 274p.)	
Third	Politiek, R. D., and J. J. Bakker. Livestock Production in Europe: Perspectives and Prospects. Amsterdam and New York; Elsevier Scientific Pub. Co., 1982. 335p. (Reprinted from Livestock Production Science, vol. 9, nos. 1, 2.)	Third
Second	Pond, Wilson G., et al., eds. Conference on Animal Agriculture, Boyne Mountain, Mich., 1980. Animal Agriculture; Research to Meet Human Needs in the 21st Century. Sponsored by the American Association for the Advancement of Science, and others. Boulder, Colo.; Westview Press, 1980. 355p.	Second
First	Pond, Wilson G., and Katherine A. Houpt. The Biology of the Pig. Ithaca, N.Y.; Comstock Pub. Associates, 1978. 371p. (Available in Spanish as Biologia del Cerdo. Zaragoza; Acribia, 1981.)	First
First	Pond, Wilson G., and J. H. Maner. Swine Production and Nutrition. Westport, Conn.; Avi Pub. Co., 1984. 731p.	First
Second	Pond, Wilson G., and J. H. Maner. Swine Production in Temperate and Tropical Environments. San Francisco; W. H. Freeman and Co., 1974. (Available in Spanish as Produccion de Cerdos en Climas Templados y Tropicales. Zaragoza; Acribia, 1976.)	First
Third	Ponting, Kenneth G. Sheep of the World. Poole, England; Blandford Press, 1980. 155p.	Third
	Popesko, Peter. Atlas of Topographical Anatomy of the Domestic Animals. Translation of Atlas Topografickej Anatomie Hospodarskych. 2d ed. Philadelphia; Saunders, 1977. 3 vols. (1st ed., English, 1971.) (Available in Spanish as Atlas de Anatomia Topografica de los Animales Domesticos. Barcelona; Salvat.)	Third
	Poppensiek, George C. Foreign Animal Diseases, VM 518. New ed. rev. and edited by Paul G. Rudenberg. Ithaca, N.Y.; Cornell University, 1985. 324p.	Third
Second	Pork Industry Handbook. West Lafayette, Ind.; Cooperative Extension Service, Purdue University, 1980+. 1 vol. (Select parts available on microcomputer disk.)	

Developed countries ranking		Third World ranking
Third	Porter, Arthur R., C. F. Foreman, and John A. Sims. Dairy Cattle in American Agriculture. Ames; Iowa State University Press, 1965. 328p.	
Third	Porter, Ruth, and Julie Whelan, eds. Symposium on Biology of Vitamin E, CIBA Foundation, London, March 1983. London; Pitman, 1983. 260p. (CIBA Foundation Symposium no. 101)	Third
Third	Portsmouth, John I. Commercial Rabbit-Keeping. 3d ed. Nimrod, 1987. 142p. (1st ed. as Commercial Rabbit Meat Production. London; Iliffe, 1962. 153p.) (Available in Spanish as Produccion Comercial de Conejos para Carne. Zaragoza; Acribia, 1975.)	
	Poultry Science Symposium, 9th, 1973, Harper Adams Agricultural College. Energy Requirements of Poultry; Proceedings. . . . Edinburgh; British Poultry Science Ltd., 1974. 199p.	Third
Third	Poultry Science Symposium, 14th, 1978, Edinburgh. Food Intake Regulation in Poultry; Proceedings . . . edited by K. N. Boorman and B. M. Freeman. Edinburgh; British Poultry Science, 1979. 469p.	
Second	Poultry Science Symposium, 17th, 1982, Edinburgh. Reproductive Biology of Poultry; Proceedings . . . Organized by the joint Standing Committee of British Poultry Science Ltd., and World's Poultry Science Association (United Kindgom) Ltd.; edited by F. J. Cunningham, P. E. Lake and D. Hewitt. Edinburgh; British Poultry Science Ltd.; Harlow, Essex, 1984. 225p.	Second
Third	Poultry Science Symposium, 18th, 1983, Edinburgh. Poultry Genetics and Breeding; Proceedings . . . Harlow, Essex, U.K.; British Poultry Science, 1985. 178p. (Poultry Science Symposium no. 18)	Third
	Poultry Science Symposium, 20th, 1985, Harper Adams Agricultural College. Egg Quality—Current Problems and Recent Advances by R. G. Wells and C. G. Belyavin. London and Boston; Butterworths, 1987. 302p. (Poultry Science Symposium no. 20)	Third
Third	Prasad, Ananda S., ed. Clinical, Biochemical, and Nutritional Aspects of Trace Elements. New York; A. R. Liss, 1982. 577p. (Current Topics in Nutrition and Disease no. 6)	Third
	Pratt, D. J., and M. D. Gwynne. Rangeland Management and Ecology in East Africa. London; Hodder and Stoughton, 1977. 310p.	Second
Second	Pratt, William B. Chemotherapy of Infection. New York; Oxford University Press, 1977. 462p. (Revision of Fundamentals of Chemotherapy, Oxford University Press, N.Y., 1973.) (Available in Spanish as Quimioterapia de la Infeccion. Mexico; Addison, 1981.)	Third

Developed countries ranking		Third World ranking
	Preston, T. R., and R. A. Leng. Matching Ruminant Production Systems with Available Resources in the Tropics and Sub-Tropics. Armidale, N.S.W., Australia; Penambul Books, 1987. 245p.	Second
First	Preston, T. R., and Malcolm B. Willis. Intensive Beef Production. 2d ed. Oxford and New York; Pergamon Press, 1974. 566p. (1st ed., 1970. 544p.) (Available in Spanish as Produccion Intensiva de Carne. Mexico; Diana, 1975.)	First
	Preston, T. R., et al., eds. Better Utilization of Crop Residues and By-Products in Animal Feeding; Research Guidelines; Proceedings of the FAO/ILCA Expert Consultation, Addis Ababa, March 1984. Rome; Food and Agriculture Organization, 1985. 1 vol. (FAO Animal Production and Health Paper no. 50)	Second
Second	Price, James F., and Bernard S. Schweigert, eds. The Science of Meat and Meat Products. 3d ed. Westport, Conn.; Food & Nutrition Press, 1987. 639p. (Previous eds. issued by the American Meat Institute Foundation, 1st, 1962.)	
Third	Price, Kent S., et al., eds. Proceedings of the First International Conference on Aquaculture Nutrition, October 1975, Lewes/Rehoboth, Delaware; Sponsored by the Delaware Sea Grant College Program in Cooperation with the U.S./Japan Aquaculture Panel. . . . Newark; College of Marine Studies, University of Delaware, 1976. 323p.	
	Pullin, Roger S. V., and Ziad H. Shehadeh, eds. Integrated Agriculture-Aquaculture Farming Systems; Proceedings of the ICLARM-SEARCalif. Conference on Integrated Agriculture-Aquaculture Farming Systems, Manila, August 1979. Metro Manila; International Center for Living Aquatic Resources Management; and Los Banos, Laguna, Philippines; Southeast Asian Regional Center for Graduate Study and Research in Agriculture, 1980.	Third
Third	Puls, Robert. Mineral Levels in Animal Health: Diagnostic Data. Clearboork, B.C., Canada; Sherpa International, 1988. 240p.	Third
	Purchase, I. F. H., ed. Mycotoxins. Amsterdam and New York; Elsevier Scientific Pub. Co., 1974. 443p.	Third
Third	Putnam, Frank W., ed. The Plasma Proteins: Structure, Function, and Genetic Control. 2d ed. New York; Academic Press, 1975. 5 vols. (1st ed., 1960. 2 vols.)	
	Putt, S. N. H., et al. Veterinary Epidemiology and Economics in Africa: A Manual for Use in the Design and Appraisal of Livestock Health Policy. Reading, U.K. and Addis Ababa, Ethiopia; Veterinary Epidemiology and Economics Research Unit, Dept. of Agriculture, University of Reading and International Livestock Centre for Africa, 1987. 130p. (ILCA Manual no. 3) (Available in French.)	Second

Developed countries ranking		Third World ranking
	Q	
Second	Qureshi, A. W., and H. A. Fitzhugh. Small Ruminants in the Near East; Expert Consultation on Small Ruminant Research and Development in the Near East. Rome; Food and Agriculture Organization, 1987–1989. 3 vols. (FAO Animal Production and Health Paper no. 54, 55, 74)	Second
	R	
First	Radostits, Otto M., and D. C. Blood. Herd Health: A Textbook of Health and Production Management of Agricultural Animals. Philadelphia; Saunders, 1985. 456p.	
First	Randall, C. J. Color Atlas of Diseases of the Domestic Fowl & Turkey. Ames, Iowa; Iowa State University Press, 1985. 116p.	Second
Second	Ranjhan, S. K. Animal Nutrition in Tropics. 2d ed. New Delhi; Vikas; New York; Advent Books, 1981. 446p.	Second
	Rathore, G. S. Camels and Their Management. New Delhi; Indian Council of Agricultural Research, 1986. 228p.	Third
Second	Read, Clark P. Animal Parasitism. Englewood Cliffs, N.J.; Prentice-Hall, 1972. 182p. (Available in Spanish as Parasitismo Animal. Mexico; CECSA, 1981.)	Third
Third	Rebell, Gerbert, and David Taplin. Dermatophytes: Their Recognition and Identification. Rev. ed. Coral Gables, Fla.; University of Miami Press, 1974. 124p. (1st ed., 1964, Miami, Fla.; Dermatology Foundation of Miami. 58p.)	Third
Second	Rechcigl, Miloslav, ed. Carbohydrates, Lipids, and Accessory Growth Factors. Basel and New York; S. Karger, 1976. 223p. (Comparative Animal Nutrition no. 1)	Third
Second	Rechcigl, Miloslav, ed. Effect of Nutrient Deficiencies in Animals. Cleveland; CRC Press, 1978. 548p.	Second
Third	Rechcigl, Miloslav, ed. Effect of Nutrient Excesses and Toxicities in Animals and Man. Cleveland; CRC Press, 1978. 518p.	Third
Third	Rechcigl, Miloslav, ed. Nitrogen, Electrolytes, Water and Energy Metabolism. Basel and New York; Karger, 1979. 260p. (Comparative Animal Nutrition no. 3)	Second
Third	Rechcigl, Miloslav, ed. Nutritional Requirements. Cleveland; CRC Press, 1977+. Vol.1, Comparative and Qualitative Requirements. (CRC Handbook Series in Nutrition and Food, Section D)	Third
Third	Rechcigl, Miloslav, ed. Physiology of Growth and Nutrition. Basel and New York; Karger, 1981. 341p. (Comparative Animal Nutrition no. 4)	Second
Second	Reece, William O. Physiology of Domestic Animals. Philadelphia and London; Lea & Febiger, 1990. 370p.	Second
Third	Reed, Jess D., Brian S. Capper, and Paul J. H. Neate, eds. Plant Breeding and the Nutritive Value of Crop Residues: Pro-	First

Developed countries ranking		Third World ranking
	nosis of Mycotoxicoses of Importance in the United States and Japan, sponsored by U.S.-Japan Cooperative Program on Development and Utilization of Natural Resources, Joint Panel on Toxic Microorganisms, and the National Animal Disease Center, USDA, ARS, Ames, Iowa, October 1984. Dordrecht; Boston and Hingham, Mass.; M. Nijhoff, 1986. 411p. (Current Topics in Veterinary Medicine and Animal Science no. 33)	
	Rico, Andre G., ed. Drug Residues in Animals. Orlando, Fla.; Academic Press, 1986. 233p.	Third
Second	Riemann, Hans, and M. J. Burridge, eds. Impact of Diseases on Livestock Production in the Tropics; International Conference . . . Kissimmee, Florida, May 1983. Amsterdam and New York; Elsevier, 1984. 632p. (Reprinted from Preventive Veterinary Medicine, vol. 2, nos. 1–4.)	Second
First	Riis, P. M. Dynamic Biochemistry of Animal Production. Amsterdam and New York; Elsevier, 1983. 501p.	Second
Second	Ristic, Miodrag. Babesiosis of Domestic Animals and Man. Boca Raton, Fla.; CRC Press, 1988. 255p.	Second
Second	Ristic, Miodrag, and Ian McIntyre. Diseases of Cattle in the Tropics: Economic and Zoonotic Relevance. The Hague; Boston and Hingham, Mass.; M. Nijhoff Publishers, 1981. 662p.	Second
Second	Robards, G. E., and R. G. Packham, eds. Feed Information and Animal Production; Proceeding of the 2d Symposium on the International Network of Feed Information Centres. Farnham Royal, U.K.; Blacktown, N.S.W., Australia; Commonwealth Agricultural Bureaux and INFIC, 1983. 516p.	Second
	Roberts, Ronald J. Fish Pathology. 2d ed. London and Philadelphia; Bailliere Tindall, 1989. 467p. (1st ed., 1978.) (Available in Spanish as Patologia de los Peces. Madrid; Mundi-Prensa, 1981.)	Second
Third	Roberts, Ronald J. Microbial Diseases of Fish; Based on Symposium of the Pathogenicity Group of the S. G. M., Edinburgh, Sept. 1981. London and New York; Published for the Society for General Microbiology by Academic Press, 1982. 305p.	Second
Second	Roberts, Stephen J., Donald H. Lein, Robert H. Foote, and Maarten Drost. Veterinary Obstetrics and Genital Diseases (Theriogenology). 3d ed. Woodstock and North Pomfret, Vt.; The author, 1986. 981p. (Available in Spanish as Ostetricia Veterinaria y Patologia de la Reproduccion (Teriogenologia). Buenos Aires; Hemisferio Sur, 1979.)	First
Second	Robertson, Alan, ed. Selection Experiments in Laboratory and Domestic Animals; Proceedings of a Symposium, Harrogate, July 1979. Farnham Royal and Slough, U.K.; Commonwealth Agricultural Bureaux, 1980. 245p.	
	Robinson, N. E., ed. Current Therapy in Equine Medicine 2. Philadelphia; Saunders, 1987. 761p. (1st ed., 1983.)	Second

Developed countries ranking		Third World ranking
Third	Robinson, T. J., ed. The Control of the Ovarian Cycle in the Sheep. Sydney; Sydney University Press, 1967. 258p. ceedings of a Workshop, ILCA, Addis Ababa, Ethiopia, December 1987. Addis Ababa; International Livestock Centre for Africa, 1988. 334p.	Third
Third	Reid, H. W. The Management and Health of Farmed Deer: A Seminar in the CEC Programme of Coordination of Research in Animal Husbandry, Edinburgh, December 1987. Dordrecht; Boston and Norwell, Mass.; Kluwer Academic Publishers for the Commission of the European Communities, 1988. 206p.	
	Reutlinger, Shlomo, and Marcelo Selowsky. Malnutrition and Poverty: Magnitude and Policy Options. Baltimore; Published for the World Bank by Johns Hopkins University Press, 1976. 82p.	Third
Third	Rhodes, Douglas N., ed. Meat Production from Entire Male Animals; Proceedings of a Symposium, Meat Research Institute, April 1969. London; Churchill, 1969. 332p.	Third
Second	Richard, J. L., and J. R. Thurston, eds. Diagnosis of Mycotoxicoses: A Publication Based on the Symposium on the Diag-	Second
	Robinson, Wayne F., and Clive R. R. Huxtable. Clinicopathologic Principles for Veterinary Medicine. Cambridge and New York; Cambridge University Press, 1988. 440p.	Third
Second	Roche, J. F., and D. O'Callaghan, eds. Follicular Growth and Ovulation Rate in Farm Animals: A Seminar in the CEC Programme of Coordination of Research in Animal Husbandry, Dublin, October 1985. Dordrecht and Boston; M. Nijhoff, 1987. 265p.	
Third	Roche, J. F., and D. O'Callaghan, eds. Manipulation of Growth in Farm Animals: A Seminar in the CEC Programme of Coordination of Research on Beef Production, Brussels, December 1982. Boston and Hingham, Mass.; M. Nijhoff for the Commission of the European Communities, 1984. 306p.	
	Roitt, Ivan M., Jonathan Brostoff, and David K. Male. Immunology. London, New York and St. Louis, Mo.; Gower Medical Pub. and C. V. Mosby, 1985. 320p.	Third
Third	Rollinson, D., and R. M. Anderson, eds. Ecology and Genetics of Host-Parasite Interactions: Papers Presented at an International Symposium Organized by the Linnean Society of London and the British Society for Parasitology, Keele University, July 1984. London and Orlando, Fla.; Academic Press, 1985. 266p. (Published for the Linnean Society of London.)	Second
Third	Romanoff, Alexis L. The Avian Embryo; Structural and Functional Development. New York; Macmillan, 1960. 1305p.	Third
	Romanoff, Alexis L. Biochemistry of the Avian Embryo; A Quantitative Analysis of Prenatal Development. New York; Interscience Publishers, 1967. 398p.	Third

Developed countries ranking		Third World ranking
Second	Romanoff, Alexis L., and Anastasia J. Romanoff. The Avian Egg. New York; J. Wiley, 1949. 918p.	Third
Second	Romans, John R., and P. Thomas Ziegler. The Meat We Eat. 12th ed. Danville, Ill.; Interstate Printers & Publishers, 1985. (1st–9th eds., by P. T. Ziegler.)	
Second	Rook, J. A. F., and P. C. Thomas. Nutritional Physiology of Farm Animals. London and New York; Longman, 1983. 704p.	Second
First	Rosenberger, Gustav, and Gerrit Dirksen. Clinical Examination of Cattle. Translation of the 2d ed. of Die klinische Untersuchung des Rindes, 1977. Berlin; Parey, 1979. 453p. (Available in Spanish as Exploracion Clinica de los Bovinos. Buenos Aires; Hemisferio Sur, 1981.)	
Third	Ross, C. V. Sheep Production and Management. Englewood Cliffs, N.J.; Prentice-Hall, 1989. 481p.	Third
	Rossdale, Peter D., and S. W. Ricketts. The Practice of Equine Stud Medicine. Philadelphia; Lea & Febiger, 1980. 564p. (1st ed., London; Bailliere Tindall, 1974. 421p.)	Second
Third	Rouse, John E. The Criollo: Spanish Cattle in the Americas. 1st ed. Norman; University of Oklahoma Press, 1977. 303p.	Third
Second	Rouse, John E. World Cattle. 1st ed. Norman; University of Oklahoma Press, 1970–1973. 3 vols.	Second
Second	Roy, J. H. B. The Calf. 5th ed. London and Boston; Butterworths, 1990. Vol. 1 has 258p. (3d ed., London; Iliffe Books, 1970. 2 vols.)	First
Third	Ruckebusch, Yves. Physiologie, Pharmacologie, Therapeutique Animales. Paris; Maloine, 1977. 424p.	Third
Third	Ruckebusch, Yves, Louis-Philippe Phaneuf, and Robert Dunlop. Physiology of Small and Large Animals. Philadelphia; B. C. Decker, 1991. 672p.	Third
Third	Ruckebusch, Yves, Pierre-Louis Toutain, and Gary D. Koritz. Veterinary Pharmacology and Toxicology: Proceedings . . . European Association for Veterinary Pharmacology and Toxicology Congress, 2d, 1982, Toulouse. Westport, Conn.; Avi Pub. Co., 1983. 838p.	Third
Second	Ruitenberg, E. J., and P. W. J. Peters. Laboratory Animals: Laboratory Animal Models for Domestic Animal Production. Amsterdam and New York; Elsevier, 1986. 350p.	Third
Third	Russell, K., and S. Slater. The Principles of Dairy Farming. 10th ed. Ipswich, UK; Farming Press, 1985. 316p. (3d ed., 1962, Ipswich; Dairy Farmer.) (Available in Spanish as Principios de Produccion Lechera. 9th ed. trans. by Ingrid Adam. Buenos Aires; Ateneo, 1986.)	
	Ruthenberg, Hans, and J. D. MacArthur. Farming Systems in the Tropics. 3d ed. Oxford and New York; Clarendon Press & Oxford University Press, 1980. 424p. (1st ed., 1971. 313p.)	First

<table>
<tr><td>Developed
countries
ranking</td><td></td><td>Third
World
ranking</td></tr>
<tr><td>Third</td><td>Ryder, Michael L., and Stuart K. Stephenson. Wool Growth. London and New York; Academic Press, 1968. 805p.</td><td></td></tr>
<tr><td colspan="3" align="center">S</td></tr>
<tr><td></td><td>SABRAO Workshop on Animal Genetic Resources in Asia and Oceania, 1979, University of Tsukuba. Animal Genetic Resources in Asia and Oceania; Proceedings . . . Tsukuba, Japan; Tropical Agriculture Research Center, Ministry of Agriculture, Forestry and Fisheries, 1980. 555p. (Nekken Shiryo no. 47)</td><td>Third</td></tr>
<tr><td></td><td>Sack, W. O. Pig Anatomy and Atlas. Ithaca, N.Y.; Veterinary Textbooks, 1982. 192p. (Also issued as Essentials of Pig Anatomy.)</td><td>Third</td></tr>
<tr><td>Third</td><td>Sadleir, R. M. F. S. The Ecology of Reproduction in Wild and Domestic Mammals. London; Methuen, 1969. 321p.</td><td></td></tr>
<tr><td>Third</td><td>Sainsbury, David. Animal Health: Health, Disease and Welfare of Farm Livestock. London and New York; Granada, 1983. 232p.</td><td>Second</td></tr>
<tr><td>Third</td><td>Sainsbury, David. Farm Animal Welfare: Cattle, Pigs and Poultry. London; Collins, 1986. 175p.</td><td></td></tr>
<tr><td>Third</td><td>Sainsbury, David. Poultry Health and Management. 2d ed. London and New York; Granada, 1984. 186p. (1st ed., 1980. 168p.) (Available in Spanish as Aves: Sanidad y Manejo . . . trans. by Francisco L. Crespo. Zaragoza; Acribia, 1987.)</td><td></td></tr>
<tr><td>Third</td><td>Sainsbury, David, and Peter Sainsbury. Livestock Health and Housing. 3d ed. London; Bailliere Tindall, 1988. 319p. (Earlier ed., 1967 as Animal Health and Housing.) (Available in Spanish as Sanidad y Alojamiento Para Animales. Mexico; CECSA, 1971.)</td><td>First</td></tr>
<tr><td></td><td>Saliki, J. T., E. Thiry, and P. P. Pastoret. La Peste Porcine Africaine. Maison-Alfort, France; Institut d'Elvage et de Medecine Veterinaire des Pays Tropicaux, 1985. (Etudes et Syntheses de l'I.E.M.V.T. no. 11)</td><td>Third</td></tr>
<tr><td>First</td><td>Salisbury, Glenn W., N. L. VanDemark, and J. R. Lodge. Physiology of Reproduction and Artificial Insemination of Cattle. 2d ed. San Francisco; W. H. Freeman, 1978. 798p. (1st ed., 1961. 639p.) (Available in Spanish as Fisiologia de la Reproduccion, Inseminacion Artificial de los Bovinos. Zaragoza; Acribia, 1964.)</td><td>First</td></tr>
<tr><td>Third</td><td>Sambrus, Hans H., ed. Nutztierethologie: Das Verhalten Landwirtschaftlicher Nutztiere: Eine Angewandte Verhaltenskunde fur die Praxis (Ethology of Animals of Economic Importance: Behavior of Farm Animals and Practical Applications of Ethology). Berlin; Paul Parey, 1978. 315p. (In German.)</td><td></td></tr>
<tr><td>Second</td><td>Sanchez, Pedro A., and Luis E. Tergas, eds. Pasture Production</td><td>Second</td></tr>
</table>

Developed countries ranking		Third World ranking
	in Acid Soils of the Tropics: Proceedings of a Seminar, CIAT, Cali, Colombia, April 1978. Cali, Colombia; Centro Internacional de Agricultura Tropical, 1979. 488p. (Available in Spanish.)	
Third	Sandford, J. C. The Domestic Rabbit. 4th ed. London and Dobbs Ferry, N.Y.; Collins, 1986. 272p. (3d ed., New York; Wiley, 1979. 258p.)	Second
	Sandford, Stephen. Management of Pastoral Development in the Third World. Chichester, West Sussex, U.K. and New York; J. Wiley, 1983. 316p. (In association with the Overseas Development Institute, London.)	Second
Second	Sands, Michael W., and Robert E. McDowell. A World Bibliography on Goats. Ithaca, N.Y.; Cornell University, 1979. 112p. (Cornell International Agriculture Mimeograph no. 70)	Second
Third	Sansoucy, Rene, G. Aarts, and T. R. Preston, eds. Sugarcane as Feed: La Cana de Azucar Como Pienso: Proceedings of an FAO Expert Consultation, Santo Domingo, Dominican Republic from July 1986. Rome; Food and Agriculture Organization, 1988. 319p. (FAO Animal Production and Health Paper no. 72)	First
Second	Sansoucy, Rene, T. R. Preston, and R. A. Leng, eds. Proceedings of the FAO Expert Consultation on the Substitution of Imported Concentrate Feeds in Animal Production Systems in Developing Countries: Held in the FAO Regional Office for Asia and the Pacific, Bangkok, September 1985. Rome; Food and Agriculture Organization, 1987. 242p. (FAO Animal Production and Health Paper no. 63)	Second
Third	Sasimowski, Ewald. Animal Breeding and Production: An Outline . . . trans. from Polish by Magdalena Bibrich. Amsterdam and New York; Elsevier, 1987. 782p. (Translation of Zarys Szczegoowej Hodowli Zwierzat.)	Third
Third	Say, Ralph, translator. Manual of Poultry Production in the Tropics. Wallingford, U.K.; Commonwealth Agriculture Bureaux, 1987. 119p. (Translation of Manuel d'Aviculture en Zone Tropicale, 1983.)	Second
	Scanlan, Charles M. Introduction to Veterinary Bacteriology. 1st ed. Ames; Iowa State University Press, 1988. 457p.	Second
Second	Scaramuzzi, R. J., D. W. Lincoln, and Barbara J. Weir, eds. Reproductive Endocrinology of Domestic Ruminants; Proceedings of a Symposium, Leura, New South Wales, Australia, February 1980. Cambridge, U.K.; Journal of Reproduction & Fertility, 1981. 263p. (Journal of Reproduction and Fertility. Supplement, 1981.)	Third
Second	Schalm, Oscar W., E. J. Carroll, and Nemi C. Jain. Bovine Mastitis. Philadelphia; Lea & Febiger, 1971. 360p.	Third
Third	Scheele, C. W., and C. H. Veerkamp, eds. World Poultry Pro-	Third

<table>
<tr><td>Developed
countries
ranking</td><td></td><td>Third
World
ranking</td></tr>
</table>

Developed countries ranking		Third World ranking
	duction: Where and How? Proceedings of the Jubillee Symposium on the Occasion of the 60th Anniversary of the Spelderholt Institute for Poultry Research, Orpheus Theatre, Apeldoorn, May 1981. Beekbergen, Netherlands; Spelderholt Institute for Poultry Resarch, 1981. 119p.	
Third	Scheelje, Reinhard, Heinrich Niehaus, and Klaus Werner. Kaninchenmast. Zucht und Haltung der Fleischkaninchen. Stuttgart; Ulmer, 1967. 179p. (Available in Spanish as Conejos para Carne: Sistema de Produccion Intensiva. 2d ed. Zaragoza; Mundi-Prensa, 1976.)	
Third	Schiemann, R., et al. Energetische Futterbewertung und Energienormen; Dokumentation der Wissenschaftlichen Grundlagen eines neuen Energetischen Futterbewertungssystems. Berlin; Deutscher Landwirtschaftsverlag, 1971. 344p.	
Third	Schlesinger, Milton J., Michael Ashburner, and Alfred Tissieres, eds. Heat Shock, from Bacteria to Man; Papers presented at a Meeting, May 1982. Cold Spring Harbor, N.Y.; Cold Spring Harbor Laboratory, 1982. 440p.	
Second	Schmidt, G. H., and L. D. Van Vleck. Principles of Dairy Science. 2d ed. Englewood Cliffs, N.J.; Prentice-Hall, 1988. 466p. (1st ed., San Francisco; Freeman, 1974. 558p.) (Available in Spanish as Bases Cientificas de la Produccion Lechera. Zaragoza; Acribia, 1976.)	
Second	Schmidt, Gerald D. CRC Handbook of Tapeworm Identification. Boca Raton, Fla.; CRC Press, 1986. 675p.	Third
Second	Schmidt, P. J., and Neil T. Yeates. Beef Cattle Production. 2d ed. Sydney; Butterworths, 1985. 338p. (1st ed., Chatswood, Australia; 1974. 323p.)	Second
Second	Schmidt-Nielsen, Knut. Animal Physiology: Adaptation and Environment. 4th ed. Cambridge and New York; Cambridge University Press, 1990. 602p. (1st ed., Englewood Cliffs, N.J.; Prentice-Hall, 1960. 118p.) (Available in Spanish as Fisiologia Animal. Mexico; Uteha.)	First
Second	Schneider, Burch H., and William P. Flatt. The Evaluation of Feeds Through Digestibility Experiments. Athens; University of Georgia Press, 1975. 423p.	Third
	Schneider, Harold K. Livestock and Equality in East Africa: The Economic Basis for Social Structure. Bloomington; Indiana University Press, 1979. 291p.	Third
Second	Schneider, Jurgen, Kurt E. Lindner, and Arnulf Burckhardt. Animal Diseases in Tropical and Subtropical Regions: Fundamentals of Control . . . trans. by Herbert Liebscher. Leipzig; Edition Leipzig, 1972. 176p.	Third
First	Schnurrenberger, Paul R., Robert S. Sharman, and Gilbert H. Wise. Attacking Animal Diseases: Concepts and Strategies for	Second

174   Wallace C. Olsen

Developed countries ranking		Third World ranking
	Control and Eradication. 1st ed. Ames; Iowa State University Press, 1987. 200p.	
Third	Schorger, Arlie William. The Wild Turkey; Its History and Domestication. 1st ed. Norman; University of Oklahoma Press, 1966. 625p.	Third
	Schultz, Theodore W., ed. Distortions of Agricultural Incentives. Bloomington; Indiana University Press, 1978. 343p.	Third
First	Schurch, A., and C. Wenk, eds. Energy Metabolism of Farm Animals; Proceedings of the 5th Symposium, Vitznau, Switzerland, September 1970. Zurich; Juris Druck and Verlag, 1970. 259p. (European Association for Animal Production; EAAP Publication no. 13.)	
Third	Schwabe, Calvin W. Veterinary Medicine and Human Health. 3d ed. Baltimore; Williams & Wilkins, 1984. 680p. (2d ed., 1969. 713p.)	Third
First	Schwabe, Calvin W., Hans P. Riemann, and Charles E. Franti. Epidemiology in Veterinary Practice. Philadelphia; Lea & Febiger, 1977. 303p.	Third
	Scott, Danny W. Large Animal Dermatology. Philadelphia; W. B. Saunders, 1988. 487p.	Third
Second	Scott, G. R., W. P. Taylor, and P. B. Rossiter. Manual on the Diagnosis of Rinderpest. Rome; Food and Agriculture Organization, 1986. 187p. (FAO Animal Production and Health Series no. 23)	Third
Third	Scott, George, and Hudson A. Glimp. The Sheepman's Production Handbook. Revised. Denver; For Sheep Industry Development Program by Abegg Printing Co., 1982. 1 vol. (1st ed., 1970, Prepared in cooperation with American Sheep Producers Council et al.)	
Second	Scott, Milton L. Nutrition of Humans and Selected Animal Species. New York; Wiley, 1986. 537p.	First
First	Scott, Milton L., Malden C. Nesheim, and Robert J. Young. Nutrition of the Chicken. 3d ed. Ithaca, N.Y.; M. L. Scott, 1982. 562p. (2d ed., 1976. 555 p.)	First
Third	Searle, A. G. Comparative Genetics of Coat Colour in Mammals. London; Logos Press; New York; Academic Press, 1968. 308p.	Second
Second	Searle, S. R. Linear Models. New York; Wiley, 1971. 532p.	Second
Third	Seidel, George E., and R. Peter Elsden. Embryo Transfer in Dairy Cattle. Fort Atkinson, Wis.; Hoard's Dairyman, 1989. 101p.	Third
Second	Seiden, Rudolph. Livestock Health Encyclopedia; The Control of Diseases and Parasites in Cattle, Sheep and Goats, Swine, Horses and Mules. 2d ed. In association with W. James Gough.	

<table>
<tr><td>Developed
countries
ranking</td><td></td><td>Third
World
ranking</td></tr>
<tr><td></td><td>New York; Springer Pub. Co., 1961. 628p. (1st ed., 1951. 613p.)</td><td></td></tr>
<tr><td>Third</td><td>Sejrsen, K., M. Vestergaard, and Neimann-Sorensen, eds. Use of Somatotropin in Livestock Production; Seminar on Use of Somatotropin in Livestock Production, Brussels, Belgium, 1988. London and New York; Elsevier, 1989. 333p.</td><td>Third</td></tr>
<tr><td></td><td>Seminar on Potential to Increase Beef Production in Tropical America, 1974, Cali, Colombia. Proceedings . . . El Potencial para la Produccion de Ganado de Carne en America Tropical: Seminario. Cali; Centro Internacional de Agricultura Tropical, 1975. 307p. (Centro Internacional de Agricultura Tropical; CE no. 10)</td><td>Second</td></tr>
<tr><td>Third</td><td>Semple, Arthur T. Grassland Improvement. London; Leonard Hill, 1970. 400p. (Available in Spanish as Avanos en Pasturos Cultivados y Naturales, 1974.)</td><td></td></tr>
<tr><td>Second</td><td>Sen, K. C., S. N. Ray, and S. K. Rahjahn. Nutritive Values of Indian Cattle Feeds and the Feeding of Animals. 6th ed. New Delhi; Indian Council of Agricultural Research, 1978. 92p. (1st ed., 1938.)</td><td>Second</td></tr>
<tr><td></td><td>Serres, H. Manual of Pig Production in the Tropics . . . trans. by Julian Wiseman. Wallingford, U.K.; CAB International, 1992. 300p.</td><td>Third</td></tr>
<tr><td></td><td>Setchell, Brian P. The Mammalian Testis. Ithaca, N.Y.; Cornell University Press, 1978. 450p.</td><td>Third</td></tr>
<tr><td></td><td>Shaner, W. W., P. F. Philipp, and W. R. Schmehl. Farming Systems Research and Development: Guidelines for Developing Countries. Boulder, Colo.; Westview Press, 1982. 414p.</td><td>Second</td></tr>
<tr><td></td><td>Sharp, J. M., and R. Hoff-Jorgensen, eds. Slow Viruses in Sheep, Goats and Cattle: In Particular Maedi Visna, Jaagsiekte, and in Caprines, Arthritis, Encephalitis and Pneumonitis; Proceedings of Two Workshops, Reykjavik, July 1982, Edinburgh, Sept. 1983. Luxembourg; Commission of the European Communities, 1985. 361p.</td><td>Third</td></tr>
<tr><td>Second</td><td>Shaw, A. M., and C. H. Hoste. Trypanotolerant Cattle and Livestock Development in West and Central Africa. Rome; Food and Agriculture Organization, 1987. 2 vols. (FAO Animal Production and Health Paper no. 67) (1st ed., 1980. 2 vols. FAO Animal Production and Health Paper no. 20/1–20/2.)</td><td>First</td></tr>
<tr><td>Third</td><td>Shaw, James H. Introduction to Wildlife Management. New York; McGraw-Hill, 1985. 316p.</td><td>Second</td></tr>
<tr><td>Third</td><td>Shaw, N. H., and W. W. Bryan, eds. Tropical Pasture Research; Principles and Methods. Farnham Royal, U.K.; Commonwealth Agricultural Bureaux, 1976. 454p. (Commonwealth Bureau of Pastures and Field Crops Bulletin no. 51)</td><td>First</td></tr>
</table>

<table>
<tr><td>Developed
countries
ranking</td><td></td><td>Third
World
ranking</td></tr>
<tr><td></td><td>Shepherd, C. Jonathan, and Niall R. Bromage. Intensive Fish Farming. Oxford; Blackwell Scentific Publishers, 1988. 404p.</td><td>Third</td></tr>
<tr><td>First</td><td>Shirley, Ray L. Nitrogen and Energy Nutrition of Ruminants. Orlando, Fla.; Academic Press, 1986. 358p.</td><td>Second</td></tr>
<tr><td>Third</td><td>Signoret, J. P. Welfare and Husbandry of Calves: Seminar in the CEC Programme of Coordination of Research on Animal Welfare, Brussels, July 1981. The Hague; Boston and Hingham, Mass.; M. Nijhoff for the Commission of the European Communities, 1982. 248p.</td><td>Third</td></tr>
<tr><td>Third</td><td>Silhavy, Thomas J., Michael L. Berman, and Lynn W. Enquist. Experiments with Gene Fusions. Cold Spring Harbor, N.Y.; Cold Spring Harbor Laboratory, 1984. 303p.</td><td></td></tr>
<tr><td></td><td>Simpson, James R. The Economics of Livestock Systems in Developing Countries: Farm and Project Level Analysis. Boulder, Colo.; Westview Press, 1988. 297p.</td><td>Third</td></tr>
<tr><td>Third</td><td>Simpson, James R., and Phylo Evangelou, eds. Livestock Development in Subsaharan Africa: Constraints, Prospects, Policy. Boulder, Colo.; Westview Press, 1984. 407p.</td><td>Third</td></tr>
<tr><td>Third</td><td>Simpson, James R., and Donald E. Farris. The World's Beef Business. 1st ed. Ames; Iowa State University Press, 1982. 334p.</td><td>Third</td></tr>
<tr><td>Second</td><td>Sindermann, Carl J., and Donald V. Lightner. Disease Diagnosis and Control in North American Marine Aquaculture. 2d ed., rev. Amsterdam and New York; Elsevier, 1988. 431p. (1st ed., 1977.)</td><td></td></tr>
<tr><td>Third</td><td>Singh, Harbans. Livestock and Poultry Production. New Delhi; Prentice-Hall of India, 1978. 550p.</td><td></td></tr>
<tr><td>Third</td><td>Singh, K. S., and B. Panda. Poultry Nutrition. New Delhi-Ludhiana; Kalyani Publishers, 1988. 322p.</td><td>Third</td></tr>
<tr><td></td><td>Sinn, R. Raising Goats for Milk and Meat. Little Rock, Ark.; Winrock International Institute, Heifer Project International, 1985. 110p.</td><td>Second</td></tr>
<tr><td>First</td><td>Sisson, Septimus. Sisson and Grossman's The Anatomy of the Domestic Animals. 5th ed. Philadelphia; Saunders, 1975. 2 vols. 2095p. (1st ed., 1911, as A Text-Book of Veterinary Anatomy. 826p.) (5th ed. available in Spanish as: Anatomia de los Animales Domisticos. Mexico City; Salvat, 1983.)</td><td>Third</td></tr>
<tr><td></td><td>Skerman, P. J., and F. Riveros. Tropical Grasses. Rome; Food and Agriculture Organization, 1990. 832p. (FAO Plant Production and Protection Series no. 23)</td><td>Third</td></tr>
<tr><td></td><td>Sloss, Margaret W., and Russell L. Kemp. Veterinary Clinical Parasitology. 5th ed. Ames; Iowa State University Press, 1978. 274p. (1st ed., 1948, by E. A. Benbrook and Sloss.)</td><td>Third</td></tr>
<tr><td>Third</td><td>Smidt, Diedrich. Indicators Relevant to Farm Animal Welfare:</td><td>Third</td></tr>
</table>

Developed countries ranking		Third World ranking
	A Seminar in the CEC Programme of Coordination of Research on Animal Welfare, Mariensee, November 1982. Boston and Hingham, Mass.; M. Nijhoff for the Commission of the European Communities, 1983. 251p.	
Second	Smith, A. J., ed. Beef Cattle Production in Developing Countries: Proceedings of the Conference, Edinburgh, September 1974. Edinburgh; University of Edinburgh, The Centre for Tropical Veterinary Medicine, 1976. 487p.	First
	Smith, A. J., and R. G. Gunn, eds. Intensive Animal Production in Developing Countries; Proceedings of a Symposium Organized by the British Society of Animal Production, Harrogate, Nov. 1979. London; Thames Ditton, 1980. 481p.	First
First	Smith, C., J. W. B. King, and J. C. McKay. Exploiting New Technologies in Animal Breeding: Genetic Developments: Proceedings of a Seminar in the CEC Animal Husbandry Research Programme, Edinburgh, June 1985. Oxford and New York; Published for the Commission of the European Communities by Oxford University Press, 1986. 202p.	Second
	Smith, E. Brian. Basic Chemical Thermodynamics. 4th ed. Oxford; Clarendon Press, 1990. 166p. (1st ed., by Jurg Waser. New York; W. A. Benjamin, 1966. 278p.)	Third
Second	Smith, John B., and Soesanto Mangkoewidjojo. The Care, Breeding and Management of Experimental Animals for Research in the Tropics. Canberra; International Development Program of Australian Universities and Colleges, 1987. 257p.	Second
First	Smith, Louis D. S., and Betsy L. Williams. The Pathogenic Anaerobic Bacteria. 3d ed. Springfield, Ill.; Thomas, 1984. 331p. (1st ed., 1968. 423p.)	Third
Third	Smith, O. B., and H. G. Bosman, eds. Goat Production in the Humid Tropics: Proceedings of the International Workshop on Goat Production in the Humid Tropics, University of Ife, Nigeria, July 1987. Wageningen; Centre for Agricultural Publishing and Documentation (PUDOC), 1988. 187p. (Summaries in English and French.)	Second
Third	Smith, Page, and Charles Daniel. The Chicken Book. San Francisco; North Point Press, 1982. 380p. (1st ed., Boston; Little, Brown, 1975. 384p.)	
	Smith, W. J., D. J. Taylor, and R. H. C. Penny. A Color Atlas of Diseases and Disorders of the Pig. London; Wolfe Medical Publications; Ames; Iowa University Press, 1990. 192p. (Earlier ed., by W. J. Smith and D. J. Taylor, London; Wolfe Medical, 1989. 200p.)	Third
Third	Snieszko, Stanislas F., and Herbert R. Axelrod. Diseases of Fishes. Neptune City, N.J.; T. F. H. Publications, 1970–1980. 6 vols.	Third

Developed countries ranking		Third World ranking
	Soltys, M. A. Introduction to Veterinary Microbiology. Serdang; Penerbit Universiti Pertanian Malaysia, 1979. 496p.	Third
Third	Somes, Ralph G., Jr. International Registry of Poultry Genetic Stocks. A Directory of Specialized Lines and Strains, Mutations, Breeds and Varieties of Chickens, Japanese Quail and Turkeys. Storrs; Storrs Agricultural Experiment Station, University of Connecticut, 1988. 98p. (Bulletin no. 476) (5th ed., 1984. 96p.)	
Third	Sorensen, Anton M. Animal Reproduction, Principles and Practices. New York; McGraw-Hill, 1979. 496p. (Available in Spanish as Reproduccion Animal . . . trans. by Ramon Elizondo Mata. Mexico; McGraw-Hill, 1982.)	
First	Soulsby, E. J. L. Helminths, Arthropods and Protozoa of Domesticated Animals. 7th ed. Philadelphia; Lea & Febiger, 1982. 809p. (1st ed. as Veterinary Helminthology and Entomology.)	Second
Second	Spallholz, Julian E., John L. Martin, and Howard E. Ganther, eds. Selenium in Biology and Medicine; Proceedings of the 2d International Symposium on Selenium in Biology and Medicine, Texas Tech University, Lubbock, 1980. Westport, Conn.; Avi Pub. Co., 1981. 573p.	Third
	Speedy, Andrew, and Rene Sansoucy, eds. Feeding Dairy Cows in the Tropics; Proceedings of the FAO Expert Consultation held in Bangkok . . . July 1989. Rome; Food and Agriculture Organization, 1991. 244p. (FAO Animal Production and Health Paper no. 86)	Third
	Speedy, Andrew. Sheep Production: Science into Practice. London; Longman, 1980. 195p.	Third
Second	Spedding, Colin R. W. The Biology of Agricultural Systems. London and New York; Academic Press, 1975. 261p.	Second
Second	Spedding, Colin R. W. Sheep Production and Grazing Management. 2d ed. London; Bailliere Tindall, 1970. 435p. (1st ed., Baltimore; Williams & Wilkins, 1965. 380p.) (Available in Spanish as Produccion Ovina. Leon; Academia, 1968.)	Second
	Sprague, Howard B. Combined Crop/Livestock Farming Systems for Developing Countries of the Tropics and Sub-Tropics. Washington, D.C.; Office of Agriculture, Bureau of Technical Assistance, Agency for International Development, 1976. 30p. (U.S. Agency for International Development, Office of Agriculture Technical Series Bulletin no. 19)	Second
Second	Squires, Victor. Livestock Management in the Arid Zone. Melbourne; Inkata Press, 1981. 271p.	Second
Second	Sreenan, J. M., and M. G. Diskin. Embryonic Mortality in Farm Animals: A Seminar in the EEC Programme of Coordination of Research on Livestock Productivity and Management.	Third

Developed countries ranking		Third World ranking
	Dordrecht; Boston and Hingham, Mass.; M. Nijhoff for the Commission of the European Communities, 1986. 280p.	
	Stableforth, Arthur W., and Ian A. Galloway, eds. Infectious Diseases of Animals: Diseases Due to Bacteria. London; Butterworth, 1959. 2 vols.	Third
Second	Stadelman, William J., and Owen J. Cotterill, eds. Egg Science and Technology. 3d ed. Westport, Conn.; Avi Pub. Co., 1986. 449p. (1st ed., 1973. 314p.)	Second
Third	Starkey, Paul, and Fadel Ndiame, eds. Animal Power in Farming Systems: Proceedings of the 2d West Africa Animal Traction Networkshop, Sept. 1986, Freetown, Sierra Leone. Braunschweig; Vieweg, 1988. 363p.	First
First	Steel, Robert G. D., and James H. Torrie. Principles and Procedures of Statistics: A Biometrical Approach. 2d ed. New York; McGraw-Hill, 1980. 633p. (1st ed., 1960.)	Third
Second	Steele, James H., ed. CRC Handbook Series in Zoonoses. West Palm Beach, Fla.; CRC Press, 1979. 1 vol.	
	Steiner, Charles V., and Richard B. Davis. Caged Bird Medicine: Selected Topics. 1st ed. Ames; Iowa State University Press, 1981. 176p.	Third
	Stephen, Lorne E. Trypanosomiasis: A Veterinary Perspective. 1st ed. Oxford and New York; Pergamon Press, 1986. 551p.	Second
Third	Stevens, Lewis. Genetics and Evolution of the Domestic Fowl. Cambridge; Cambridge University Press, 1991. 306p.	
Third	Stevenson, John P. Trout Farming Manual. 2d ed. Farnham, U.K. and Great Neck, N.Y.; Fishing News Books, 1987. 259p. (1st ed., 1980. 186p.)	Third
	Stewart, D. J., ed. Footrot in Ruminants: Proceedings of a Workshop, Melbourne 1985. Glebe, New South Wales; Commonwealth Scientific and Industrial Research Organization, 1986. 283p.	Third
Third	Stickney, Robert R. Culture of Nonsalmonid Freshwater Fishes. Boca Raton, Fla.; CRC Press, 1986. 201p.	Third
Second	Stoddart, Laurence A., Arthur D. Smith, and Thadis W. Box. Range Management. 3d ed. New York; McGraw-Hill, 1975. 532p. (1st ed., 1943.)	First
Third	Stolen, Joanne S., Douglas P. Anderson, and Willem B. van Muiswinkel. Fish Immunology: Papers Presented at an International Meeting, Sandy Hook, New Jersey, September 1985. Amsterdam and New York; Elsevier, 1986. 443p. (Reprinted from Veterinary Immunology and Immunopathology, vol. 12.)	Third
	Storz, Johannes. Chlamydia and Chlamydia-Induced Diseases. Springfield, Ill.; Thomas, 1971. 358p.	Third
	Strange, L. R. N. African Pastureland Ecology: With Particular	Third

Developed countries ranking		Third World ranking
	Reference to the Pastoral Environment of Eastern Africa. Rome; Food and Agriculture Organization, 1980. 188p. (FAO Pasture and Fodder Crop Studies no. 7)	
Third	Straub, O. C., ed. Fifth International Symposium on Bovine Leukosis. A Symposium in the EEC Programme of Coordination of Research on Animal Pathology, Tubingen, Germany, October 1982. Luxembourg; Commission of the European Communities, 1984. 657p.	Third
Third	Straub, O. C., organizer and ed., and G. Gentile, organizer. Fourth International Symposium on Bovine Leukosis: A Seminar in the EEC Programme of Coordination of Research on Animal Pathology, Bologna, November 1980. The Hague; Boston and Hingham, Mass.; M. Nijhoff for the Commission of the European Communities, 1982. 614p.	Third
Third	Strauch, D. Animal Production and Environmental Health. Amsterdam and New York; Elsevier, 1987. 324p.	Second
	Strombeck, Donald R. Small Animal Gastroenterology. Davis, Calif.; Stonegate Pub., 1979. 564p.	Third
First	Sturkie, Paul D., ed. with C. A. Benzo. Avian Physiology. 4th ed. New York; Springer-Verlag, 1986. 516p. (1st ed., Ithaca, N.Y.; Comstock Pub., 1954. 423p.) (Available in Spanish as Fisiologia Aviar. Zaragoza; Acribia, 1968.)	Second
Second	Sumberg, J. E., and K. Cassaday, eds. Sheep and Goats in Humid West Africa; Proceedings of the Workshop on Small Ruminant Production Systems in the Humid Zone of West Africa, Ibadan, Nigeria, January 1984. Addis Ababa, Ethiopia; International Livestock Centre for Africa, 1985. 74p.	Second
Third	Summerfelt, Robert C., and Gordon E. Hall, eds. Age and Growth of Fish; Proceedings of an International Symposium . . . Des Moines, Iowa, June 1985. 1st ed. Ames; Iowa State University Press, 1987. 544p.	Third
Third	Summers, John D., and Steven Leeson. Poultry Nutrition Handbook. Rev. ed. Guelph, Ontario; Dept. of Animal and Poultry Science, Ontario Agricultural College, University of Guelph, 1985. 230p.	Third
Third	Sundlof, Stephen F., J. Edmond Riviere, and Arthur L. Craigmill. Food Animal Residue Avoidance Databank, Trade Name File: A Comprehensive Compendium of Food Animal Drugs. 2d ed. Gainesville, Fla.; Institute of Food and Agricultural Sciences, University of Florida, 1988. 609p.	Second
Second	Sundstol, F., and E. Owen. Straw and Other Fibrous By-Products as Feed. Amsterdam and New York; Elsevier, 1984. 604p.	Second
Third	Sutherland, T. M., J. R. McWilliam, and R. A. Leng, eds. From Plant to Animal Protein; Proceedings of a Symposium, University of New England, Armidale, Australia, August 1975.	

Developed countries ranking		Third World ranking
	Armidale; University of New England Pub. Unit, 1976. 187p.	
Second	Swan, Henry, and W. H. Broster, eds. Principles of Cattle Production; 23d Easter School in Agricultural Science. London and Boston; Butterworths, 1976. 438p. (Available in Spanish as Principios para la Produccion Ganadera. Buenos Aires; Hemisferio Sur, 1982.)	Second
Second	Swatland, H. J. Structure and Development of Meat Animals. Englewood Cliffs, N.J.; Prentice-Hall, 1984. 436p.	Second
Third	Sybesma, W. The Welfare of Pigs: A Seminar in the EEC Programme of Coordination of Research on Animal Welfare, Brussels, November 1980. The Hague; Boston and Hingham, Mass.; M. Nijhoff for the Commission of the European Communities, 1981. 334p.	
Third	Sybesma, W., P. G. van der Wal, and P. Walstra, eds. Recent Points of View on the Condition and Meat Quality of Pigs for Slaughter; Proceedings of an International Symposium . . . Schoonoord, Zeist, Netherlands, May 1968. Zeist; Research Institute for Animal Husbandry, 1968. 300p.	
Third	Syme, G. J., and L. A. Syme. Social Structure in Farm Animals. Amsterdam and New York; Elsevier Scientific Pub. Co., 1979. 200p.	Third
	Symons, L. E. A. Pathophysiology of Endoparasite Infetion: Compared with Ectoparasite Infestation and Microbial Infection. Sydney; Academic Press, 1989. 331p.	Second
Third	Symposium on Biological Roles of Copper, 1980, London. Biological Roles of Copper. Amsterdam; Excerpta Medica; New York; Elsevier/North Holland, 1980. 343p. (Ciba Foundation Symposium no. 79)	
First	Symposium on Energy Metabolism, 3d, 1964, Troon, Scotland. Energy Metabolism; Proceedings . . . edited by K. L. Blaxter. Organized by the European Association for Animal Production, the British Society of Animal Production, and the Hannah Dairy Research Institute, Ayr. London and New York; Academic Press, 1965. 450p. (EAAP Pub. no. 11)	
Second	Symposium on Energy Metabolism, 8th, 1979, Cambridge. Energy Metabolism; Proceedings . . . edited by Laurence E. Mount. London and Boston; Butterworths, 1980. 484p. (EAAP Publication no. 26)	Second
First	Symposium on Energy Metabolism, 9th, 1982, Lillehammer, Norway. Energy Metabolism of Farm Animals: Proceedings . . . edited by A. Ekern and F. Sundstol. Aas, Norway; Dept. of Animal Nutrition, Agricultural University of Norway, 1982. 330p. (EAAP Publication no. 29)	
First	Symposium on Energy Metabolism, 10th, 1985, Airlie, Virginia. Energy Metabolism of Farm Animals: Proceedings of the	Second

Developed countries ranking		Third World ranking
	10th Symposium . . . edited by P. W. Moe, H. F. Tyrrell, and P. J. Reynolds. Totowa, N.J.; Rowman & Littlefield, 1987. 381p. (EAAP Publication no. 32)	
First	Symposium on Energy Metabolism, 11th, 1988, Lunteren, Netherlands. Energy Metabolism of Farm Animals: Proceedings . . . compiled by Y. van der Honing and W. H. Close. Wageningen; Pudoc, 1989. 414p. (EAAP Publication no. 43)	Second
Second	Symposium on the Effect of Processing on the Nutritional Value of Feeds, 1972, Gainesville, Fla. Proceedings . . . Sponsored by the Committee on Animal Nutrition, Agricultural Board, National Research Council; Center for Tropical Agriculture and the Department of Animal Science, University of Florida. Washington, D.C.; National Academy of Sciences, 1973. 494p.	
	Symposium on the Physiology and Biochemistry of Muscle as a Food, 2d, 1969, University of Wisconsin. Proceedings . . . edited by E. J. Briskey, R. G. Cassens and B. B. Marsh. Madison; University of Wisconsin Press, 1970. 843p.	Third
Third	Szabo, Kalman T. Congenital Malformations in Laboratory and Farm Animals. San Diego; Academic Press, 1989. 313p.	Third

T

Developed countries ranking		Third World ranking
	Taiganides, Eliseos Paul, ed. Animal Wastes; Proceedings of a Seminar . . . Organized by the Regional Office for Europe of the World Health Organization, held at the Czechoslovak Research and Development Centre for Environmental Pollution Control, Bratislava. London; Applied Science, 1977. 429p.	Third
Third	Talbot, Richard B., A. Haydee Fernandez, and Luis V. Melendez, eds. List of FDA Approved Animal Drug Products. Blacksburg; Laboratory of Veterinary Medical Informatics, Virginia-Maryland Regional College of Veterinary Medicine, Virginia Polytechnic Institute and State University, 1987. 1 vol. (various pagings).	
Third	Tarrant, P. V., G. Eikelenboom, and G. Monin. Evaluation and Control of Meat Quality in Pigs: A Seminar in the EEC Agricultural Research Programme, Dublin, November 1985. Dordrecht and Boston; M. Nijhoff, 1987. 498p.	Third
First	Taylor, D. J. Pig Diseases. 4th ed. Glasgow; D. J. Taylor, 1986. 300p. (1st ed., 1979. 176p.)	Second
Third	Taylor, Lewis W., ed. Fertility and Hatchability of Chicken and Turkey Eggs. New York; J. Wiley, 1949. 423p.	
Second	Taylor, Robert E. Scientific Farm Animal Production: An Introduction to Animal Science. 4th ed. New York, etc.; Macmillan, 1991. (1st ed., by Ralph Bogart, Minneapolis; Burgess Pub. Co., 1977. 420p.)	Second

Developed countries ranking		Third World ranking
Third	Thacker, P. A., and R. N. Kirkwood, eds. Nontraditional Feed Sources for Use in Swine Production. Boston; Butterworths, 1990. 515p.	Second
Third	Thear, Katie. Goats and Goatkeeping. London; Merehurst, 1988. 176p.	Second
First	Thedford, Thomas R. Sheep Health Handbook: A Field Guide for Producers with Limited Veterinary Services. Morrilton, Ark.; Winrock International, 1983. 132p.	Third
	Thickett, Bill, Dan Mitchell, and Bryan Hallows. Calf Rearing. 2d ed. Farming Press, 1988. 180p. (1st ed., 1986. 139p.)	Second
Third	Thomas, D. G. M., D. G. Beynon, T. G. G. Herbert, and J. Lloyd Jones. Animal Husbandry. 3d ed. London; Bailliere Tindall, 1983. 257p. (1st ed., London; Cassell, 1963.)	Second
Third	Thomas, Verl M. Beef Cattle Production: An Integrated Approach. Philadelphia; Lea & Febiger, 1986. 270p.	Third
Second	Thompson, G. B., and C. C. O'Mary. Commercial Beef Cattle Production. 3d ed. Philadelphia; Lea & Febiger, 1986. 414p. (1st ed., 1972; 3d ed., 1978 by G. B. Thompson, C. C. O'Mary, and I. A. Dwyer)	
Second	Thompson, G. B., and C. C. O'Mary, eds. The Feedlot. 3d ed. Philadelphia; Lea & Febiger, 1983. 306p. (1st ed., by Irwin A. Dyer and C. C. O'Mary, 1972. 224p.)	Second
Third	Thomson, D. J., D. E. Beever, and R. G. Gunn, eds. Forage Protein in Ruminant Animal Production; Proceedings of a Symposium organized by the British Society of Animal Production, and the British Grassland Society, University of Leeds, Sept. 1981. Thames Ditton; British Society of Animal Production, 1982. 193p. (BSAP Occasional Publication no. 6)	Second
Third	Thomson, E. F., and F. S. Thomson, eds. Increasing Small Ruminant Productivity in Semi-Arid Areas: Proceedings of a Workshop, International Center for Agricultural Research in the Dry Areas, Aleppo, Syria, November-December 1987. Dordrecht and Boston; Kluwer Academic Publishers, 1988. 296p.	Second
	Thomson, R. G. General Veterinary Pathology. 2d ed. Philadelphia; W. B. Saunders, 1984. 463p. (1st ed., 1978. 444p.) (Available in Spanish as Anatomia Patologica General Veterinaria. 1st ed. trans. by Juan Jose Badiola Diez. Zaragoza; Acribia, 1986.)	Second
Third	Thornton, Keith. Practical Pig Production. 3d ed. Ipswich, U.K.; Farming Press, 1981. 234p. (1st ed., 1973. 190p.)	Second
	Thrall, Donald E. Textbook of Veterinary Diagnostic Radiology. Philadelphia; Saunders, 1986. 563p.	Third
	Thrusfield, Michael V. Veterinary Epidemiology. London and Boston; Butterworths, 1986. 280p.	Third
Third	Timon, V. M., and R. P. Baber, eds. La Production de Viande	Third

Developed countries ranking		Third World ranking
	Ovine et Caprine Dans les Regions Tropicales Humides de l'Afrique de l'Ouest: Compte Rendu d'un Seminaire Qui s'est Tenu a Yamoussoukro, Cote d'Ivoire, Septembre 1987 = Sheep and Goat Meat Production in the Humid Tropics of West Africa: Proceedings of a Seminar . . . Rome; Food and Agriculture Organization, 1989. 260p. (FAO Animal Production and Health Paper no. 70; Etude FAO Production et Sante Animales no. 70)	
Third	Titus, Harry W., and James C. Fritz. The Scientific Feeding of Chickens. 5th ed. Danville, Ill.; Interstate, 1971. 336p. (1st ed., by H. W. Titus, 1941. 110p.) (Available in Spanish as Alimentacion Cientifica de las Gallinas. Zaragoza; Acribia, 1960.)	Second
	Tizard, Ian R. Veterinary Immunology: An Introduction. 3d ed. Philadelphia; Saunders, 1987. 401p. (1st ed., 1977, as An Introduction to Veterinary Immunology.)	Second
Third	Toivanen, Auli, and P. Toivanen. Avian Immunology: Basis and Practice. Boca Raton, Fla.; CRC Press, 1987. 2 vols.	Third
	Tomek, William G., and Kenneth L. Robinson. Agricultural Product Prices. 3d ed. Ithaca, N.Y.; Cornell University Press, 1990. 360p. (1st ed., 1972. 376p.)	Second
	Tomes, G. J., R. J. Robertson, R. J. Lightfoot, and William Haresign, eds. Sheep Breeding; International Sheep Breeding Congress. 2d ed. London and Boston; Butterworths, 1979. 580p. (Earlier ed., 1976, as the Proceedings of the International Sheep Breeding Congress with title: Sheep Breeding.)	Second
Second	Topley, W. W. C., Graham Wilson, and Ashley Miles. Principles of Bacteriology, Virology, and Immunity. Baltimore; Williams & Wilkins, 1983–1984. 3 vols. 2563p. (1st-2d eds. as The Principles of Bacteriology and Immunity. 6th ed., Topley and Wilson's Principles of Bacteriology, Virology, and Immunity.)	Third
	Tothill, J. C., and J. J. Mott, eds. Ecology and Management of the World's Savannas; Proceedings of the International Savanna Symposium, Brisbane, Queensland, 1984. Canberra and Farnham Royal, U.K.; Australian Academy of Science and Commonwealth Agricultural Bureaux, 1985. 384p.	Third
Third	Toussaint, Raven E. Cattle Footcare and Claw Trimming. Ipswich, U.K.; Farming Press, 1985. 126p. (Translation of Klauwverzorging Bij Het Rund.)	Second
	Tribe, D. E., ed. Carcase Composition and Appraisal of Meat Animals; Selected Papers, from Technical Conference . . . University of Melbourne, 1963. East Melbourne, Australia; Commonwealth Scientific and Industrial Research Organization, 1964. 1 vol.	Second

Developed countries ranking		Third World ranking
	Tribe, D. E., and G. J. R. Coles. Prime Lamb Production. Melbourne, Australia; F. W. Cheshire, 1966. 239p.	Third
	Trigo Tavera, F. Patologia General Veterinaria. Mexico City; Universidad Nacional Autonoma de Mexico, 1986. 379p.	Third
Third	Trimberger, George W., W. M. Etgen, and David M. Galton. Dairy Cattle Judging Techniques. 4th ed. Englewood Cliffs, N.J.; Prentice-Hall, 1987. 356p. (1st ed., 1958. 304p.)	
Third	Tropical Products Institute (Great Britain). Proceedings of the Conference on Animal Feeds of Tropical and Subtropical Origin, London School of Pharmacy, April 1974. London; Tropical Products Institute, 1975. 347p. (Summaries in English, French, and Spanish.)	Second
Third	Tucker, C. S. Channel Catfish Culture. Amsterdam and New York; Elsevier, 1985. 657p.	
	Turner, A. Simon, C. Wayne McIlwraith, and Bruce L. Hull. Techniques in Large Animal Surgery. 2d ed. Philadelphia; Lea & Febiger, 1989. 381p. (1st ed., by A. S. Turner and C. W. McIlwraith, 1982. 333p.)	Second
Third	Turner, Charles W. The Mammary Gland: I. The Anatomy of the Udder of Cattle and Domestic Animals; A revision and enlargement of his The Comparative Anatomy of the Mammary Glands. Columbia, Mo.; Lucas Bros., 1952. 389p. (Vol. 2 never published.)	
Second	Turner, Helen N., and Sydney S. Y. Young. Quantitative Genetics in Sheep Breeding. Ithaca, N.Y.; Cornell University Press; Melbourne; Macmillan, 1969. 332p.	First
Third	Turner, Mary. Goat Care: A Complete Handbook. Jefferson, N.C.; McFarland, 1984. 186p.	Second

U

Developed countries ranking		Third World ranking
First	Underwood, Eric J. The Mineral Nutrition of Livestock. 2d ed. Farnham Royal, U.K.; Commonwealth Agricultural Bureaux, 1981. 180p. (1st ed., 1966. 237p.) (Available in Spanish as Los Minerales en la Nutricion del Ganado. 2d ed. Zaragoza; Acribia, 1983.)	First
	UNESCO, UNEP, and FAO. Tropical Grazing Land Ecosystems; State-of-Knowledge Report. Paris; UNESCO, 1979. 655p. (Natural Resources Research no. 16)	Second
Third	United Nations Development Programme/FAO Regional Project. Research on Tick-borne Diseases and Tick Control; East Coast Fever and Related Tick-Borne Diseases: Selected Reprints of Papers. Rome; Food and Agriculture Organization, 1980. 982p.	Second

Developed countries ranking		Third World ranking
	United States Animal Health Association. Committee on Foreign Animal Diseases. Foreign Animal Diseases; Their Prevention, Diagnosis and Control. 3d ed. Richmond, Va.; The Committee, 1975. 360p. (Previous eds. by U.S. Livestock Sanitary Association.)	Third
Third	United States. Dept. of Agriculture. Production and Marketing Administration. Handbook of Official Hay and Straw Standards. Washington, D.C.; USDA and U.S. Govt. Print. Off., 1958. 55p.	
	Upson, D. W. Handbook of Clinical Veterinary Pharmacology. 3d ed. Manhattan, Kans.; Ian Upson Enterprises, 1989. 729p. (1st ed., Bonner Springs, Kans.; Vin Pub. Co., 1981.)	Second
First	Urquhart, G. M. Veterinary Parasitology. Essex, U.K.; Longman Scientific & Technical, 1987. 286p.	Third

V

Third	Vahouny, George V., and David Kritchevsky, eds. Dietary Fiber in Health and Disease. New York; Plenum Press, 1982. 330p.	Third
Second	Vallentine, John F. Range Development and Improvements. 3d ed. San Diego; Academic Press, 1989. 524p. (1st ed., Provo, Utah; Brigham Young University Press, 1971. 516p.)	Second
First	Van Vleck, L. Dale, E. John Pollak, and E. A. Branford Oltenacu. Genetics for the Animal Sciences. New York; W. H. Freeman, 1987. 391p.	First
Second	Van Vleck, L. Dale, and Shayle R. Searle, eds. Variance Components and Animal Breeding; Proceedings of a Conference in honor of C. R. Henderson, July 1979. Ithaca, N.Y.; Cornell University, 1979. 227p.	
Second	Vandeplassche, M. Reproductive Efficiency in Cattle: A Guideline for Projects in Developing Countries. Rome; Food and Agriculture Organization, 1982. 118p.	Second
First	VanSoest, Peter J. Nutritional Ecology of the Ruminant: Ruminant Metabolism, Nutritional Strategies, the Cellulolytic Fermentation and the Chemistry of Forages and Plant Fibers. Ithaca, N.Y.; Comstock Pub. Associates, 1987. 373p. (Reprint; originally published, Corvallis, Oreg.; O & B Books, 1982. 2d rev. ed. in press.)	First
Second	Verstegen, M. W. A., and A. M. Henken. Energy Metabolism in Farm Animals: Effects of Housing, Stress, and Disease. Dordrecht; Boston and Hingham, Mass.; M. Nijhoff, 1987. 500p.	Second
	Villemin, M. Dictionnaire des Termes Veterinaires et Zootechniques. 3d ed. Paris; Vigot, 1984. 472p. (1st ed., 1963.)	Third

Developed countries ranking		Third World ranking
Third	Voisin, Andre. Grass Tetany; Translation of Tetanie d'Herbe. Springfield, Ill.; Charles C. Thomas, 1963. 262p.	
Third	Von Bergen, Werner, ed. Wool Handbook; A Text and Reference Book for the Entire Wool Industry. 3d ed., enl. New York; Interscience Publishers, 1963–1970. 2 vols. (1st ed., 1938, as American Wool Handbook.)	

W

Third	Wachtel, Stephen S. Evolutionary Mechanisms in Sex Determination; Proceedings of an International Conference . . . Memphis, Tenn., May 1987. Boca Raton, Fla.; CRC Press, 1989. 322p.	
Second	Wadsworth Anaerobic Bacteriology Manual. 4th ed. edited by Vera L. Sutter et al. Belmont, Calif.; Star Pub. Co., 1985. 152p. (3d ed., St. Louis; Mosby, 1980.)	Third
Third	Walker, B. H. Management of Semi-Arid Ecosystems. Amsterdam and New York; Elsevier Scientific Pub. Co., 1979. 398p.	Third
Second	Walker, Warren F. Anatomy and Dissection of the Fetal Pig. 4th ed. New York; W. H. Freeman, 1988. 116p. (1st ed., San Francisco; 1964. 45p.)	
Third	Wallach, Joel D. Diseases of Exotic Animals: Medical and Surgical Management. Philadelphia; Saunders, 1983. 1159p.	Second
	Walton, John R. A Handbook of Pig Diseases. 2d ed. Liverpool; Liverpool University Press, 1987. 166p.	Second
	Wannamaker, Lewis W., and John M. Matsen. Streptococci and Streptococcal Diseases; Recognition, Understanding, and Management. New York; Academic Press, 1972. 635p.	Third
	Waring, George H. Horse Behavior: The Behavioral Traits and Adaptations of Domestic and Wild Horses, Including Ponies. Park Ridge, N.J.; Noyes Publications, 1983. 292p.	Third
Third	Warner, Carol M., Max F. Rothschild, and Susan J. Lamont, eds. The Molecular Biology of the Major Histocompatibility Complex of Domestic Animal Species; Papers Presented at a Symposium, Iowa State University, October 1987. Ames; Iowa State University Press, 1988. 193p.	
First	Waterlow, J. C., P. J. Garlick, and D. J. Millward. Protein Turnover in Mammalian Tissues and in the Whole Body. Amsterdam and New York; North-Holland Pub. Co., 1978. 804p.	
Second	Watson, James D., et al. Molecular Biology of the Gene. 4th ed. Menlo Park, Calif.; Benjamin/Cummings, 1987. 2 vols. (1st ed., New York; W. A. Benjamin, 1965. 494p.) (Available in Spanish as Biologia Molecular del Gen. 3d ed. Mexico; Addison, 1978.)	Second
	Watson, Peter R. Animal Traction. Summit, N.J.; Artisan Pub-	Third

Developed countries ranking		Third World ranking

	lications, 1983. 151p. (1st ed. prepared for the Peace Corps Information Collection & Exchange Office by the TransCentury Corporation.)	
Third	Weatherley, A. H., H. S. Gill, and J. M. Casselman. The Biology of Fish Growth. London and Orlando, Fla.; Academic Press, 1987. 443p.	Third
Third	Weber, W. T., and D. L. Ewert, eds. Avian Immunology: Proceedings of the 2nd International Conference on Avian Immunology, Philadelphia, July 1986. New York; A. R. Liss, 1987. 351p.	Third
	Webster, C. C., and P. N. Wilson. Agriculture in the Tropics. 2d ed. London; Longman, 1980. 640p. (1st ed., 1966.)	Second
Third	Webster, John. Calf Husbandry, Health, and Welfare. London and New York; Granada, 1984. 202p.	Second
Third	Webster, John. Understanding the Dairy Cow. Oxford and Boston; BSP Professional Books, 1987. 357p.	Third
Third	Wegner, Rose-Marie, ed. 2nd European Symposium on Poultry Welfare; Proceedings. . . . Celle, Germany; World Poultry Science Assocation, German Branch, 1985. 360p.	
	Weisbroth, Steven H., Ronald E. Flatt, and Alan L. Kraus. The Biology of the Laboratory Rabbit. New York; Academic Press, 1974. 496p.	Third
Third	Wells, R. G., and C. G. Belyavin, eds. Egg Quality—Current Problems and Recent Advances. Papers from the 20th Poultry Science Symposium, Harper Adams Agricultural College, Newport, Shropshire, September 1985. London and Boston; Butterworths, 1987. 302p. (Poultry Science Symposium no. 20)	
Third	Wenkoff, M. S. The Evaluation of Bulls for Breeding Soundness. Ottawa; Canadian Veterinary Medical Association, 1987. 48p.	Second
First	Wheeler, J. L., and Richard D. Mochrie, eds. Forage Evaluation: Concepts and Techniques; Proceedings of a Workshop. Lexington, Ky.; East Melbourne, Victoria; American Forage and Grassland Council, and CSIRO, 1981. 582p.	First
	Whitaker, John R., and Steven R. Tannenbaum, eds. Food Proteins; Papers from a Symposium Sponsored by the Institute of Food Technologists and the International Union of Food Science and Technology. Westport, Conn.; Avi Pub. Co., 1977. 603p.	Third
Second	White, Edwin G., and F. T. W. Jordan. Veterinary Preventive Medicine. Baltimore; Williams & Wilkins, 1963. 334p.	Second
First	Whiteman, C. E., and A. A. Bickford. Avian Disease Manual. 3d ed. Dubuque, Iowa; Kendall/Hunt; Kennett Square, Pa.; American Association of Avian Pathologists, 1989. 209p. (1st ed., 1980, Ft. Collins, Colo. 193p.)	Third

Developed countries ranking		Third World ranking
	Whiteman, Peter C., et al. Tropical Pasture Science. Oxford; Oxford University Press, 1980. 398p.	Third
	Whittaker, Robert H. Communities and Ecosystems. 2d ed. New York; Macmillan, 1975. 385p. (1st ed., London, 1975.)	Second
Second	Whittemore, Colin T. Elements of Pig Science. Harlow, U.K.; Longman Scientific & Technical; New York; Wiley, 1987. 181p.	Second
Third	Whittemore, Colin T. Pig Production: The Scientific and Practical Principles. London; Longman, 1980. 145p. (Available in Spanish as Produccion del Cerdo. 1st ed. Barcelona; Aedos, 1987.)	Third
Third	Whittemore, Colin T., and F. W. H. Elsley. Practical Pig Production. 2d ed., 2d impression (with amendments). Ipswich, U.K.; Farming Press, 1979. 190p. (1st ed., 1976.) (Available in Spanish as Alimentacion Practica del Cerdo. 1st ed. Barcelona; Aedos, 1978.)	Second
Third	Wiener, Gerald, ed. Animal Genetic Resources: A Global Programme for Sustainable Development; Proceedings of an FAO Expert Consultation, Rome, Sept. 1989. Rome; Food and Agriculture Organization, 1990. 300p. (FAO Animal Production and Health Paper no. 80)	Third
Second	Wiepkema, P. R., and P. W. M. van Adrichem, eds. Biology of Stress in Farm Animals: An Integrative Approach: A Seminar in the EEC Programme of Coordination Research on Animal Welfare, April 1986, Pietersberg Conference Centre, Oosterbeek, the Netherlands. Dordrecht and Boston; M. Nijhoff for the Commission of the European Communities, 1987. 198p.	Third
	Wierenga, H. K., and D. J. Peterse, eds. Cattle Housing Systems, Lameness and Behaviour: Proceedings of a Seminar . . . Brussels, June 1986. Dordrecht and Boston; M. Nijhoff for the Commission of the European Communities, 1987. 187p.	Third
	Wiggins, Geoffrey S., and Andrew Wilson. Color Atlas of Meat and Poultry Inspection. New York; Van Nostrand Reinhold, 1976. 68p. (Available in Spanish as Inspeccion de Carnes y Aves. Bogota; Interamericana, 1976.)	Third
First	Wilcox, C. J., et al., eds. Large Dairy Herd Management; Proceedings of a Symposium, Gainesville, January 1976. Gainesville; University Press of Florida, 1978. 1046p.	
Third	Wilkinson, J. M. Beef Production from Silage and Other Conserved Forages. London and New York; Longman, 1985. 140p.	Second
Third	Wilkinson, J. M., and Barbara A. Stark. Commercial Goat Production. Oxford and Boston; BSP Professional Books, 1987. 159p.	
Third	Williams, Ralph E. Livestock Entomology. New York; Wiley, 1985. 335p.	Second

Developed countries ranking		Third World ranking
Second	Wilson, Andrew. Practical Meat Inspection. 4th ed. Oxford, Boston, St. Louis, Mo.; Blackwell Scientific Publications, 1985. 289p. (1st ed., 1968.)	Second
Third	Wilson, James A. Principles of Animal Physiology. 2d ed. New York; Macmillan, 1979. 891p. (1st ed., 1972. 842p.)	Second
Third	Wilson, P. N., and T. D. A. Brigstocke. Improved Feeding of Cattle and Sheep: A Practical Guide to Modern Concepts of Ruminant Nutrition. London and New York; Granada, 1981. 238p.	Second
Third	Wilson, P. N., and T. D. A. Brigstocke. Improved Feeding of Pigs and Poultry: A Practical Guide to Modern Concepts of Pig and Poultry Nutrition. London; Granada, 1985. 238p.	Third
Second	Wilson, R. Trevor. The Camel. London and New York; Longman, 1984. 223p.	Second
	Wilson, R. Trevor, and D. Bourzat. Small Ruminants in African Agriculture = Les Petits Ruminants Dans l'Agriculture Africaine; Proceedings of a Conference . . . ILCA, Addis Ababa, Ethiopia, September-October 1985. Addis Ababa; International Livestock Centre for Africa, 1985. 261p.	Second
	Wilson, R. Trevor, and Azeb Melaku, eds. African Small Ruminant Research and Development; Proceedings of a Conference, Bamenda, Cameroon, January 1989. Addis Ababa, Ethiopia; ILCA, 1989. 578p.	Second
	Winrock International. Sheep and Goats in Developing Countries: Their Present and Potential Role. Washington, D.C.; World Bank, 1983. 116p.	Third
Second	Winrock International Livestock Research and Training Center, and United States Agency for International Development. Proceedings of a Workshop on the Role of Sheep and Goats in Agricultural Development, November 1976, Winrock International Center. Morrilton, Ark.; Winrock International Livestock Research Training Center, 1976. 43p.	Second
Third	Winston, Mark L. The Biology of the Honey Bee. Cambridge, Mass.; Harvard University Press, 1987.	Third
Second	Wiseman, Julian. Fats in Animal Nutrition; Proceedings of the 37th Nottingham Easter School in Agricultural Science. London and Boston; Butterworths, 1984. 521p.	Second
Third	Wiseman, Julian, translator and ed. Feeding of Non-Ruminant Livestock: Collective edited work by the Research Staff of the Departement de l'Elevage des Monogastriques, INRA, under the responsibility of Jean-Claude Blum. London and Boston; Butterworths, 1987. 214p. (Translation of L'Alimentation des Animaux Monogastriques.)	Third
Third	Wittmann, G., Rosalind M. Gaskell, and H. J. Rziha. Latent	Third

Developed countries ranking		Third World ranking
	Herpes Virus Infections in Veterinary Medicine. Boston; M. Nijhoff for the Commission of the European Communities, 1984. 522p.	
Third	Wobeser, Gary A. Diseases of Wild Waterfowl. New York; Plenum Press, 1981. 300p.	
Second	Wolf, Ken. Fish Viruses and Fish Viral Diseases. Ithaca, N.Y.; Comstock Pub. Associates, 1988. 476p.	Second
Second	Wolfe, Stephen L. Biology of the Cell. 2d ed. Belmont, Calif.; Wadsworth Pub. Co., 1981. 544p. (1st ed., 1972. 545p.) (Available in Spanish as Biologia de la Celula. Barcelona; Omega.)	Second
Third	Wong, Noble P., et al., eds. Fundamentals of Dairy Chemistry. 3d ed. New York; Van Nostrand Reinhold Co., 1988. 779p. (1st ed., 1965, by Byron H. Webb and A. H. Johnson, as Fundamentals of Dairy Science.)	Second
Second	Wood, Dennis W. Principles of Animal Physiology. 3d ed. London; E. Arnold, 1983. 348p. (1st ed., 1968. 332p.) (Available in Spanish as Fisiologia Animal. Leon; Academia, 1976.)	Second
Third	Wood-Gush, D. G. M. The Behaviour of the Domestic Fowl. London; Heinemann Educational, 1971. 147p.	
Second	Wood-Gush, D. G. M. Elements of Ethology: A Textbook for Agricultural and Veterinary Students. London and New York; Chapman & Hall, 1983. 240p.	Second
Third	Woolcock, J. B. Bacterial Infection and Immunity in Domestic Animals. Amsterdam and New York; Elsevier Scientific, 1979. 254p.	Third
Third	Woolcock, J. B., ed. Microbiology of Animals and Animal Products. Amsterdam, etc.; Elsevier, 1991. 278p.	Third
	Worden, Alastair N., Kenneth C. Sellers, and Derek E. Tribe, eds. Animal Health, Production and Pasture. London; Longmans, 1963. 786p. (Available in Spanish as Salud Animal: Produccion y Pasturas. Universidad de Argentina, 1977.)	Second
Third	Workman, John P. Range Economics. New York and London; Macmillan Collier Macmillan, 1986. 217p.	
	World Bank. Accelerated Development in Sub-Saharan Africa: An Agenda for Action. Washington, D.C.; World Bank, 1981. 198p.	Second
Third	World Conference on Animal Production, 3d, 1973, University of Melbourne. Proceedings . . . edited by R. L. Reid. Sponsored by the World Association of Animal Production, the Australian Society of Animal Production, and the Commonwealth and State Governments of Australia. Sydney; Sydney University Press, 1975. 694p.	Second
Second	World Conference on Animal Production, 4th, 1978, Buenos	Second

Developed countries ranking		Third World ranking

	Aires, Argentina. IV Conferencia Mundial de Produccion Animal = IV World Conference on Animal Production: Memorias, Sponsored by the World Association for Animal Production and Others. Edited by Luis S. Verde and Angel Fernandez. Buenos Aires; Asociacion Argentina de Produccion Animal, 1980. 2 vols.	
	World Conference on Animal Production, 5th, Tokyo, August 1983; Proceedings. . . . Tokyo; Japanese Society of Zootechnical Science, 1983. 2 vols.	Third
	World Congress on Animal Feeding, 2d, 1972, Madrid. II Congreso Mundial de Alimentacion Animal = 2d World Congress on Animal Feeding = II Congres Mondial d'Alimentation Animale = II. Tierernaehrungs-Weltkongress; Proceedings . . . Octubre 1972. Madrid; Industrias Graficas Espana, 1972. 3 vols.	Third
Third	World Congress on Diseases of Cattle, 12th, 1982, Amsterdam. Proceedings . . . International Congrescentrum RAI, Amsterdam; World Association for Buiatrics. Utrecht, Netherlands; Groep Geneeskunde van het Rund van de Koninklijke Nederlandse Maatschappij voor Diergeneeskunde, 1982. 2 vols. (Summaries in English, French and German.)	Third
Second	World Congress on Diseases of Cattle, 14th, 1986, Dublin, Ireland. Proceedings . . . and the World Association for Buiatrics . . . edited by P. J. Hartigan, M. L. Monaghan. Dublin; Irish Cattle Veterinary Association; Ballsbridge, Dublin; Available from M. Monaghan, Faculty of Veterinary Medicine, University College Dublin, 1986. 2 vols. (Articles or summaries in English, French or German.)	Third
Second	World Congress on Genetics Applied to Livestock Production, 1st, 1974, Madrid; Proceedings. . . . Madrid; Editorial Garsi, 1974–1978. 4 vols.	
Second	World Congress on Genetics Applied to Livestock Production, 2d, 1982, Madrid. 2d World Congress on Genetics Applied to Livestock Production = II Congreso Mundial de Genetica Aplicada a la Produccion Ganadera; Proceedings . . . edited by C. L. de Cuenca. Madrid; Editorial Garsi, 1982. 4 vols. (Zootechnia; v. 31, nos. 7–9)	Second
Second	World Congress on Genetics Applied to Livestock Production, 3d, 1986, Lincoln, Nebraska. 3d World Congress . . . July 1986. Lincoln; University of Nebraska, Institute of Agriculture and Natural Resources, 1986. 4 vols.	Second
Third	World Congress on Sheep and Beef Cattle Breeding, 2d, 1984, Pretoria, South Africa. Proceedings . . . edited by J. H. Hofmeyr and E. H. H. Meyar. Bloemfontein, South Africa;	

Developed countries ranking		Third World ranking
	South African Stud Book and Livestock Improvement Association, 1984. 803p.	
Second	World's Poultry Congress and Exhibition, 17th, 1984, Helsinki, Finland. Proceedings and Abstracts = Actes et Abstraits, Helsinki Exhibition and Congress Centre, August 1984. Hameenlinna, Finland; The Branch, 1984. 800p. (English, French, German, Russian, and Spanish.)	Third
	Woynarovich, Elekne, and L. Horvath. The Artificial Propagation of Warm-Water Finfishes: A Manual for Extension. Rome; Food and Agriculture Organization, 1980. 183p. (FAO Fisheries Technical Paper no. 201)	Third
	Wrathall, Anthony E. Reproductive Disorders in Pigs. Farnham Royal, U.K.; Commonwealth Agricultural Bureaux, 1975. 311p.	Third
	Wright, I. G., ed. Veterinary Protozoan and Hemoparasite Vaccines. Boca Raton, Fla.; CRC Press, 1989. 242p.	Second
	Wright, Peter, Peter G. Caryl, and David M. Vowles, eds. Neural and Endocrine Aspects of Behaviour in Birds; Papers from a Conference sponsored by the Dept. of Psychology, University of Edinburgh, 1974. Amsterdam and New York; Elsevier Scientific Pub. Co., 1975. 408p.	Third
Second	Wright, Sewall. Evolution and the Genetics of Populations; A Treatise. Chicago; University of Chicago Press, 1968–1978. 4 vols.	Third
Second	Wright, Sewall. Evolution: Selected Papers of Sewall Wright; edited . . . by William B. Provine. Chicago; University of Chicago Press, 1986. 649p.	Third
	Wyllie, Thomas D., and Lawrence G. Morehouse. Mycotoxicoses of Domestic and Laboratory Animals, Poultry, and Aquatic Invertebrates and Vertebrates. New York; M. Dekker, 1978. 570p.	Third

Y

Developed countries ranking		Third World ranking
Third	Yagil, R. Camels and Camel Milk. Rome; Food and Agriculture Organization, 1982. 69p.	Second
Third	Yagil, R. The Desert Camel: Comparative Physiological Adaptation. Basel and New York; Karger, 1985. 163p.	Second
	Yeates, Neil, T. N. Edey, and Mervyn K. Hill. Animal Science: Reproduction, Climate, Meat, Wool. Rev. ed. Rushcutters Bay, New South Wales and Elmsford, N.Y; Pergamon Press, 1975. 389p. (1st ed., 1965, as Modern Aspects of Ani-	Third

Developed countries ranking		Third World ranking
	mal Production.) (Available in Spanish as Avances en Zootecnia. Zaragoza; Acribia, 1967.)	
Third	Yerex, David, and Ian Spiers. Modern Deer Farm Management. Carterton, N.Z.; Ampersand Pub. Associates, 1987. 168p.	Third
	Youdeowei, Anthony, and M. W. Service. Pest and Vector Management in the Tropics: With Particular Reference to Insects, Ticks, Mites, and Snails. London and New York; Longman, 1983. 399p.	Third
	Youmans, Guy P., Philip Y. Paterson, and Herbert M. Sommers. The Biologic and Clinical Basis of Infectious Diseases. 2d ed. Philadelphia; W. B. Saunders, 1980. 849p. (Available in Spanish as Infectologia Clinica . . . trans. by Ramon Elizondo Mata. Mexico; Interamericana, 1982.)	Second
Third	Youngner, V. B., and C. M. McKell, eds. The Biology and Utilization of Grasses. New York; Academic Press, 1972. 426p.	
Third	Yousef, Mohamed K., ed. Animal Production in the Tropics. Proceedings of a Symposium, February 1981, University of Gezira, Sudan. New York; Praeger Scientific, 1982. 376p.	Second
Second	Yousef, Mohamed K., ed. Stress Physiology in Livestock. Boca Raton, Fla.; CRC Press, 1985. 3 vols.	Second

Z

Developed countries ranking		Third World ranking
Third	Zaneveld, Lourens J. D., and Robert T. Chatterton, eds. Biochemistry of Mammalian Reproduction. New York; Wiley, 1982. 561p.	Third
	Zaslow, Ira M., and A. J. Cawley. Veterinary Trauma and Critical Care. Philadelphia; Lea & Febiger, 1984. 584p.	Third
Third	Zayan, Ren, and Ian J. H. Duncan. Cognitive Aspects of Social Behaviour in the Domestic Fowl. Amsterdam and New York; Elsevier, 1987. 492p.	
Second	Zemjanis, Raimunds. Diagnostic and Therapeautic Techniques in Animal Reproduction. 3d ed. Baltimore; Williams & Wilkins, 1984. (1st ed., 1962. 238p.) (Available in Spanish as Reproduccion Animal: Diagnostico y Tecnicas Terapeuticas. 11th ed. trans. by Daniel P. Leal. Mexico; Limusa-Noriega, 1989.)	

D. The Top Twenty Monographs

The top ranking monographs for both the developed countries and the Third World countries are displayed here in their ranking order. Eleven of the titles are in both lists, which demonstrates enormous agreement on which books are most valuable. Five of these eleven are the famous multi-edition farm animal nutrition reports of the U.S. National Academy of Science; group committee activity which has been well received. A related farm livestock nutrition three-volume set from the British Agricultural Research Council rates 10–12 in the developed countries but is the most highly ranked monograph in the Third World. The top eight monographs for the developed countries are all within the top 11 of the Third World monographs, with the exception of the Leman, which is ranked 19–20 in the Third World, and the ARC nutrition work, which is first in the Third World, but 10–12th in the developed countries.

Twenty Top-Ranked Monographs for Developed Countries and Third World

Developed countries ranking		Third World ranking
1	Dukes, H. H., and Melvin J. Swenson, eds. Dukes' Physiology of Domestic Animals. 10th ed. Ithaca, N.Y.; Comstock Pub. Associates, 1984. 922p. (Available in Spanish as Fisiologia de los Animales Domesticos. 4th ed., Madrid; Aguilar, 1977.)	7–8
2	Leman, Allen D., et al. Diseases of Swine. 6th ed. Ames; Iowa State University Press, 1986. 930p.	19–20
3–4	National Research Council (U.S.). Subcommittee on Beef Cattle Nutrition. Nutrient Requirements of Beef Cattle. 6th ed., rev. Washington, D.C.; National Academy Press, 1984. 90p. (5th ed., 1976. 56p.) (Available in Spanish as Necesidades Nutritivas del Ganado Vacuno de Carne. 2d ed. Buenos Aires; Hemisferio Sur, 1980.)	5–6
3–4	National Research Council (U.S.). Subcommittee on Dairy Cattle Nutrition. Nutrient Requirements of Dairy Cattle. 6th ed., rev. Washington, D.C.; National Academy of Sciences, 1988. 157p. (1st ed., 1958.) (Available in Spanish as Necesidades Nutritivas del Ganado Lechero. Buenos Aires; Hemisferio Sur, 1982.)	2
5–7	Hafez, E. S. E. Reproduction in Farm Animals. 5th ed. Philadelphia; Lea & Febiger, 1987. 649p. (1st ed., 1962.) (Available	5–6

Developed countries ranking		Third World ranking

<table>
<tr><td></td><td>in Spanish as Reproduccion e Insemination Artificial en Animales. 4th ed. Mexico City; Interamericana, 1985.)</td><td></td></tr>
<tr><td>5–7</td><td>National Research Council (U.S.). Subcommittee on Poultry Nutrition. Nutrient Requirements of Poultry. 8th ed. Washington, D.C.; National Academy of Sciences, 1984. 71p. (Editions for 1954, 1960, and 1966 as National Academy of Sciences-National Research Council Publications no. 301, 827 & 1345.)</td><td>7–8</td></tr>
<tr><td>5–7</td><td>National Research Council (U.S.). Subcommittee on Swine Nutrition. Nutrient Requirements of Swine. 9th ed., rev. Washington, D.C.; National Academy of Sciences, 1988. 93p. (Title varies slightly. 1st ed., 1953.) (Available in Spanish as Necesidades Nutritivas del Cerdo. Buenos Aires; Hemisferio Sur, 1980.)</td><td>4</td></tr>
<tr><td>8</td><td>National Research Council (U.S.). Subcommittee on Sheep Nutrition. Nutrient Requirements of Sheep. 6th ed., rev. Washington, D.C.; National Academy of Sciences, 1985. 72p. (Available in Spanish as Necesidades Nutritivas de los Ovinos. Buenos Aires; Hemisferio Sur, 1979.)</td><td>11</td></tr>
<tr><td>9</td><td>Larson, Bruce L., ed. Lactation: A Comprehensive Treatise. Ames; Iowa State University Press, 1985. 276p. (Earlier ed., 1974, edited by B. Larson and Vearl Smith. 3 vols.)</td><td></td></tr>
<tr><td>10–12</td><td>Agricultural Research Council (Great Britain). The Nutrient Requirements of Farm Livestock. 2d ed. London; Agricultural Research Council, 1980–1981. 3 vols. (1st ed., 1965–1975.)</td><td>1</td></tr>
<tr><td>10–12</td><td>Calnek, B. W., et al., eds. Diseases of Poultry. 9th ed. Ames; Iowa State University Press, 1991. 929p. (1st ed., edited by Harry E. Biester et al., 1943. 1005p. Earlier eds. by Grahame Williamson.)</td><td>14–17</td></tr>
<tr><td>10–12</td><td>VanSoest, Peter J. Nutritional Ecology of the Ruminant: Ruminant Metabolism, Nutritional Strategies, the Cellulolytic Fermentation and the Chemistry of Forages and Plant Fibers. Ithaca, N.Y.; Comstock Pub. Associates, 1987. 373p. (Reprint; originally published in Corvallis, Oreg.; O & B Books, 1982.)</td><td></td></tr>
<tr><td>13</td><td>Morrison, Frank B. Feeds and Feeding; A Handbook for the Student and Stockman. 22d ed., unabridged. Ithaca, N.Y.; Morrison Pub. Co., 1956. 1207p. (1st-9th eds. edited by W. A. Henry; 10th-14th eds. by W. A. Henry assisted by F. B. Morrison; 15th-21st eds. revised and rewritten by F. B. Morrison.) (Available in Spanish as Alimentos y Alimentacion del Ganado. Mexico City; UTEHA, 1980.)</td><td></td></tr>
<tr><td>14</td><td>Agricultural Research Council (Great Britain). The Nutrient Requirements of Ruminant Livestock: Technical Review. Farnham Royal, U.K.; Commonwealth Agricultural Bureaux, 1980. 351p. (Enlarged ed., 1965, of The Nutrient Requirements of Farm Livestock. no. 2: Ruminants.)</td><td></td></tr>
</table>

<table>
<tr><td>Developed
countries
ranking</td><td></td><td>Third
World
ranking</td></tr>
</table>

Developed countries ranking		Third World ranking
15–16	International Symposium on Ruminant Physiology, 3d, 1969, Cambridge, England. Physiology of Digestion and Metabolism in the Ruminant; Proceedings . . . edited by A. T. Phillipson et al. Newcastle upon Tyne; Oriel, 1970. 636p.	
15–16	International Symposium on Ruminant Physiology, 5th, 1979, Clermont-Ferrand, France. Digestive Physiology and Metabolism in Ruminants; Proceedings . . . edited by Y. Ruckebusch and P. Thivend. Lancaster, U.K.; MTP Press, 1980. 854p.	
17	Hagan, William A., Dorsey W. Bruner, and John F. Timoney. Microbiology and Infectious Diseases of Domestic Animals. 8th ed. Ithaca, N.Y.; Comstock Pub. Associates, 1988. 951p. (Rev. ed. of Hagan and Bruner's Infectious Diseases of Domestic Animals. 7th ed., 1981. 1st ed., 1943, by Hagan and Bruner.) (3d English ed. trans. to 2d Spanish ed. as Enfermedades Infecciosas de los Animales Domesticos. Mexico City; Prensa Medica Mexicana, 1961.)	
18	Blood, D. C., and Otto M. Radostits. Veterinary Medicine: A Textbook of the Diseases of Cattle, Sheep, Pigs, Goats and Horses. 7th ed. London and Philadelphia; Bailliere Tindall, 1989. 1502p. (Available in Spanish as Medicina Veterinaria. 5th ed. Bogota; Interamericana, 1982.)	14–17
19–20	Hall, Harold T. B. Diseases and Parasites of Livestock in the Tropics. 2d ed. London and New York; Longman, 1985. 328p. (1st ed., 1977. 288p.)	
19–20	Haresign, William, and D. J. A. Cole, eds. Recent Advances in Animal Nutrition, 1991. London; Butterworth-Heinemann, 1991. 255p. (W. Haresign and Dyfed Lewis, eds., 1964–1984.)	
	Loosli, John K., Victor A. Oyenuga, and Gabriel M. Babatunde, eds. Animal Production in the Tropics; Proceedings of an International Symposium . . . Ibadan; Published for the Dept. of Animal Science, University of Ibadan, Nigeria by Heinemann Educational Books, 1974. 402p.	3
	Devendra, C., and Marca Burns, eds. Goat Production in the Tropics. 2d ed. Farnham Royal, U.K.; Commonwealth Agricultural Bureaux, 1983. 183p. (1st ed., 1970. 184p.) (CAB Bureau of Animal Breeding & Genetics Technical Communication no. 19)	9–10
	McDowell, R. E. Improvement of Livestock Production in Warm Climates. San Francisco; W. H. Freeman, 1972. 711p. (Available in Spanish as Bases Biologicas de la Produccion Animal en Zonas Tropicales. Trans. by Pedro Ducar Malvenda. Zaragoza; Acribia, 1975.)	9–10
	Church, David C., ed. The Ruminant Animal: Digestive Physiology and Nutrition. Englewood Cliffs, N.J.; Prentice-Hall, 1988. 564p. (Previously published as Digestive Physiology and Nutri-	12–13

Developed countries ranking		Third World ranking

tion of Ruminants. 2d ed., vol. I, 1969, 1976, and vol. II, 1971, 1979, O & B Books.)

Mason, I. L. A World Dictionary of Livestock Breeds, Types and Varieties. 3d ed. Wallingford, Oxon, U.K.; CAB International, 1988. 348p. (1st ed., 1951. 272p.) — 12–13

Hacker, J. B., ed. Nutritional Limits to Animal Production from Pastures; Proceedings of an International Symposium, St. Lucia, Queensland, Australia, August 1981. Farnham Royal, U.K.; Commonwealth Agricultural Bureaux, 1982. 536p. — 14–17

Underwood, Eric J. Trace Elements in Human and Animal Nutrition. 4th ed. New York; Academic Press, 1977. 595p. (1st ed., 1956. 430p.) — 14–17

Butterworth, M. H. Beef Cattle Nutrition and Tropical Pastures. London and New York; Longmans, 1985. 500p. — 18

Kleiber, Max. The Fire of Life; An Introduction to Animal Energetics. Rev. ed. Huntington, N.Y.; R. E. Krieger Pub. Co., 1975. 453p. (1st ed., Wiley, 1961. 454p.) (Available in Spanish as Bioenergetica Animal. Zaragoza; Acribia, 1973.) — 19–20

Of the twenty-nine monographs in this composite list, only six had not been published before in variant titles or editions. In fact, seven of the twenty-nine were second editions, and the remaining sixteen ranged from the third edition through the twenty-second. These appear to be tried and lasting publications of great reputation and value. Seven of the twenty-nine are used extensively as textbooks while an additional half-dozen are used widely for supplemental classroom readings or as reference tools.

In these top twenty from developed and Third World countries, thirteen, or 45%, are currently published by commercial presses; ten, or 34.5%, are published by government agencies including the CAB International and the National Academy of Sciences (U.S.). The remaining six titles are equally published by Iowa State University Press and Comstock Publishing Associates, a unit of Cornell University Press. The six university press titles continue works begun years before which are now in second, sixth, eighth, ninth and tenth editions. The most remarkable book is Morrison's *Feeds and Feeding,* last published in 1956 in its twenty-second edition, and translated as recently as 1980 into Spanish. Morrison's association with the publication ended years ago, but the succeeding editors and authors kept it as Morrison's work.

Eleven of these titles were published or originated in England; the remainder bear U.S. imprints although one of these was published for the Department of Animal Science, University of Ibadan. Eleven of the titles have been translated into Spanish. The median age of the merged top twenty titles is 1984.5, or less than six years from the time this study was done. However, the range is great with one title from 1959, and five from the 1970s. One conclusion is that a title must be upgraded and issued in a new edition fairly often in animal science and health, or it will be quickly downgraded. One can probably also conclude that animal scientists tend to stick with tried and true literature and known names.

E. Nature of the Core Monograph Titles

Because the Third World titles included veterinary medicine and because of the differing orientation of Third World literature, there would be some logic in assuming differing publication patterns. Even with half the titles (47.7%) appearing in one list only, the diversity of sources of publication and publishers is not great, as demonstated in Figure 5.3. Commercial presses issued half again as many titles in animal science and health for the developed and developing countries as the other types of publishers combined. Academic, Elsevier, and Butterworths ranked in that order in both groups. The top sixteen publishers which are identical in both groups accounted for 59.8% of all titles in the developed countries and 57.7% of the Third World titles. This demonstrates the strong influence of the 631 titles which are common to both groups. Iowa State was the most represented university press in both groups, in fact, nearly equal to its three closest competitors combined, Cambridge, Cornell and Oxford. Academic departments, institutes and experiment stations accounted for only 21–25% of all university publications.

Publications from governments or international governmental agencies constitute a sizable number of publications; greater in the Third World as might be expected. FAO and the U.S. government have thirty-four and thirty-five, respectively, in the developed countries listing, while they have fifty-two and thirty-one, respectively, in the Third World list. The Commonwealth Agricultural Bureau International ranks third in both cases with twenty-two and twenty-one publications. French government publications ranked fourth in the Third World publications. In all, twenty-two governments or international governmental agencies are publishers in the core list.

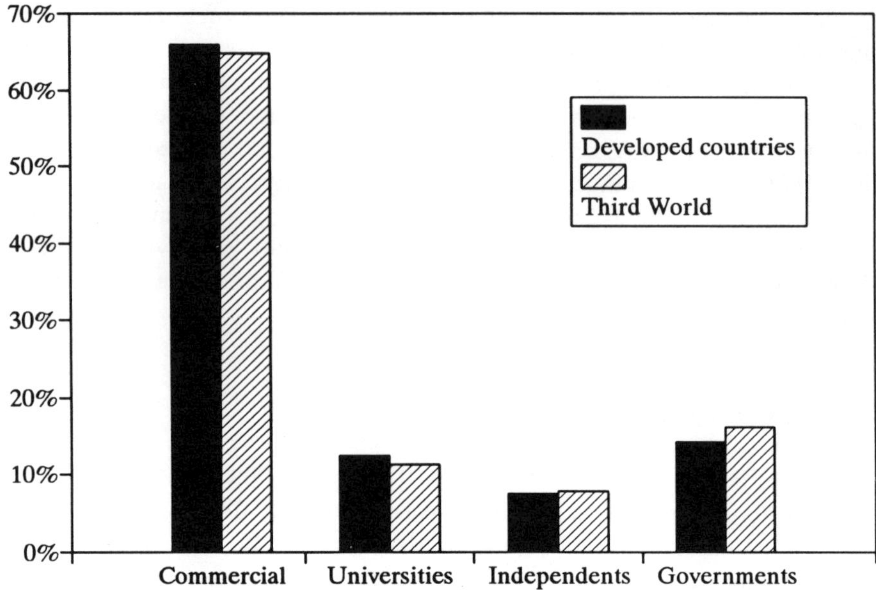

Figure 5.3. Types of publishers of core monographs.

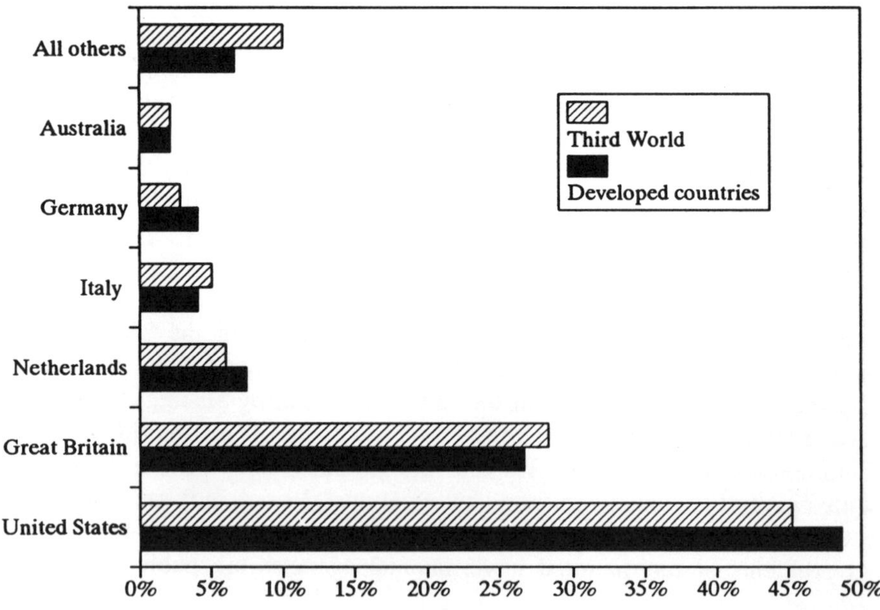

Figure 5.4. Place of publication of core monographs.

Table 5.2. Summary characteristics of core monographs

	Developed countries list N = 959	Third World countries list N = 1,033
Type of publisher		
Commercial press	65.9%	64.7%
Government (including FAO, UN)	14.0	16.1
University (press, department, institute)	12.4	11.3
Independent organization or society	7.7	7.9
Place of publication		
United States	48.9%	45.1%
United Kingdom	27.2	28.9
Netherlands	82.	6.1
Italy	4.9	5.1
Germany	4.8	3.1
Australia	2.5	2.5
Primary publisher		
Academic Press	6.8%	6.4%
Elsevier	5.2	4.2
Butterworths	4.0	3.6
Food and Agriculture Organization	3.7	4.9
U.S. Government	3.6	3.1
Iowa State University Press	2.7	2.9
Prentice-Hall	2.7	2.6
Non-English publications	1.8%	1.9%
Non-English publications and translations to English	4.6	2.6
Median age of publications	1982.8	1983.2

The independents in Figure 5.3 are societies, independent institutes, and international agricultural research centers. The top three publishers with this ranking in both groups are Winrock Institute, International Livestock Centre for Africa, and the British Poultry Society, although all of the independents have only seventy-one to eighty titles in the core listing.

Figure 5.4 indicates the country of publication for titles in the core monograph list. They have been divided by developed countries and Third World for purpose of comparison. Country was chosen on the basis of the first city or country mentioned in the imprint of the publication. Although many large publishers have offices on nearly every continent, the data reflects the origin of most of the publishcations since publishers tend to list the place of origination first.

The titles in the core monographic lists are characterized in Table 5.2.

F. Relationship of Core to Four Libraries

One of the purposes of these efforts is to determine the improvements that can be expected when the compact disks with full text are issued. To assist in these determinations, the Core Agricultural Literature Project asked four libraries to check the core monograph lists against their library collections. Two were chosen to contrast data from library collections in the developed world, and two provide data on strong collections in the Third World. The data are these:

N = 1,286 (both lists)	Owned	Earlier eds. only
University of California, Davis	94.4%	1.9%
South Australia Dept. of Agriculture Library, Adelaide	25.0	NA
Universiti Pertanian Malaysia, Selangor Darul Ehsan	57.3	6.8
Universidad Nacional Autonoma de México, Facultad de Medicina Veterinaria y Zootecnia	31.4	19.1

"Earlier editions" indicates that although the title was counted as being on the campus, only an earlier edition was available. This tends to show lack of currency. It can be argued that a third edition is probably nearly as valuable as a fifth edition by the same author and with the same title. It must also be noted that the 1,286 titles searched were to all of the titles determined as core for both the developed countries and the Third World. Therefore, it is somewhat illogical to expect a larger registration than 31.4% from the UNAM. UNAM had 341 of the 1,030 Third World titles, or 33.1%, slightly higher than for the total list. Of all the titles owned by UNAM, 12.6% were to Spanish titles only, a very logical conclusion in a Spanish language educational institution.

Of the seventy-two titles not owned by the University of California, Davis, libraries, twenty-five were Third World titles only, which they might logically not need or own. The number of missing developed world titles only were about an equal number, nineteen. The University of California, Davis, depends on the resources of its other campuses to some degree; when these other campus holdings were included, the total coverage in the university libraries was 99.8%. However, these works were ninety to 400 miles away.

Mann Library (Agriculture) and Flower Library (Veterinary Medicine), both on the Cornell University campus, own 97.7% of the titles, and only 0.5% of these are older editions.

6. Primary Journals and the Core List

WALLACE C. OLSEN

Mann Library, Cornell University

Quantitative studies during the past twenty years concerned with the journal literature of animal science are not common. Most studies are concerned with listings of monograph and journals or examinations of very specific subjects within the field. These generally do not give much assistance today because the titles and their importance change, and many listings are not evaluative. However, there are two general sources which are helpful.[1]

Veterinary medicine offers some enlightenment, and because the Third World aspect of the listings in this and the preceding chapter includes veterinary science, one recent study has relevance. The title of the article refers to primary literature of veterinary science, but deals only with veterinary journals.[2] The author uses published reports and data coupled with questionnaires to reach his consensus. Data are provided on veterinary science journal half-life (7.5 years), methodologies and pa ameters, and a core list of fifteen journals for veterinary sciences of which nine are in the Core Journals for Developed and Third World Countries in section C of this chapter. These nine are long-standing journals basic to both animal science and health, and the veterinary sciences. Houston also provides interesting data about the growth of veterinary science journals from the early 1800s until 1980. The literature of this subject does not show an astounding growth, rather, "about 15% of the presently available veterinary science primary literature has become available in the past ten years."[3]

1. (a) Ann E. Kerker and Henry T. Murphy, compilers, *Comparative and Veterinary Medicine; A Guide to the Resource Literature* (Madison: University of Wisconsin, 1973). (b) Mike Gibb, *Keyguide to Information Sources in Veterinary Medicine* (London and New York: Mansell Pub., 1990).

2. W. Houston, "The Application of Bibliometrics to Veterinary Science Primary Literature," *IAALD Quarterly Bulletin* 28 (1) (1983): 6–13.

3. Ibid, p. 6.

A. Source Documents and Methodology

The nineteen monographs and twenty-five journal articles used as Source Documents for the citation analysis for monographs (compare Chapter 5) were also used to obtain data on journals, periodicals, serials and report series. The same methods, definitions, and caveats apply to the journal and serial data as outlined for monographs in section B of Chapter 5. All journals, annuals, and select serials cited in the Source Documents were recorded and tabulated by title and date of publication. In these cases, each time an article within a journal was cited, a count was made for the journal or serial title. This provided a count of each time a journal or serial was cited in the entire 25,533 citations analyzed.

Proceedings volumes listed as journals or serials require clarification. Of the numerous proceedings identified, approximately 65% were tallied and evaluated as monographs because they had distinctive titles, short term or non-continuous editors, or concentrated on a specialized aspect of some area of animal science and health. Proceedings volumes were counted as journals or serials when they represented the continuing deliberations of an organization or society, with no varying subject focus or title other than *Proceedings* or *Transactions*. An example is the *Proceedings of the Nutrition Society*, which runs consistently under the same title each year and includes technical papers on a variety of subjects as well as happenings at annual meetings and societal operations.

B. Literature Cited in Journals

Table 5.1 and Figure 5.1 (Chapter 5) indicate that 75% of the references in the analyzed documents were to journal articles. This is close to the 82.4% of journal items in the CABI database for animal science. Within the journal source documents analyzed, the percentage of journal literature cited went higher, to 81%. This is a rather dramatically higher ratio of journal to monograph citations when compared to two other subject areas analyzed and represented in Table 5.1, Chapter 5. In contemporary literature of a science field, any representation of journal literature under 75% is unusual. It appears that the journal animal science literature is on the same norm as that in most scientific fields.

Of the 25,533 citations resulting from analyses of the Sources of Citations (Chapter 5), 19,150 were to journals or serials. This immense database of journals included references to 696 distinct titles. The monographs alone yielded a scatter with 659 distinct titles; the distinct titles cited in the journals analyzed were nearly 100 fewer. This scatter pattern with 100 to 150 journals garnering nearly all the citations is common, particularly in an application science such as agriculture. The top 114 journals and proceedings accounted for 71% of all the citations to journals and serials. These 114 top titles are shown in the following list in order of descending numerical importance.

Citation Analysis Ranking on Top 114 Journals in Descending Order

1. Journal of Animal Science
   Journal of Dairy Science
   Poultry Science
   Animal Production
   Journal of Agricultural Science
   Journal of Nutrition
   British Journal of Nutrition
   Journal of Food Science
   Nutrition Abstract Review
10. Endocrinology
   British Poultry Science
   Journal of Reproduction and Fertility
   Australian Journal of Agricultural
     Research
   Veterinary Record
   Canadian Journal of Animal Science
   Biology of Reproduction
   Australian Journal of Exp. Agriculture
     and Animal Husbandry
   Nature
   Tropical Grasslands
20. American Journal of Physiology
   Biochemical Journal
   Journal of Endocrinology
   American Journal of Veterinary
     Research
   Journal of Biological Chemistry
   Proceedings of the Nutrition Society
   Science
   World Animal Review
   Journal of Agricultural Science
     (Cambridge)
   FED Proceedings
30. Journal of Science, Food and
     Agriculture
   Journal of the American Veterinary
     Medical Association

   Livestock Production Science
   Feedstuffs
   Animal Breeding Abstracts
   Journal of Dairy Research
   Australian Veterinary Journal
   Animal Production in Australia
   Avian Diseases
   Agricultural Systems
40. General and Comparative
     Endocrinology
   Journal of Physiology
   Archiv fur Tierernahrung
   Tropical Animal Health and Production
   Animal Feed Science and Technology
   Journal of Range Management
   Meat Science
   Proceedings of the National Academy
     of Sciences (U.S.)
   Journal of Heredity
   Journal of Food Technology
50. World Review of Animal Production
   Annales de Zootechnie
   World's Poultry Science
   Biochimica et Biophysica Acta
   Proceedings of the Society for
     Experimental Biology and Medicine
   Theriogenology
   British Veterinary Journal
   Rhodesian Journal of Agricultural
     Research
   American Society of Animal Science
     Meeting Abstracts
   East African Agricultural and Forestry
     Journal
60. Food Technology
   Applied Animal Ethology
   Acta Agriculturae Scandinavica

Agronomy Journal
Journal of the Australian Institute of
    Agricultural Science
Biometrics
Cornell Veterinarian
Revue d'Elevage et de Medecine
    Veterinaire des Pays Tropicaux
Journal of Agricultural and Food
    Chemistry
Genetics
70. Journal of Molecular Biology
Tropical Agriculturalist
Archives of Biochemistry and
    Biophysics
Proceedings of the New Zealand
    Society of Animal Production
Indian Veterinary Journal
Tropical Animal Production
Annual Report, Division of
    Agriculture, Rhodesia
Biophysical Journal
Journal of Cell Biology
American Journal of Anatomy
80. FAO Production Yearbook
Physiological Reviews
Transactions of the American Society
    of Agricultural Engineers
American Journal of Agricultural
    Economics
Avian Pathology
Journal of Applied Bacteriology
Journal of Lipid Research
Agronomia Tropical
Applied Environmental Microbiology

Archiv fur Geflugelkunde
90. Journal of Agricultural Research
Journal of the British Grassland
    Society
The Philippine Agriculturalist
South African Journal of Animal
    Science
Queensland Agricultural Journal
Tropical Agriculture (Trinidad) Food
    Research
Indian Journal of Animal Science
Acta Veterinaria Scandinavica
Anatomical Record
100. Developments in Biological
    Standardization
International Journal of
    Biometeorology
Malaysian Agriculturalist
Nutrition Reports International
Zeitschrift fur Tierpsychol.
Cereal Chemistry
Research Veterinary Science
Zeitschrift fur Tierzuchtung and
    Zuchtungsbiologie
Acta Endocrinologica
Comparative Biochemistry and
    Physiology
110. Genetical Research
Immunogenetics
Journal de la Recherches Porcines en
    France
Journal of Experimental Biology and
    Medicine
Prostaglandins

The significance of the top three journals is demonstrated in Figure 6.1.

Within the 114 journals there is considerable spread of literature in non-animal science titles. Two related areas show a concentration: science and general agriculture journals number twenty-three, and food science six. Within the more closely allied animal science subjects the specialities are:

Biology, biochemistry, and biophysics	17
Veterinary medicine, including physiology and anatomy	17
Nutrition, feedstuff, and crops	12
Breeding, genetics, and reproduction	8
Animal diseases	7

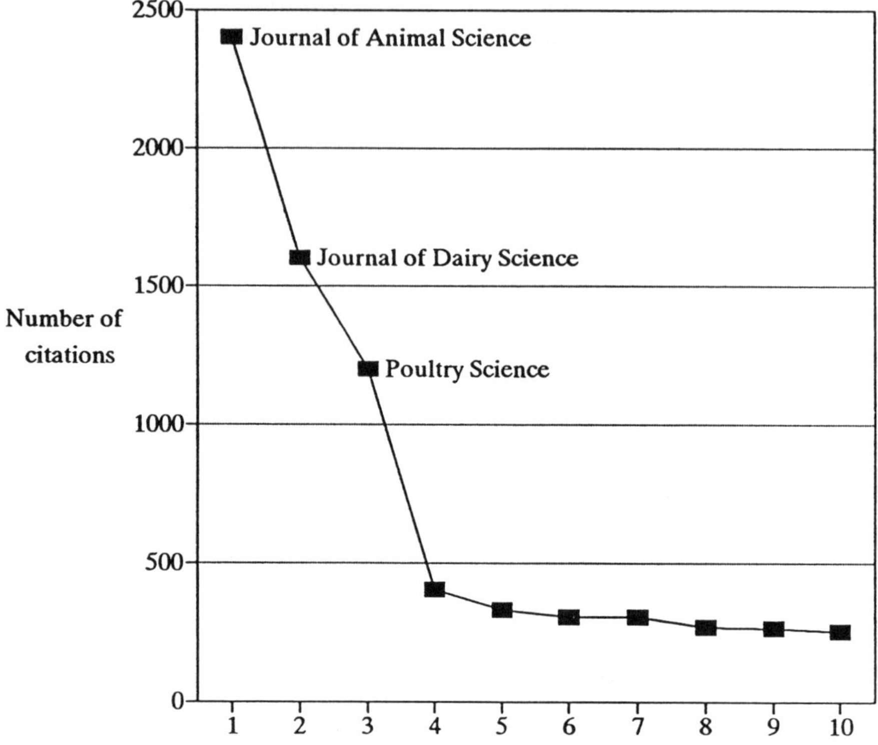

Figure 6.1. Distribution of top ten journals and serials.

Of course, the greatest number deal with animal science, its major species, and commodity areas. This scattering is more accentuated when all of the 659 titles are examined. The proportion of journals dealing with general agriculture, statistical compilations, food technology, and more extraneous subjects is far greater than with the 114 listed.

Table 6.1 provides indicators or rankings of the journals from different data and points of comparison. COLUMN 1 is the ranking in two groups of the composite numbers resulting from the citation analysis. This involves citations to the journal or serial from both the monographs and journals in the source documents. The ranking of the titles in the list is based on these numbers, which are numerically ranked to the left of the titles. In all of the columns, the rankings have been broken into two groups: A = top-ranked journals, B = those of lesser rank and statistically valid within that column. COLUMN 2 demonstrates the influence of the citations coming from jour-nals only, which accounted for 66% of the total journal citations in COL-

UMN 1. The influence of the journal source documents is provided in order to examine any possible skews. Journal citations with heavy rankings for journals tend to indicate a research-oriented journal. COLUMN 3 is a ranking of the total citations to these journals cited in specific Third World titles, of which there were ten monographs and two journal articles. COLUMN 4 covers the same titles as COLUMN 1, but ranked on the basis of the number of times cited by other publications, 1981 through 1988, in *Science Citation Index*.[4] The *SCI* indexes articles in approximately 5,000 journals as well as the number of times a journal is cited in any of those 5,000 journals. The citations in articles of each journal are totaled each year and provided in summary tables. The database indexes a quantity of animal science and health journals, thus providing more data than if one were examining economic or general agricultural journals. *SCI* does not have citing information which is statistically valid for all titles, for example, the *Proceedings of the Nutrition Society*, overall ranked twenty-six. Considering the scope of the titles included in the *SCI* database, it is rather surprising that only fifteen have inadequate data; this includes some titles which are deceased, such as USDA's *Journal of Agricultural Research*.

One aim of this study was to determine the animal science and health journals most valuable for Third World teaching and research. To accomplish this, a subset of monographs and journals articles which were written about or aimed at Third World animal science were analyzed. Ten of these source documents were monographs and two were journal articles. The rankings of these journals are shown in COLUMN 3 of Table 6.1.

From comparisons in Table 6.1, other observations, and data accumulated from other sources, these conclusions can be made:

(1) The Third World journals have a match of thirty-two of the total seventy-two statistically valid journals from the citation analysis for developed and Third World titles. This represents a 44% agreement. Only about half of the thirty-two have the same ranking in both Columns 1 and 3.

(2) Third World animal science literature has not gotten into the mainstream, or it is too site-specific to be cited by primary monographs and journals outside a country or region. This is demonstrated by citations to journals from only a few developing countries: India, Kenya, Rhodesia, and Trinidad. Of great interest is the fact that so many Australian journals are heavily cited in Third World literature. There are four Australian-published journals in this category. Most Third World journals group around the word "tropical."

(3) As a corollary, the journal literature in animal science from the Third World is

4. *Science Citation Index Citation Report*. Ranking was on the average of the sums of eight years for each title, 1981–1988.

Table 6.1. Top journals cited by rank

Rank	Journal title	1	2	3	4
1	Journal of Animal Science	A	A	A	A
2	Journal of Dairy Science	A	A	A	A
3	Poultry Science	A	A	A	A
4	Animal Production	A	A	A	B
5	Journal of Agricultural Science	A	A	A	—
6	Journal of Nutrition	A	A	—	A
7	British Journal of Nutrition	A	A	A	B
8	Journal of Food Science	A	—	—	A
9	Nutrition Abstract Review	A	—	B	—
10	Endocrinology	A	A	—	B
11	Journal of Reproduction and Fertility	A	A	B	A
12	British Poultry Science	A	—	B	B
13	Australian Journal of Agricultural Research	A	B	A	B
14	Veterinary Record	A	A	A	A
15	Canadian Journal of Animal Science	A	B	B	B
16	Biology of Reproduction	A	A	—	A
17	Australian Journal of Experimental Agriculture and Animal Husbandry	A	—	A	B
18	Nature	A	B	B	A
19	Tropical Grasslands	A	—	A	B
20	American Journal of Physiology	A	B	—	B
21	Biochemical Journal	A	B	—	A
22	Journal of Endocrinology	A	A	—	A
23	American Journal of Veterinary Research	A	A	B	A
24	Science	A	A	—	A
25	Journal of Biological Chemistry	A	B	—	A
26	Proceedings of the Nutrition Society	A	B	—	—
27	World Animal Review	A	B	A	B
28	Journal of Agricultural Science (Cambridge)	A	B	A	B
29	FED Proceedings	B	B	—	—
30	Journal of Science, Food and Agriculture	B	—	—	B
31	Journal of the American Veterinary Medical Association	B	B	—	A
32	Livestock Production Science	B	B	—	B
33	Feedstuffs	B	—	—	—
34	Journal of Dairy Research	B	B	—	B
35–36	Australian Veterinary Journal	B	—	A	B
35–36	Proceedings of the Australian Society of Animal Production	B	—	A	—
37	Avian Diseases	B	—	—	B
38	Agricultural Systems	B	—	B	B
39	General and Comparative Endocrinology	B	B	—	A
40–41	Journal of Physiology	B	—	—	A
40–41	Tropical Animal Health and Production	B	—	A	B
42	Archiv fur Tierernahrung	B	—	A	B
43	Animal Feed Science and Technology	B	—	—	B
44–45	Journal of Range Management	B	—	A	B
44–45	Meat Science	B	—	—	B
46	Proceedings of the National Academy of Sciences	B	B	—	—

47	Journal of Heredity	B	—	—	B
48	Journal of Food Technology	B	—	—	B
49	World Review of Animal Production	B	—	A	—
50	Annales de Zootechnie	B	—	—	B
51	World's Poultry Science	B	—	—	B
52–54	Biochimica et Biophysica Acta	B	—	—	B
52–54	Proceedings of the Society for Experimental Biology and Medicine	B	B	—	—
52–54	Theriogenology	B	B	—	B
55	Animal Breeding Abstracts	B	B	—	—
56–57	Rhodesian Journal of Agricultural Research	B	—	A	—
56–57	British Veterinary Journal	B	—	—	B
58–59	East African Agricultural and Forestry Journal	B	—	B	—
58–59	Food Technology	B	—	—	B
60	Applied Animal Ethology	B	B	—	—
61–63	Acta Agriculturae Scandinavica	B	—	—	B
61–63	Agronomy Journal	B	—	B	A
61–63	Journal of the Australian Institute of Agricultural Science	B	—	B	B
64	East African Journal of Agriculture	B	—	B	—
65–67	Biometrics	B	B	—	B
65–67	Cornell Veterinarian	B	B	—	B
65–67	Revue d'Elevage et de Medecine Veterinaire des Pays Tropicaux	B	—	B	—
68	Journal of Agricultural and Food Chemistry	B	—	—	A
69	Genetics	B	B	—	A
70–72	Archives of Biochemistry and Biophysics	B	—	—	B
70–72	Journal of Molecular Biology	B	—	—	A
70–72	Tropical Agriculture (Trinidad)	B	—	B	B

heavily in non-animal science journals which tend to be general agricultural journals. This is probably a logical pattern of development.

The literature also indicates that many Third World authors who wish to be recognized as good scientists within the mainstream of animal science publish outside their home countries. This intermixing of Third World and developed countries literature in international journals may stymie quality animal science publication in the Third World for some time. The most active subjects of Third World journal literature seem to be animal diseases, veterinary medicine, and feeding.

Other bibliometric studies of publication patterns suggest that the majority of Third World researchers continue to publish in national journals, because of the difficulties of publishing in a foreign language and meeting the editorial standards of international journals.[5] The abstracting services of in-

5. J. M. Russell and C. S. Galina, "Research and Publishing Trends in Cattle Reproduction in the Tropics: Part 2. A Third World Prerogative," *Animal Breeding Abstracts* 55 (11) (Nov. 1987): 819–826.

ternational and regional databases make Third World research literature more accessible to a wider audience, although the problem of translation remains.

C. Current Core Journal List

This recommended core list does not match the top 114 titles listed earlier. The primary reason for dropping a title is that it is no longer published. Table 6.1 ranks by the number of citations to the journal from literature published over a twenty-five-year period, the latest being 1990. The following list identifies and ranks those journals or serials currently published which constitute the core today. Each list has been divided into top ranked title (1) and second-ranked (2).

Core Journals for Developed and Third World Countries

	Developed countries	Third World
Acta Agriculturae Scandinavica. Vol. 1. (1950)+. Copenhagen, Munksgaard; Official journal of the Scandinavian Association of Agricultural Scientists and the Royal Swedish Academy of Agriculture and Forestry. In 1992 available in Pt. A, Animal Science and Pt. B, Soil and Plant Science. Each part has 4 issues/year.	2	—
Agricultural Systems. Vol. 1. (Jan. 1976)+. Barking, Eng.; Elsevier Applied Science. Monthly.	2	2
Agronomy Journal. Vol. 1. (1907/09)+. Madison, Wis.; American Society of Agronomy. 6 issues/yr. (Proceedings of the American Society of Agronomy, 1907–12; Journal of the American Society of Agronomy, 1913–48.)	—	2
American Journal of Physiology. Vol. 1. (Jan. 1898)+. Bethesda, Md.; American Physiological Society. Bimonthly.	1	—
American Journal of Veterinary Research. Vol. 1. (Oct. 1940)+. Chicago; American Veterinary Medical Association. Monthly.	1	2
Animal Feed Science and Technology. Vol. 1. (April 1976)+. Amsterdam; Elsevier Scientific. Quarterly.	2	—
Animal Production. Vol. 1. (Mar. 1959)+. British Society of Animal Production. Bimonthly.	1	1
Animal Production in Australia: Proceedings of the Australian Society of Animal Production. Vol. 13. (1980)+. Australia; Pergamon Press. Annual. (Continues Proceedings of the Australian Society of Animal Production, 1956–1978.)	—	1

	Developed countries	Third World
Archiv fur Tierernahrung. Vol. 1. (July/Aug. 1950)+. Berlin; Akademie Verlag. (Parallel title: Archives of Animal Nutrition, Vol. 30—.) Irregular.	—	2
Archives of Biochemistry and Biophysics. Vol. 31. (Mar. 1951)+. New York; Academic Press. 14 nos./year. (Continues Archives of Biochemistry.)	2	—
Australian Journal of Agricultural Research. Vol. 1. (Jan. 1950)+. Melbourne; Commonwealth Scientific and Industrial Research Organization. Bimonthly, 1974—.	2	1
Australian Journal of Experimental Agriculture. Vol. 25 (1985)+. East Melbourne; Commonwealth Scientific and Industrial Research Organization. 5 nos./year. (Continues Australian Journal of Experimental Agriculture and Animal Husbandry.)	—	1
Australian Veterinary Journal. Vol. 1. (Mar. 1925)+. Brunswick, Victoria; Australian Veterinary Association. Monthly. (Vol. 1–2, 1925–26 as the Association's Journal.)	2	1
Avian Diseases. Vol. 1. (May 1957)+. Kennett Square, Pa.; American Association of Avian Pathologists. 5 nos./year.	2	—
Biochemical Journal. Vol. 1. (Jan. 1906)+. London; The Biochemical Journal. Monthly, 1935—. For 1973–83 odd and even numbered vols.	1	—
Biology of Reproduction. Vol. 1. (April 1969)+. Champaign, Ill.; Society for the Study of Reproduction. Monthly (except Jan. and July), June 1976—.	1	—
British Journal of Nutrition. Vol. 1. (Sept. 1947)+. Cambridge and New York; Cambridge University Press for the Nutrition Society. Bimonthly.	1	1
British Poultry Science. Vol. 1. (April 1960)+. Edinburgh; Longmans. Bimonthly.	1	2
British Veterinary Journal. An Anglo-American Monthly Review of Veterinary Science. Vol. 105. (1949)+. London; Balliere Tindall. Monthly. (Continues Veterinary Journal.)	2	—
Canadian Journal of Animal Science. Vol. 37. (June 1957)+. Ottawa; Agricultural Institute of Canada. Quarterly, 1972—. (Continues Canadian Journal of Agricultural Science.)	1	2
East African Agricultural and Forestry Journal. Vol. 26. (July 1960)+. Nairobi, Kenya; East African Agriculture and Forestry Research Organization. Quarterly, 1940/41—. Continues East African Agricultural Journal of Kenya, Tanganyika, Uganda and Zanzibar. Vol. 1–25. (July 1935–April 1960).	—	2
Endocrinology. Vol. 1. (1917)+. Philadelphia; Published for the Endocrine Society by J. B. Lippincott. Biannual.	1	—
Feedstuffs. Vol. 1. (May 1929)+. Minneapolis; Miller Pub.	2	—

	Developed countries	Third World
Co. Weekly (except semiweekly during third week of Sept.).		
Food Technology. Vol. 1. (Jan. 1947)+. Chicago; Institute of Food Technologists. Monthly.	2	—
General and Comparative Endocrinology. Vol. 1. (Apr. 1961)+. New York; Academic Press. Bimonthly.	2	—
Genetics. Vol. 1. (1916)+. Austin, Tex.; Genetics Society of America. Monthly.	2	—
Indian Veterinary Journal. Vol. 1. (1924)+. Madras; Indian Veterinary Association. Biannual.	—	2
International Journal of Food Science and Technology. Vol. 22. (1987)+. Oxford, Eng.; Blackwell Scientific for the Institute of Food Science and Technology (U.K). Bimonthly. (Supersedes Journal of Food Technology.)	2	—
Journal of Agricultural Science (Cambridge). Vol. 1. (1905/06)+. Cambridge; Cambridge University Press. Bimonthly.	2	1
Journal of Agricultural and Food Chemistry. Vol. 1. (April 1953)+. Washington, D.C.; American Chemical Society. Bimonthly, 1960—.	2	—
Journal of Animal Science. Vol. 1. (Feb. 1942)+. Champaign, Ill.; American Society of Animal Science. Monthly, Dec. 1975—.	1	1
Journal of Biological Chemistry. Vol. 1. (Oct. 1905)+. Baltimore; American Society of Biological Chemists. 3 times/month.	1	—
Journal of Dairy Research. Vol. 1. (Nov. 1929)+. Cambridge; Cambridge University Press. Irregular.	2	—
Journal of Dairy Science. Vol. 1. (May 1917)+. Champaign, Ill.; American Dairy Science Association. Monthly, 1934—.	1	1
Journal of Endocrinology. Vol. 1. (June 1939)+. Bristol, Eng.; Journal of Endocrinology. Monthly.	1	—
Journal of Food Science. Vol. 26. (1961)+. Chicago; Institute of Food Technologists. Bimonthly. (Continues Food Research, 1936–60.)	1	—
Journal of Heredity. Vol. 1. (1910)+. New York; Oxford University Press for the American Genetic Association. Bimonthly. (Continues American Breeder's Magazine.)	2	—
Journal of Molecular Biology. Vol. 1. (April 1959)+. London; Academic Press. Twice/month.	2	—
Journal of Nutrition. Vol. 1 (Sept. 1928)+. Bethesda, Md.; American Institute of Nutrition. Monthly.	1	—
Journal of Physiology. Vol. 1. (1878/79)+. London; Cambridge University Press for the Physiological Society. Thirteen times/year.	2	—

	Developed countries	Third World
Journal of Range Management. Vol. 1. (Oct. 1948)+. Denver, Colo.; American Society of Range Management. Bimonthly.	—	1
Journal of Reproduction and Fertility, and its Supplement. Vol. 1. (Feb. 1960)+. Cambridge; Journal of Reproduction and Fertility. Bimonthly, 1962—.	1	2
Journal of the Science of Food and Agriculture. Vol. 1. (1950)+. London; Blackwell Scientific. Sponsored by Society of Chemical Industry. 12 issues/year in 3 vols.	2	—
Journal of the American Veterinary Medical Association. Vol. 48. (Oct. 1915)+. Chicago; American Veterinary Medical Association. Monthly. (Continues American Veterinary Review, 1877–1915.)	2	—
Livestock Production Science. Vol. 1. (1974)+. Amsterdam; Elsevier Scientific. Quarterly. (Official journal of the European Association for Animal Production.)	2	—
Meat Science. Vol. 1. (Jan. 1977)+. Barking, Essex; Elsevier Applied Science. Quarterly.	2	—
Nature. Vol. 229. (Jan. 1971)+. London; Macmillan Magazines. Weekly.	1	2
Nutrition Abstracts and Reviews, B; Livestock Feeds and Feeding. Vol. 47. (Jan. 1977)+. Farnham Royal; Commonwealth Agricultural Bureaux. Monthly. (Continues Nutrition Abstracts and Review, 1931–1976.)	—	2
Poultry Science. Vol. 1. (Oct. 1921)+. Champaign, Ill.; Poultry Science Association. Monthly. (Supersedes American Association of Instructors and Investigators in Poultry Husbandry. Journal.)	1	1
Proceedings of the National Academy of Sciences (U.S.). Vol. 1. (Jan. 1915)+. Washington, D.C.; National Academy of Sciences. Biweekly.	2	—
Proceedings of the Nutrition Society. Vol. 1. (1944)+. Cambridge; Cambridge University Press for the Nutrition Society. 3 issues/year.	1	—
Proceedings of the Society for Experimental Biology and Medicine. Vol 1. (1903/04)+. New York; Academic Press. Monthly, except Aug.	2	—
Revue d'Elevage et de Medecine Veterinaire des Pays Tropicaux. Vol. 1. (Jan./Mar. 1947)+. Paris; Vigot Freres for Institut d'Elevage et de Medecine Veterinaire des Pays Tropicaux. Quarterly. (Supersedes Recueil de Medecine Veterinaire Exotique.)	—	2
Science. Vol. 1. (Jan. 1895)+. Washington, D.C.; American Association for the Advancement of Science. Weekly, except last week in Dec.	1	—
South African Journal of Animal Science; Proceedings of the	—	2

	Developed countries	Third World
South African Society of Animal Production. Vol. 1. (1971)+. Pretoria; South African Society of Animal Production. 2 nos./year.		
Theriogenology; An International Journal of Animal Reproduction. Vol. 1. (Jan. 1974)+. Los Altos, Calif.; Geron-X. Monthly.	2	—
Tropical Agriculture. Vol. 1. (Jan. 1924)+. Surrey, Eng.; IPC Science & Technology Press for the Imperial College of Tropical Agriculture (Trinidad and Tobago). Quarterly.	—	2
Tropical Animal Health and Production. Vol. 1. (Aug. 1969)+. Edinburgh; Scottish Academic Press for University of Edinburgh. Quarterly.	—	1
Tropical Grasslands. Vol. 1. (May 1967)+. Brisbane; Tropical Grassland Society of Australia. 3 nos./year.	—	1
Veterinary Record. Vol. 1. (1888/89)+. London; British Veterinary Association. Weekly. (Supersedes Veterinary Record and Transactions of the Veterinary Medical Association.)	1	1
World Animal Review. Vol. 1. (1972)+. Rome; Food and Agriculture Organization. Quarterly.	—	1
World Review of Animal Production. Vol. 1. (1965)+. Lugano; International Pub. Enterprises for the World Association for Animal Production. Quarterly.	—	1
World's Poultry Science Journal. Vol. 1. (Spring 1945)+. London; Butterworths for the World's Poultry Science Association. Quarterly.	2	—
Zimbabwe Journal of Agricultural Research. Vol. 18 (1980)+. Salisbury; R. & S. S. Information Services, Dept. of Research and Specialist Services, Ministry of Agriculture. Biannual. (Continues Rhodesian Journal of Agricultural Research, 1963–1979.)	—	1

These points must be noted about the Core list of journals.

(1) The Core list is not a match of the overall rankings in Table 6.1, left side of the table, or any other columns. Additional influences had to be incorporated, such as the inordinate weight caused by research journals, lack of substantive data to make correlations between the developed countries and the Third World, shifts in subject coverage in the last decade, and reactions of collaborating educators in the field. Influential titles which have not been published for five years were not included as core. The five to ten years of active journal life for many titles seem to make this a moot consideration.

(2) A total of sixty-one journals are identified as core for the two combined groups. Fourteen of these, which constitute the most valuable core to both communities, are only 23% of all the titles. An additional sixteen titles are identified as core for the Third World but not for developed countries. It must be empha-

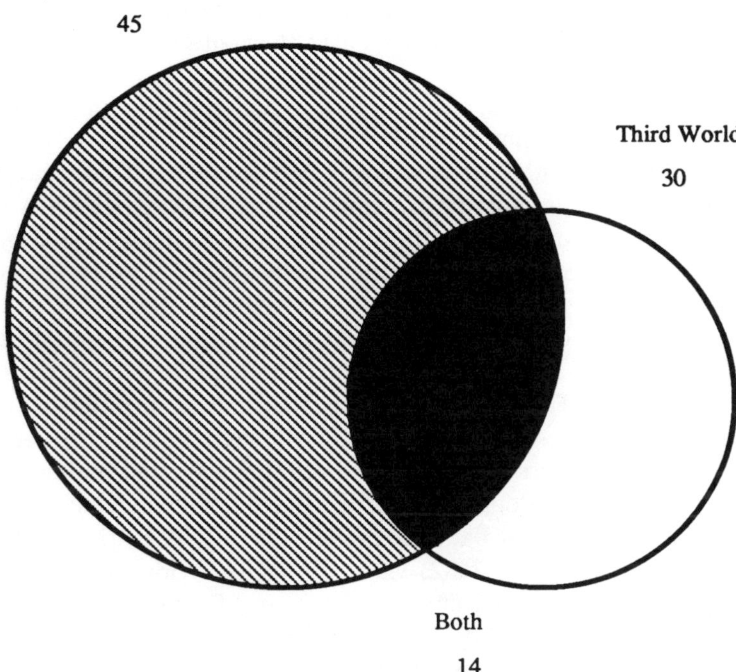

Figure 6.2. Influence and commonality of journals.

sized that the literature of animal science and health in developing countries is relatively site-specific, small in quantity, and dispersed in several formats, especially reports. The small number of fourteen journals valuable to both communities should not be surprising.

(3) The subject areas of the fourteen common journals demonstrate a rather limited scope of animal science and health:

Animal production and science	5 titles
General agriculture	4
Diseases and veterinary medicine	3
Nutrition	1
Reproduction	1

The subject breakdown for all sixty-one journals is:

Animal science and production	20 titles
General agriculture, and science	15
Biology, biochemistry, and biophysics	8
Nutrition, feedstuff, and crops	7
Veterinary medicine and diseases	7
Breeding, genetics, and reproduction	5

These show a remarkably close mask of each other although the sixty-one give a much more balanced representation of the total field.

(4) The influence of Australian publications should be noted for both the Third
World and the developed countries. This strong showing is remarkable and
appears to be a reflection of a national interest and investment.

Figure 6.2 is a Venn diagram of Third World and developed countries
journals showing the common core of fourteen.

The sixty-four core titles are completely indexed by CAB International in
one or more of its abstracting or indexing services. The AGRICOLA file of
the National Agricultural Library fully indexes thirty-eight of the sixty-four
cover to cover, and an additional thirteen selectively. Thirteen are not indexed in any way.[6]

The first known journal concerned with animal science to appear only in
electronic form was announced in 1991 and entitled *Livestock Research for
Rural Development*. The journal was launched because of problems in disseminating livestock research information. Although the principal language
is English, papers are also accepted in French, Spanish, and Portugese. The
journal is distributed on floppy disk for IBM-compatible microcomputers by
Convenio Interinstitucional para las Produccion Agropecuaria en el Valle
del Cauca, Apartado Aéro 7482, Calí, Colombia. Wide distribution was
made of 1300 disks to African, Caribbean and Pacific countries of the
Lomé Convention sponsored by Technical Centre for Agricultural and Rural
Cooperation (CTA), Ede, Netherlands.

Phenomena in agricultural research in the Third World are the networking arrangements among scientists in specific disciplines or commodities
such as peanuts, soil management, and selective dissemination of information. These prospered in the 1970s and 1980s and are widespread, often
organized by the international agricultural research centers, members of the
Consultative Group on International Agricultural Research (CGIAR). *International Agricultural Research: A Database of Networks* lists over sixty-
five of these informal networks.[7] They are important because they tie researchers together, and most issue newsletters or proceedings of value.
These relate to animal science:

African Livestock Policy Analysis Network (ALPAN), begun 1985, issues *ALPAN
    Network Paper*.
African Network on Rural Poultry Development, begun 1985, issues a newsletter.

6. Data taken from *List of Journals Indexed in AGRICOLA, 1991*, compiled and edited by
Carol L. Dowling and Thor Lehnert (Beltsville, Md.: National Agricultural Library, 1991).

7. Donald L. Plucknett, Nigel J. H. Smith, and Selcuk Ozgediz, *International Agricultural
Research: A Database of Networks* (Washington, D.C.: The World Bank, 1990 [*CGIAR Study
Paper* no. 26]). A detailed book on this topic was written by the same authors and published by
Cornell University Press in 1990 as *Networking in International Agricultural Research*.

Animal Traction Research Network, begun 1988, issues a newsletter.

Cattle Milk and Meat Network, begun 1988, issues occasional proceedings volumes.

Collaborative Research Support Program—Pond Dynamics, begun 1982.

Forage Network in Ethiopia, begun 1983, issues a newsletter.

International Center for Living Aquatic Resources Management, begun 1977, issues newsletter and proceedings.

Pasture Network for Eastern and Southern Africa, begun 1984, issues *PANESA Newsletter*.

Rede de Investigaccion en Sistemas de Produccion Animal en Latinoamerica—Latin American Research Network for Animal Production Systems, formally established 1986, issues *Carta de RISPAL*, proceedings and workshop volumes.

Small Ruminant and Camel Group Research Network, begun 1986; issues a newsletter.

South East Asia/Pacific Forage Research and Development Program, begun 1986, issues *Forage Research Newsletter*.

Trypanotolerant Livestock Network, begun 1983, issues occasional manuals, proceedings, and evaluative studies.

All but five of these networks and programs are coordinated at the International Livestock Centre for Africa (ILCA) in Addis Ababa, Ethiopia. The networks are subject to budget changes, disbanding, or reorganization which does not favor continuity of effort.

The International Livestock Centre for Africa (ILCA) has a very active documentation and library program, as noted in Chapter 2. The librarians at ILCA maintain a large, interactive database with all of the citations from their microfilming project, plus references to journal articles pertinent to African animal science from major journals around the world, especially those published in Africa. ILCA recently surveyed its scientific staff concerning the 603 journals to which the library subscribes. Exclusive of three currently popular computer journals, the most important journals were ranked in this order:

1. *Animal Production*
2. *New Scientist*
3. *Journal of Animal Science*
4. *Journal of Dairy Science*
5. *Tropical Animal Health and Production*
6. *Livestock Production Science*
7. *Indian Journal of Animal Science*

The bibliographic database (ILCABIB) created by the Centre for its use includes references to articles in journals with emphases on application in

Africa. The numbers of records in the databases were counted for primary journals, a process which provided this ranking for the top twelve:

1. *Journal of Animal Science*
2. *Journal of Dairy Science*
3. *Revue d'Elevage et de Medecine Veterinaire*
4. *Animal Production*
5. *East African Agricultural and Forestry Journal*
6. *Indian Journal of Animal Science*
7. *Veterinary Record*
8. *Tropical Animal Health and Production*
9. *Journal of Range Management*
10. *Australian Journal of Agricultural Research*
11. *Sudan Journal of Veterinary Science & Animal Husbandry*
12. *South African Journal of Animal Science*

This is a ranking by number of citations for each in the database. The *Journal of Animal Science* has nearly twice the number of entries as the second journal.[8]

ILCA announced publication of a quarterly journal, *African Livestock Research*, in 1992 which is available free of charge to libraries of national agricultural research systems within Africa, while other libraries must pay U.S. $120. This will probably be a very important animal science journal for the Third World.

A study of the use of journals by veterinary practicioners and researchers in a Third World country is of interest.[9] Citations in the published works (1971–1980) of the scientists of the National Veterinary Research Institute, Vom, Nigeria were examined to determine which journals were most heavily cited. Of the 754 citations in the study, 85% were to journal articles. The top ten journals provided 39% of the citations to the journal literature. Nigerian journals did not register well. Of the top twenty journal cited, nine were from the United Kingdom, eight from the United States and one each from Australia, India and Kenya. Fourteen of these nineteen extant journals are in the *Core Journals for Developed and Third World Countries* in Section C of this chapter. The research and application work of the Nigerian institute appears to be a close match with the general animal science and health activites, and literature citings in the Third World.

Ikpaahindi comments that the age of the core journals and their status might explain the poor performance of Nigerian journal titles.[10] The death

8. Personal communication from Sirak Teklu, ILCA librarian, Nov. 1992.

9. L. N. Ikpaahindi, "Journal Use by Nigerian Veterinary Practitioners: The National Veterinary Research Institute," *IAALD Quarterly Bulletin* 27 (4): 116–120.

10. Ibid, p. 117.

rate of journals in many developing countries is very high. Another scholar comments on Nigerian science and technology journals: "Outright mortality rate of Nigerian journals is high and this is vexing. It is, however, an economic issue."[11] The Nigerian experiences are replicated in many countries and tend to force a quantity of Third World literature into the international literature arena.

D. New Journals

Citation analysis was used to identify the core journals listed in Section C. These analysis procedures do not record information on very recent titles since they have not been around long enough to have been cited. Therefore, very recent journal titles often do not make a core list. The major journals which began publication in 1980 or after are listed here for information. This is a selective list of the more substantive or influential journals excluding many less scholarly publications such as newsletters. Titles which have only slightly changed title are not listed, nor are veterinary titles.

Animal Science and Health Scholarly Journals Begun 1980+

Advances in Meat Research. Vol. 1. (1985)+. Westport, Conn.; Avi Pub. Co. Annual.

Animal and Human Health. Vol. 1, no. 1. (1988)+. New York; Animal and Human Health, Inc. Quarterly.

Animal Biotechnology. Vol. 1, no. 1. (1990)+. New York; M. Dekker. Semiannual.

Animal Husbandry and Breeding. Vol. 1. (1986)+. Athens, Greece; Agrotechnical Pub.

Annual Review of Fish Diseases. Vol. 1. (1991)+. New York; Pergamon Press. Annnual.

Cahiers d'Ethologie Appliquée. Vol. 1, no. 1. (1981)+. Liege, Belgium; Service d'Ethologie Institute de Zoologie de l'Université. Quarterly.

Coastal Aquaculture. Vol. 1. (1984)+. College Station; Texas Agricultural Extension Service. Biannual.

Critical Reviews in Poultry Biology. Vol. 1, issue 1. (1987)+. Boca Raton, Fla.; CRC Press. Quarterly.

Current Concepts of Animal Growth. Vol. 1. (1985)+. Champaign, Ill.; American Society of Animal Science.

11. I. Adamson, "Access and Retrieval of Information as Coordinates of Scientific Development and Achievement in Nigeria," *Scientometrics* 23 (1) (1992): 191–199.

Domestic Animal Endocrinology. Vol. 1, no. 1. (Jan. 1984)+. Auburn, Ala.; Domendo, Inc. Quarterly.

Experimental and Applied Acarology. Vol. 1, no. 1. (Mar 1985)+. Amsterdam and New York; Elsevier. Quarterly.

Fish Physiology and Biochemistry. Vol. 1, no. 1. (Jan. 1986)+. Amsterdam and Berkeley; Kugler. 6 nos./year.

Genomics. Vol. 1. (1987)+. San Diego, Calif.; Academic Press. 8 issues/year, in 2 vols.

International Dairy Journal. Vol. 1. (1991)+. Amsterdam; Published in association with the International Dairy Federation by Elsevier Applied Science. Quarterly.

Investigacion Agraria, Producción y Sanidad animales. Vol. 1. (1986)+. Madrid; Instituto Nacional de Investigaciones Agrarias. 3 issues/year.

Journal of Animal Production Research. Vol. 1. (1981)+. Zaria, Nigeria; National Animal Production Research Institute. Semiannual. Ahmadu Bello University.

Journal of Applied Aquaculture. Vol. 1. (1991)+. Binghamton, N.Y.; Food Products Press. Quarterly.

The Journal of Applied Poultry Research. Vol. 1. (1992)+. Athens, Ga.; Journal of Applied Poultry Research. 4 nos./year.

Journal of Aquatic Animal Health. Vol. 1. (1989)+. Bethesda, Md.; American Fisheries Society. Quarterly.

Misset World Poultry. Vol. 6, no. 4. (Aug./Sept. 1991)+. Doetinchem, Netherlands; Misset International. 6 issues/year. (Continues Poultry, 1984–1990.)

National Cattlemen. Vol. 1. (1985)+. Englewood, Colo.; National Cattlemen's Association. Monthly.

Ontario Swine Research Review. Vol. 1. (1985)+. Guelph, Ontario; Ontario Agricultural College, University of Guelph. Annual.

Pigs. Vol. 1. (Oct. 1984)+. Doetinchem, Netherlands; Misset International. 6 issues/year.

Small Ruminant Research. Vol. 1. (1988)+. Amsterdam; Elsevier Science. The Journal of the International Goat Association. (Continues in part: International Goat and Sheep Research.) Quarterly.

Trends in Genetics. Vol. 1. (1985)+. Amsterdam; Elsevier Science. Monthly.

Tropical Veterinary and Animal Science Research: TVASR. Vol. 1, no. 1 (Mar. 1983)+. New Delhi, India; Allied Publishers. Quarterly.

Western Polled Hereford Journal. Vol. 1. (1987)+. Klamath Falls, Oreg.; Klamath Pub.

World Animal Science. Amsterdam and New York; Elsevier Scientific. *A. Basic Information*. Vol. 1 (1981)+. *B. Disciplinary Approach*. Vol. 1. (1981)+. *C. Production-Systems Approach*. Vol. 1 (1982)+.

7. Reference Update

Jo Anne Boorkman

Judith Levitt

Loren D. Carlson Health Sciences Library, University of California, Davis

Keeping alert to the numerous reference or working tools that continuously appear is a difficult task. These include handbooks, cumulative indexes of long-term value, data collections and lengthy analyses of data, authoritative histories, and valuable bibliographies. Such books are not read chapter by chapter or as a reading assignment for a class. They provide reference points of authoritative data, literature citations, sources of detailed information, or some general background.

The most recent major compilation of reference sources for animal sciences and veterinary medicine was published in 1981: *Guide to Sources for Agricultural and Biological Research*, edited by J. Richard Blanchard and Lois Farrell (Berkeley, University of California, 1981). This immense work of 735 pages serves as the basic guide to the literature of the agricultural sciences. The book's chapter D, compiled by Marjan Merala, Jane Kimball, and J. Richard Blanchard, covers animal sciences in the following subdivisions: Veterinary Medicine; Animal Husbandry; Poultry Husbandry; Wildlife and Wildlife Management; Commercial Fishing and Fisheries; Entomology and Nematology.

All these topics are covered in this book and in this updating chapter with the exception of Entomology and Nematology, which will appear in a later volume concerned with crop improvement and protection. Chapter D in the Blanchard and Farrell *Guide* presented 1,164 reference or background entries. Each entry was annotated and sequentially numbered. This chapter is a supplement and complement to the *Guide*'s chapter D on animal sciences.

The research for this chapter was supported in part by a Librarians' Association of the University of California, Davis (LAUC-D) mini-grant no. 3-6005100-19900-4005-576.

223

Older materials in the *Guide* are not reproduced in this update. However, those titles which have been updated are noted in this chapter (reference by D number is made back to the item in chapter D). When a title is a direct successor, the reader may wish to consult Blanchard and Farrell for the complete annotation and description. Some important titles such as textbooks and handbooks are in the core monograph list of this book and are not included here as extensively as in Blanchard and Farrell. There is a distinct bias toward United States agriculture, although major new works with Third World application are included. As with any large compilation, some items may have been overlooked.

Contents

A. Animal Husbandry, by Judith Levitt

Items identified as Core Monographs in Chapter 6 are indicated in this section by: CORE.

Literature Guides

Cregier, Sharon E. *Farm Animal Ethology: A Guide to Sources*. North York, Ontario; Captus University Publications, 1989. 213p.

Published by arrangement with the Canadian Federation of Humane Societies; the Society for Veterinary Ethology; and the Center for Animals, Tufts University School of Veterinary Medicine.

Abstracts and Indexes

Since 1980, no new printed general services for animal husbandry have been published. Subject indexes or abstracts on specialized subjects will be described later in appropriate areas.

Bibliographies

Bebee, Charles N., and Janice Swanson, compilers and eds. *Farm Animal Welfare, January 1979–April 1989*. Beltsville, Md.; U.S. Dept. of Agriculture, National Agricultural Library, 1989. 301p. 2,737 citations from AGRICOLA. (USDA Bibliographies and Literature of Agriculture no. 84)

Vallentine, John F., ed. *U.S.-Canadian Range Management, 1978–1980: A Selected Bibliography on Ranges, Pastures, Wildlife, Livestock, and Ranching.* Phoenix, Ariz.; Oryx Press, 1981. 166p. 3,719 citations.
"Complete contents of the *Journal of Range Management* and *Rangemen's Journal* have been included in the Bibliography with the exception of the few without North American emphasis and foreign language entries."—Preface

Dictionaries

Dictionary of Animal Production Terminology: In English, French, Spanish, German, and Latin. Compiled by European Association for Animal Production. Amsterdam and New York; Elsevier, 1985. 683p. (EAAP Publication no. 30)

Revised ed. of: *Vocabulary of Animal Husbandry Terms.*   [D287]

Hurnik, J. F., A. B. Webster, and P. B. Siegel. *Dictionary of Farm Animal Behaviour.* Guelph, Ontario; University of Guelph, 1985. 176p.

Steinmetz, H. *Tierische Produktion: Mehrsprachen-Bildwortenbuch = Animal Production: Multilingual Illustrated Dictionary.* 5, aufl. Eschborn, Germany; Deutsche Gesellschaft fur Technische Zusammenarbeit (GTZ) GmbH, 1986. 550p.

In German, Chinese, English, French, Italian and Spanish.
This illustrated dictionary has evolved from a first edition published in 1962 as: *Tierfutterung und Tierhaltung.*   [D289]

Directories

Agricultural and Veterinary Sciences International Who's Who. 3d ed. Detroit, Mich.; Harlow; Longman; Distributed in the U.S. and Canada by Gale Research, 1987. 2 vols. (Reference on Research)

A companion to: *Agricultural Research Centres: A World Directory of Organizations and Programmes.* Previously published as: *Who's Who in World Agriculture.* Provides biographical details of about 7,500 senior agricultural and veterinary scientists from over 100 countries.

Agricultural Research Centres: A World Directory of Organizations and Programmes. 8th ed. Harlow, U.K., and Detroit, Mich.; Longman; Distributed exclusively in the U.S. and Canada by Gale Research, 1986. 2 vols. 1138p. (Reference on Research)

A companion to: *Agricultural & Veterinary Sciences International Who's Who.* Revised ed. of: *Agricultural Research Index.* Provides details of relevant laboratories and organizations which are carrying out or funding research and development in over 125 countries in the world. Revised ed. of: *Agricultural Research Index.*

Beaugrand, Jacques, compiler and ed. *International Directory of Ethologists.* 1st ed. Special Issue, *Behavioral Processes,* Elsevier Science Publishers B.V. (Biomedical Division). Vol. 21, no. 1, 1990. 57p.

Printed copies can be obtained by writing directly to Elsevier Science Publishers B.V., P.O. Box 211, 1000 AE Amsterdam, Netherlands. Also available on diskette for personal computers (IBM-compatible and Mac), and on magnetic tape for mainframes.

European Association for Animal Production. *Index of Teaching and Research Institutions in the Field of Animal Production.* 1977 + . Rome; EAAP, 1977. 38p. (EAAP Publication no. 20, pt. 1 +)

Who's Who in Live Animal Trade and Transport. Biennial. Fort Washington, Md; Silesia Companies, 1991. 4th ed., 252p.

Continues: *Who's Who in Animal Transportation.* 3d ed., 1989. 1991 edition contains over 5,000 listings of people and firms who are active in some form of animal trade or transportation.

Lists of Periodicals

Clingerman, Karen J. *Serials at the National Agricultural Library Relating to Animal Care, Use, and Welfare.* Beltsville, Md.; National Agricultural Library, 1990. 30p. 267 citations. (AWIC Series no. 5)

A listing of English language serials housed within the National Agricultural Library. The document will be updated periodically.

International Union List of Agricultural Serials. National Agricultural Library of the U.S. Dept. of Agriculture. Commission of the European Communities. Food and Agriculture Organization. Wallingford; CAB International, 1990. 767p.

The list is a compilation of serials indexed in AGRICOLA, AGRIS, and CABI ABSTRACTS. Four years in the making, it gives details of 11,567 publications, coming from 129 different countries, with titles in 53 languages. The entries were derived from a database of over 60,000 serial bibliographic records created and maintained by NAL. Entries are sorted alphabetically, by title, in word-by-word order. Includes a subject index and a country index.

Jensen, Richard D., Connie Lamb, and Nathan M. Smith, compilers. *Agricultural and Animal Sciences Journals and Serials: An Analytical Guide*. Westport, Conn.; Greenwood Press, 1986. 211p. (Annotated Bibliographies of Serials: A Subject Approach; 0748–5190; no. 4)

Lists 362 of the 10,000 or more agricultural titles being published (at the time of printing). Titles are English language only, contain information about agriculture and animal science and are research oriented. Some titles were included because they treat topics that received minimal coverage in other serials. Representative trade journals and magazines are included. Most state agricultural experiment station publications are excluded except for research journals. Only sixteen major U.S. Government serials, largely from the U.S. Dept. of Agriculture, are included. Includes a geographical index and an index of publishers.

Handbooks and Texts

Acker, Duane. *Animal Science and Industry*. 3d ed. Englewood Cliffs, N.J.; Prentice-Hall, 1983. 658p. CORE

Blakely, J., and D. H. Bade. *The Science of Animal Husbandry*. 5th ed. Englewood Cliffs, N.J.; Prentice-Hall, 1990. 618p. CORE

Provides information about the history, reproduction, feeding, management, and health care of the most important breeds of beef and dairy cattle, sheep, pigs, horses and poultry, each species being examined separately. Contains an appendix on the composition and nutitional value of feed.

Cole, Harold Harrison, and W. N. Garrett, eds. *Animal Agriculture: The Biology, Husbandry, and Use of Domestic Animals*. 2d ed. San Francisco; W. H. Freeman, 1980. 739p. (A Series of Books in Animal Science) CORE   [D301]

Ensminger, M. Eugene. *The Stockman's Handbook*. 6th ed. Danville, Ill; Interstate, 1983. 1192p. (Animal Agriculture Series) CORE

Reference work for those dealing with meat animals and horses. Much of the information is in tabular form.   [D302]

Farm Animal Welfare Programme: Evaluation Report 1979–83. Luxembourg; Office for Official Publications of the European Communities, 1984. 89p. (EUR: 9180EN)

Graffis, Don W., E. M. Juergenson, and Malcolm H. McVickar. *Approved Practices in Pasture Management*. 4th ed. Danville, Ill.; Interstate Printers & Publishers, 1985. 356p.

3d ed., 1974, by Malcolm H. McVickar.

Halley, R. J., and R. J. Soffe, eds. *Primrose McConnell's the Agricultural Notebook*. 18th ed. London and Boston; Butterworths, 1988. 689p.

Standard reference work on farm management. Includes sections on farm buildings and animal production (including a brief review of animal health).

Handbook of Live Animal Transport. 1986+. Irregular. Fort Washington, Md.; Silesia Companies, Inc. Vol. 5, 1988: "Aircraft Configuration." Unpaged. Supplements issued quarterly.

Continues: *Handbook (Animal Air Transportation Association)*.

International Air Transport Association. *IATA Live Animals Regulations*. 18th ed. Geneva; IATA, 1991. 234p. (IATA Resolution 620, Attachment "A")

Continues: *International Air Transport Association. IATA Live Animals Manual*.

Maton, Andre, J. Daelemans, and J. Lambrecht. *Housing of Animals: Construction and Equipment of Animal Houses*. English text, F. Lunn; drawings, A. Stevens. Amsterdam and New York; Elsevier; Distributed for the U.S. and Canada, Elsevier Science, 1985. 458p. (Developments in Agricultural Engineering no. 6) CORE

Translation of: *De Huisvesting van Dieren*. Includes the scientific aspects of animal housing in terms of animal behavior, hygiene and layout. Covers housing for cattle, swine, poultry, horses, sheep, rabbits and fur bearing animals.

Moss, R., ed. *Transport of Animals Intended for Breeding, Production and Slaughter*. Martinus Nijhoff, The Hague, 1982. 246p. CORE

Payne, William J. A. *An Introduction to Animal Husbandry in the Tropics*. 4th ed. Harlow, Essex, U.K.; Longman Scientific & Technical; New York; Wiley, 1990. 881p. (Tropical Agriculture Series)

Revised ed. of: *An Introduction to Animal Husbandry in the Tropics* by Grahame Williamson, 3d ed., 1978.

Putman, Paul A., ed. *Handbook of Animal Science*. San Diego, Calif.; Academic Press, 1991. 401p.

Radostits, O. M., and D. C. Blood. *Herd Health: A Textbook of Health and Production Management of Agricultural Animals*. Philadelphia; Saunders, 1985. 456p. CORE

Sainsbury, David. *Farm Animal Welfare: Cattle, Pigs and Poultry*. London; Collins, 1986. 175p. Bibliography, p. 171.

Universities Federation for Animal Welfare. *Management and Welfare of Farm Animals: The UFAW Handbook*. 3d ed. London and Philadelphia; Bailliere Tindall, 1988. 260p.

Rev. edition of: *The UFAW Handbook on the Care and Management of Farm Animals*.   [D305]

World Animal Science. Subseries A: Basic Information, 1983 + ; *Subseries B: Disciplinary Approach*, 1981 + ; *Subseries C: Production-System Approach*, 1982 + . Amsterdam and New York; Elsevier Scientific Pub. Co.

"A comprehensive and up-to-date review of the Animal Science literature covering the entire range of technical knowledge that is now required in animal production and development." —General Preface

History

Clutton-Brock, Juliet. *A Natural History of Domesticated Mammals*. Austin; University of Texas Press, 1987. 208p.

Published in 1981 as: *Domesticated Animals from Early Times,* by British Museum (Natural History).

Mason, Ian L. *Evolution of Domesticated Animals*. London and New York; Longman, 1984. 452p. CORE

Urquhart, Judy. *Animals on the Farm: Their History from the Earliest Times to the Present Day*. London; MacDonald, 1983. 182p. Bibliography, pp. 175–177.

Wiser, Vivian, Larry Mark, and H. Graham Purchase, eds.; Donald V. Robertson, technial ed. *100 Years of Animal Health*. Beltsville, Md.; Associates of the National Agricultural Library, 1987. 230p. (Journal of the NAL Associates, n.s., v.11, no.1/4)

Genetics

Brackett, Benjamin G., George E. Seidel, Jr., and Sarah M. Seidel, eds. *New Technologies in Animal Breeding*. New York; Academic Press, 1981. 268p. CORE

Based on papers presented at the OTA Conference on"Impacts of Applied Genetics: Animal Breeding" held in Denver, Colo., January 15–17, 1980.

Hutt, Frederick Bruce, and Benjamin A. Rasmusen. *Animal Genetics*. 2d ed. New York; Wiley, 1982. 582p. CORE

Long recognized reference text on applied genetics in relation to domestic animals.   [D311]

Jones, William Elvin. *Genetics and Horse Breeding*. Philadelphia; Lea & Febiger, 1982. 660p. CORE

Previous ed. published as: *Genetics of the Horse,* 1971.   [D313]

Lasley, John Foster. *Genetics of Livestock Improvement*. 4th ed. Englewood Cliffs, N.J.; Prentice-Hall, 1987. 477p. CORE

Aim of this book is to expound principles of qualitative and quantitative genetics, to be applied in selection and mating of farm animals by the breeder.   [D315]

Legates, James Edward, and Everett James Warwick. *Breeding and Improvement of Farm Animals*. 8th ed. New York and London; McGraw-Hill, 1990. 342p. CORE

Previous ed., 1979. 6th ed., by V. A. Rice.   [D317]

Pirchner, Franz. *Population Genetics in Animal Breeding*. Translated from German with the assistance of D. L. Frape. 2d ed. New York; Plenum Press, 1983. 414p. Bibliography, pp. 387–408. CORE

Translation of: *Populationsgenetik in der Tierzucht*.   [D316]

Smith, C., J. W. B. King, and J. C. Mckay, eds. *Exploiting New Technologies in Animal Breeding: Genetic Developments; Proceedings of a Seminar in the CEC Animal Husbandry Research Programme, held in Edinburgh, June, 1985*. Sponsored by the Commision of the European Communities, Directorate-General for Agriculture, Co-ordination of Agricultural Research. Oxford and New York; Published on behalf of the CEC by Oxford University Press, 1986. 202p. CORE

Stufflebeam, Charles E. *Genetics of Domestic Animals*. Englewood Cliffs, N.J.; Prentice-Hall, 1989. 295p.

Wiener, Gerald, ed. *Animal Genetic Resources: A Global Programme for Sustainable Development*. Proceedings of an FAO Expert Consultation, Rome, September 1989. Rome; Food and Agriculture Organization, 1990. 300p. (FAO Animal Production and Health Paper no. 80)

Reproduction

Cupps, Perry T., ed. *Reproduction in Domestic Animals*. 4th ed. San Diego; Academic Press, 1991. 670p.

Reference text; a summary of current research in reproduction of domesticated species, with individual chapters written by authorities on the various subjects.
    [D320]

Herman, Harry August, and F. W. Madden. *The Artificial Insemination and Embryo Transfer of Dairy and Beef Cattle (Including Techniques for Goats, Sheep, Horses, and Swine): A Handbook and Laboratory Manual for Students, Herd Operators, and Workers in the AI Field*. 7th ed. Danville, Ill.; Interstate Printers & Publishers, 1987. 279p. Bibliography, pp. xxi-xxii. CORE   [D322]

Johnson, Judith A. *Animal Sciences: Advances in Reproductive and Health Technologies: Report*. Prepared by the Congressional Research Service, Library of Congress for the Subcommittee on Investigations and Oversight transmitted to the Subcommittee on Science and Technology, U.S. House of Representatives, Ninety-Eighth Congress, first session. Washington, D.C.; U.S. G.P.O., 1983. 76p.

Laing, J. A., W. J. Brinley Morgan, and W. C. Wagner, eds. *Fertility and Infertility in Veterinary Practice*. 4th ed. London and Philadelphia; Bailliere Tindall, 1988. 280p. CORE

Rev. ed. of: *Fertility and Infertility in Domestic Animals*. [D324]

Lamming, G. E., ed. *Marshall's Physiology of Reproduction*. 4th ed. Edinburgh and New York; Churchill Livingstone, 1984–1990. 2 vols. CORE

Comprehensive treatise and reference work. [D325]

Feeds and Nutrition

Association of American Feed Control Officials. *Official Publication*. Annual. College Station, Tex.; The Association.

Church, D. C. *Livestock Feeds and Feeding*. 3d ed. Englewood, N.J.; Prentice-Hall, 1991. 546p. CORE [D329]

Church, D. C., ed. *The Ruminant Animal: Digestive Physiology and Nutrition*. Englewood Cliffs, N.J.; Prentice-Hall, 1988. 564p. ("*A Reston Book*") CORE

"Previously published as: *Digestive Physiology and Nutrition of Ruminants*. 2d ed., vol. 1, 1969, 1976; vol. 2, 1971, 1979, by D. C. Church et al. O & B Books, Inc." [D328]

Cullison, Arthur E., and Robert S. Lowrey. *Feeds and Feeding*. 4th ed. Englewood Cliffs, N.J.; Prentice-Hall, 1987. 645p. CORE

Handbook-text in which general information on feeds and feeding methods is consolidated, with facts and figures from several National Research Council publications. [D332]

Ensminger, M. Eugene, J. E. Oldfield, and W. W. Heinemann. *Feeds and Nutrition*. 2d ed. Clovis, Calif.; Ensminger Pub. Co., 1990. 1544p. CORE

Formerly: *Feeds and Nutrition, Complete*. [D335]

Feed Additive Compendium. 1966+. Annual. Minneapolis; Miller Pub. Co. 1991, 508p.

Published annually and updated monthly. Issued in cooperation with the Animal Health Institute, Washington, D.C., and geared to provide current information on the frequently changing regulations concerning feed additives. [D336]

Feed Industry Red Book. Annual. Edina, Minn.; Communications Marketing. 1991, 218p. Title varies.

Reference medium for companies and individuals engaged in the manufacture of livestock feeds, poultry feeds and pet foods throughout the world. [D337]

Gillespie, James R. *Animal Nutrition and Feeding*. Albany, N.Y.; Delmar, 1987. 418p. Bibliography, pp. 293–301. Includes many tables.

Gohl, Bo. *Tropical Feeds: Feed Information Summaries and Nutritive Values.* Rome; Food and Agriculture Organizations; New York; Unipub, distributor, 1981. 529p. (FAO Animal Production and Health Series no. 12)   [D338]

International Feedstuffs Institute. *Arab and Middle East Tables of Feed Composition: Nutritional Data for Algeria. . . .* Prepared by L. C. Kearl et al. Logan, Utah; International Feedstuffs Institute, Dept. of Animal, Dairy, and Veterinary Sciences, Utah Agricultural Experiment Station, Utah State University; Damascus, Syria; League of Arab States, Arab Center for the Studies of Arid Zones and Dry Lands, Dept. of Animal Science, 1979. 554p. (Research Report, Utah Agricultural Experiment Station no. 30) Bibliography, p. 13 (2d group).

Includes glossaries of technical terms in English, Arabic and Turkish.

Kearl, Leonard C. *Nutrient Requirements of Ruminants in Developing Countries.* Logan, Utah; International Feedstuffs Institute, Utah Agricultural Experiment Station, Utah State University, 1982. 381p. Bibliography, pp. 133–150.

A companion volume to *Arab and Middle East Tables of Feed Composition: Nutritional Data for Algeria. . .* prepared by L. C. Kearl et al., 1979. —From Introduction.

McDonald, Peter, R. A. Edwards, and J. F. D. Greenhalgh. *Animal Nutrition.* 4th ed. Harlow, Essex, U.K.; Longman; New York; Copublished in the U.S. with Wiley, 1988. 543p. CORE

British manual on scientific feeding of livestock.   [D342]

Mertz, Walter, ed. *Trace Elements in Human and Animal Nutrition.* 5th ed. Orlando, Fla.; Academic Press, 1986–1987. 2 vols. CORE

Rev. ed. of: *Trace Elements in Human and Animal Nutrition*, by Eric J. Underwood. 4th ed., 1977.   [D347]

National Research Council (U.S.). Commission on Natural Resources, Board on Agriculture and Renewable Resources, Committee on Animal Nutrition, Subcommittee on Feed Composition. *United States-Canadian Tables of Feed Composition: Nutritional Data For United States and Canadian Feeds.* 3d revision. Washington, D.C.; National Academy Press, 1982. 148p. Bibliography, pp. 147–148. CORE

Thompson, G. B., and Clayton C. O'Mary, eds. *The Feedlot.* 3d ed. Philadelphia; Lea & Febiger, 1983. 306p. CORE

Description of feedlot operations as cattle complete their growing and fattening preparatory for marketing for slaughter.   [D334]

Behavior

Craig, James V. *Domestic Animal Behavior: Causes and Implications for Animal Care and Management.* Englewood Cliffs, N.J.; Prentice-Hall, 1981. 364p. CORE

A basic text treating such subjects as domestication, socialization, communication, aggression, feeding, shelter, handling, and welfare. Emphasis is upon practical applications to farm animal management.

Fraser, Andrew Ferguson, ed. *Ethology of Farm Animals: A Comprehensive Study of the Behavioural Features of the Common Farm Animals.* Amsterdam and New York; Elsevier, 1985. 500p. (World Animal Science. A, Basic Information no. 5) CORE

Fraser, Andrew Ferguson, and D. M. Broom. *Farm Animal Behaviour and Welfare.* 3d ed. London and Philadelphia; Bailliere Tindall, 1990. 437p. Includes bibliographical references, pp. 392–429. CORE

Previous editions as *Farm Animal Behaviour.*   [D349]

Hart, Benjamin L. *The Behavior of Domestic Animals.* New York; W. H. Freeman, 1985. 400p. CORE

Aims to offer a biological perspective on comparative animal behavior, and to present behavioral information relevant to the care and management of livestock and companion animals.

Kiley-Worthington, M. *The Behaviour of Horses in Relation to Management and Training.* London; J. A. Allen, 1987. 265p.

Written for the horse owner to give insight into equine behaviour but includes references to the original literature.

Kilgour, Ronald, and Clive Dalton. *Livestock Behavior: A Practical Guide.* St. Albans, U.K.; Granada, 1983. 256p. Bibliography, pp. 293–294. CORE

Describes the behavior of eight main farm species—cattle, sheep, goats, deer, horses, pigs, poultry, and dogs—with special reference to how this knowledge can be used to improve management, handling, safety and welfare.

Sumner, W. Dayton. *Breaking Your Horse's Bad Habits.* 2d ed. Millwood, N.Y.; Breakthrough, 1986. 226p.   [D353]

General Livestock

Bibliographies

Clingerman, Karen J. *Transport and Handling of Livestock, January 1979–February 1991.* Beltsville, Md.; National Agricultural Library, 1991. 27p. (Quick Bibliography Series no. QB 91-143) 308 citations from AGRICOLA.

Stevens, Donald G. *The Effects of Environment on Livestock: A Bibliography.* New Orleans, La.; Agricultural Research Service, Southern Region, U.S. Dept. of Agriculture; College Station, Tex.; Available from Meat Processing and Marketing Research, 1982. 52p. (USDA Agricultural Reviews and Manuals. ARM-S no. 23) (Deposit Item 22-A-5 on microfiche.)

"Over 1,900 titles published from 1945–1978." —Preface

Dictionaries

Mason, Ian Lauder. *A World Dictionary of Livestock Breeds, Types and Varieties.* 3d ed., rev. C.A.B. International, 1988. 348p. Bibliography, pp. 344–348. CORE   [D363]

Histories

Hall, Stephen J. G., and Juliet Clutton-Brock. *Two Hundred Years of British Farm Livestock.* Foreword by H.R.H. the Prince of Wales. London; British Museum (National History), 1989. 272p. Biographical references, pp. 247–250.

International Livestock Centre for Africa. *ILCA, the First Years.* Addis Ababa, Ethiopia; ILCA, 1980. 127p.

Breeds

Briggs, Hilton M., and Dinus M. Briggs. *Modern Breeds of Livestock.* 4th ed. New York; Macmillan, 1980. 802p. CORE   [D361]

Wallis, Derek. *The Rare Breeds Handbook.* Poole, Dorset and New York; Blandford Press; Distributed in the U.S. by Sterling Pub. Co., 1986. 160p. Bibliography, p. 157.

"In association with the Rare Breeds Survival Trust."

Husbandry

Battaglia, Richard A., and Vernon B. Mayrose. *Handbook of Livestock Management Techniques.* Minneapolis; Burgess Pub. Co., CEPCO Division, 1981. 595p. CORE

Boer, F. de, and H. Bickel, eds. *Livestock Feed Resources and Feed Evaluation in Europe: Present Situation and Future Prospects.* Amsterdam and New York; Elsevier, 1988. 408p. (EAAP Publication no. 37) Contributors represent 25 specialists in the field.

Devendra, C., ed. *Small Ruminant Production Systems in South and Southeast Asia; Proceedings of a Workshop held in Bogor, Indonesia, October 6–10, 1986.* Ottawa; International Development Research Centre, 1987. 414p. (IDRC no. 256e)

Sponsored by the International Development Research Centre and the Small Ruminant Collaborative Research Support Program.

Feeding Strategies for Improving Productivity of Ruminant Livestock in Developing Countries; Proceedings of a Combined Advisory Group Meeting and a Research Coordination Meeting Organized by the Joint FAO/IAEA Division of Nuclear Techniques in Food and Agriculture, Vienna, March 13–17, 1989. Vienna, Austria; International Atomic Energy Agency Publication, 1989. 233p. (IAEA STI/PUB no. 823)

Fourteen reviews and recommendations by leading world authorities in animal production of developing countries.

Galal, E. S. E., M. B. Aboul-Ela, and M. M. Shafie, compilers. *Ruminant Production in the Dry Subtropics: Constraints and Potentials; Proceedings of the International Symposium on the Constraints and Possibilities of Ruminant Production in the Dry Subtropics, Cairo, Egypt, November 5–7, 1988.* Wageningen, Netherlands; Pudoc, 1989. 268p. (EAAP Publication no. 38, 1989)

Handbook of Medicinal Feed Additives. 1982 + . Annual. Baslow, Bakewell, Derbyshire; HGM Pub. 1986/87, 283p.

Lists the medicinal feed additives available in the U.K., details their characteristics and other relevant data, as well as the conditions of usage permitted within the EEC.

Livestock Reproduction in Latin America. Vienna, Austria; International Atomic Energy Agency (IAEA), 1990. 445p. (IAEA STI/PUB no. 833)

Proceedings of a meeting held in Bogota, Columbia, September 19–23, 1988. Papers cover a wide range of topics in animal production and reproduction.

McNitt, J. I. *Livestock Husbandry Techniques.* London and New York; Granada, 1983. 280p. Bibliography, pp. 254–255. CORE

Practical guide on the management of cattle and calves, pigs and poultry.

Nutrient Requirements of Ruminant Livestock: Technical Review by an Agricultural Research Council Working Party. Farnham Royal, U.K.; Published on behalf of the Agricultural Research Council by the Commonwealth Agricultural Bureaux, 1980. 351p. CORE

Previous ed. published in 1965 as: *The Nutrient Requirements of Farm Livestock.* Bibliography, pp. 315–347.   [D327]

Qureshi, A. W., and H. A. Fitzhugh, technical eds. *Small Ruminants in the Near East.* Rome; Food and Agriculture Organization, 1987–1989. 3 vols. (FAO Animal Production and Health Paper no. 54-[55, 74]. CORE

Raising Livestock on Small Farms. Prepared by Extension Service. Revised June 1972, slightly revised October 1983. Washington, D.C.; U.S. Dept. of Agriculture, 1983. 20p. (Farmers' Bulletin no. 2224)

Sainsbury, David, and Peter Sainsbury. *Livestock Health and Housing.* 3d ed. London and Philadelphia; Bailliere Tindall, 1988. 319p. CORE

Small Ruminant Production in the Humid Tropics. Addis, Ababa, Ethiopia; International Livestock Centre for Africa, 1979. 122p. (ILCA Systems Study no. 3) CORE

Squires, Victor. *Livestock Management in the Arid Zone.* Melbourne; Inkata Press, 1981. 271p. Bibliography, pp. 256–266. CORE

Timon, V. M., and J. P. Hanrahan, eds. *Small Ruminant Production in the Developing Countries; Proceedings of An Expert Consultation Held in Sofia, Bulgaria, July 8–12, 1985*. Rome; Food and Agriculture Organization, 1986. 234p. (FAO Animal Production and Health Paper no. 58)

Trimberger, George W., William M. Etgen, and David M. Galton. *Dairy Cattle Judging Techniques*. 4th ed. Englewood Cliffs, N.J.; Prentice-Hall, 1987. 356p. CORE   [D365]

Wilson, R. T., and D. Bourzat, eds. *Small Ruminants in African Agriculture; Proceedings of a Conference held at ILCA, Addis Ababa, Ethiopia, September 30–October 4, 1988*. Addis Ababa, Ethiopia; International Livestock Centre for Africa, 1985. 261p. Bibliography, pp. 244–255. CORE

Cattle

Bibliographies

Adams, Ramon F. *The Rampaging Herd: A Bibliography of Books and Pamphlets on Men and Events in the Cattle Industry*. Cleveland, Ohio; John Zubal, 1982. 463p. Reprint of 1959 publication, University of Oklahoma Press.   [D367]

Butterworth, M. H., et al. *Beef Cattle Production from Tropical Pastures: A Descriptive Bibliography*. Addis Ababa, Ethiopia; Documentation Centre, International Livestock Centre for Africa. 1985. 112p. 631 citations.

Swanson, Janice C.
Calf Housing and Facilities, January 1979–August 1990: 205 Citations from AGRICOLA. Beltsville, Md.; National Agricultural Library, 1990. 19p. (Quick Bibliography Series no. QB-91-13)

Dairy Cattle Housing and Facilities, January 1979–August 1990. 27p. 321 Citations from AGRICOLA. (Quick Bibliography no. QB 91-19)

Stress in Cattle, January 1979–August 1990. 37p. 386 Citations from AGRICOLA. (Quick Bibliography no. QB 91-18)

Welfare, Care and Husbandry of Cattle, January 1979–August 1990: 250 Citations from AGRICOLA. 21p. (Quick Bibliography Series no. QB 91-17)

Directories

American Association of Bovine Practitioners. *Directory*. 197-? + . Triennial. West Lafayette, Ind.; The Association, Office of Executive Secretary-Treasurer. Latest ed., January 1, 1991, 79p.

Ayrshire Cattle Society of Great Britain and Ireland. *Herd and AI Directory*. 1988 + . Ayr, Scotland; The Society. 1990 is latest ed., 100p.

National Cattle Feedlot, Meat Packer and Grain Dealers Directory. 1970 + . Biennial. Lubbock, Tex.; Tara Pub. Co., in association with Trina Caranfa Garcia, etc. 1985–1986 ed., 826p.

Title varies slightly. Frequency irregular on early issues.   [D292]

Histories and Breeds

Akerman, Joe A., Jr. *American Brahman: A History of the American Brahman*. Houston, Tex.; American Brahman Breeders Association, 1982. 384p. Bibliography, pp. 331–343.

Felius, Marleen, author and illustrator. *Genus Bos: Cattle Breeds of the World*. Rahway, N.J.; MSD AGVET, 1985. 234p. Bibliography, pp. 227–230.

Herman, Harry August. *Improving Cattle by the Millions: NAAB and the Development and Worldwide Application of Artificial Insemination*. Columbia; University of Missouri Press, 1981. 377p. Bibliography, pp. 365–366. CORE

Lewington, Peter. *Canada's Holsteins*. Markham, Ontario; Fitzhenry & Whiteside, 1983. 350p. Bibliography, pp. 340–342.

Mansfield, Richard Henry; edited by Robert H. Hastings. *Progress of the Breed: The History of U.S. Holsteins*. Centennial ed. Sandy Creek, N.Y.; Holstein-Friesian World, 1985. 362p.

National Cattle Breeders Association. *British Cattle*. Tring; The Association, 1980. 132p.

Descriptions and photographs of the breeds with details of breed societies.

Skaggs, Jimmy M. *Prime Cut: Livestock Raising and Meatpacking in the United States. 1607–1983*. College Station; Texas A&M University Press, 1986. 263p. Bibliography, pp. 219–245.

Husbandry

Bath, Donald L., et al. *Dairy Cattle: Principles, Practices, Problems, Profiles*. 3d ed. Philadelphia; Lea & Febiger, 1985. 473p. CORE [D380]

Butterworth, M. H. *Beef Cattle Nutrition and Tropical Pastures*. London and New York; Longman, 1985. 500p. Bibliography, pp. 438–489. CORE

Curtis, John L. *Cattle Embryo Transfer Procedure: An Instructional Manual for the Rancher, Dairyman, Artificial Insemination Technician, Animal Scientist, and Veterinarian*. San Diego, Calif.; Academic Press, 1991. 131p. Includes bibliographical references, pp. 130–131.

Diggins, Ronald V., Clarence E. Bundy, and Virgil W. Christensen. *Beef Production*. 4th ed. Englewood Cliffs, N.J.; Prentice-Hall, 1984. 256p. (Prentice-Hall Agriculture Series) CORE

Ensminger, M. Eugene. *Beef Cattle Science*. 6th ed. Danville, Ill.; Interstate Printers & Publishers, 1987. 1030p. (Animal Agriculture Series) CORE [D383]

Esslemont, R. J., J. H. Bailie, and M. J. Cooper. *Fertility Management in Dairy Cattle*. London; Collins, 1985. 143p.

International Stockman's School. *Beef Cattle Science Handbook*. Vol. 1, 1964+. Annual. Clovis, Calif.; Agriservices Foundation, 1991. Vol. 25, 193p.

Juergensen, Elwood M. *Approved Practices in Beef Cattle Production*. 5th ed. Danville, Ill.; Interstate Printers & Publishers, 1980. 467p. CORE

Lasley, John F. *Beef Cattle Production*. Englewood Cliffs, N.J.; Prentice-Hall, 1981. 468p. CORE

More O'Ferrall, G. J., ed. *Beef Production from Different Dairy Breeds and Dairy Beef Crosses; A Seminar in the CEC Programme of Coordination of Research on Beef Production held at Castleknock, Co. Dublin, Ireland, April 13–15, 1981*. The Hague and Boston; Martinus Nijhoff for the Commission of the European Communities; Hingham, Mass.; Distributors for the U.S. and Canada, Kluwer Boston, 1982. 395p. (Current Topics in Veterinary Medicine and Animal Science no. 21) Sponsored by the Commission of the European Communities, Directorate-General for Agriculture, Coordination of Agricultural Research.

Neumann, A. L., and K. S. Lusby. *Beef Cattle*. 8th ed. New York; John Wiley, 1986. 326p. CORE

Guide to the science and practice of beef cattle husbandry with particular reference to conditions in the United States. [D385]

National Research Council (U.S.). Subcommittee on Beef Cattle Nutrition, Committee on Animal Nutrition, Board on Agriculture. *Nutrient Requirements of Beef Cattle*. 6th rev. ed. Washington, D.C.; National Academy Press, 1984. 90p. (Nutrient Requirements of Domestic Animals). Bibliography, pp. 65–76. CORE

National Research Council (U.S.). Subcommittee on Dairy Cattle Nutrition, Committee on Animal Nutrition, Board on Agriculture. *Nutrient Requirements of Dairy Cattle*. 6th rev. ed. Washington, D.C.; National Academy Press, 1988. 157p. Includes 1 computer disk (51/4 in.) for PC or MS DOS. (Nutrient Requirements of Domestic Animals) Bibliography, pp. 116–117. CORE

Owen, John Bryn. *Cattle Feeding*. Ipswich, Suffolk; Farming Press, 1983. 170p. CORE

Putnam, Paul Adin, and Everett J. Warwick. *The Farm Beef Herd*. Prepared by Science and Education Administration, revised June 1980. Dept. of Agriculture, Science and Education Administration; For Sale by the Supt. of Docs., U.S. Govt. Print. Off., 1980. 22p. (USDA Farmers' Bulletin no. 2126)

Roy, J. H. B. *The Calf*. 5th ed. London and Boston; Butterworths, 1990. Vol.1 has 258p. CORE [D387]

240   Jo Anne Boorkman and Judith Levitt

Stansfield, Malcolm. *The New Herdsman's Book.* Ipswich; Farming Press, 1983. 179p. Basic manual of stockmanship.

Straiton, Eddie. *Calving the Cow and Care of the Calf.* 3d ed. Ipswich, Suffolk; Suffolk Farming Press, 1988. 164p. (T.V. Vet Book for Stock Farmers no. 2)

Unshelm, J., and G. Schonmuth, compilers. *Automation of Feeding and Milking: Production, Health, Behaviour, Breeding; Proceedings of the EAAP-Symposium of the Commissions on Animal Management and Health and Cattle Production, Helsinki, Finland, July 1, 1988.* Wageningen; Pudoc, 1988. 56p. (EAAP Publications no. 40)

Horses

Literature Guides

Wells, E. B. *Horsemanship: A Guide to Information Sources.* Detroit, Mich; Gale Research, 1979. 138p. (Sports, Games and Pastimes Information Guide Series no. 4)

Nearly 800 titles selected from an estimated 1,200 books and periodicals about horses, covering works that range from those published as early as 1470 through recent titles of 1972.

Abstracts and Indexes

Horse Magazine Index. Raytown, Mo. Vol. 1, no. 1, 1983 + .

Zentralblatt Pferd; Equine Abstracts. Vol. 1, 1984 + . Quarterly. Warendorf; FN-Verlag der Deutschen Reiterlichen Vereinigung.

"Collected up-to-date papers and bibliographies of scientific publications on the subject of horses." Titles are in both German and English and about ten percent have abstracts in German.

Bibliographies

American Quarter Horse Association. *Alphabetical Index of Stud Books: Book Number 1 Through Book Number 43. Registration Number 1 Through Registration Numbers 1,612,000, 1941 Through October 1980.* Amarillo, Tex.; American Quarter Horse Association, 1981. 2 vols. 1584p.

The Arabian Horse Bibliography: A Project of the Arabian Horse Trust with Special Cooperation of the W. K. Kellogg Arabian Horse Library, California State Polytechnic University, Pomona. Bibliographic research and annotations by Ruth E. Boyd and Melissa J. Paul. Westminster, Colo.; The Trust, 1985. 180p. Citations unnumbered.

Primarily includes books which focus on the Arabian horse—its heritage, characteristics, conformation, breeding, bloodlines, etc.

Clingerman, Karen J.
Equine Housing and Facilities, January 1979–August 1990: 65 Citations from AGRICOLA. Beltsville, Md.; National Agricultural Library, 1990. 7p. (Quick Bibliography Series no. QB 91-05)

Stress in Horses, January 1979–August 1990: 47 Citations from AGRICOLA. 5p. (Quick Bibliography Series no. QB 91-06)

Welfare of Horses, January 1979–August 1990. 16p. 182 Citations from AGRICOLA. (Quick Bibliography Series no. QB 91-04)

Grimshaw, Anne. *The Horse, a Bibliography of British Books, 1851–1976: With a Narrative Commentary on the Role of the Horse in British Social History, as Revealed by the Contemporary Literature*. London; Library Association; Phoenix, Ariz.; Oryx Press, 1982. 474p. 3,226 citations.

Over 3,000 entries, fully indexed and containing a commentary on the role of the horse in British social history.

Heymering, Henry, compiler. *On the Horse's Foot, Shoes and Shoeing*. Cascade, Md.; St. Elroy Publishing, 1990. 366p.

A bibliographic record of literature on the equine hoof and horseshoeing dating from 430 B.C. through 1990 A.D.

Huth, Frederick Henry. *Works on Horses and Equitation: A Bibliographical Record of Hippology*. Hildesheim; Olms, 1981. 439p.

Chronological system of arrangement, covering 430 B.C. to 1879. Magazine articles or articles from sporting journals not included. Citations unnumbered. Reprint of the 1887 ed. published by Quadritch, London.

Wells, E. B. *Horsemanship: A Bibliography of Printed Materials from the Sixteenth Century Through 1974*. New York; Garland Pub., 1985. 282p. 8,577 citations. (Garland Reference Library of the Humanities no. 474)

Directories

American Association of Equine Practitioners. *Membership Directory*. 1991. 201p.

Continues: *American Association of Equine Practitioners. A.A.E.P. Directory*.

American Horse Council in cooperation with American Horse Publications. *Horse Industry Directory*. 1976+. Annual. 1991/92, 140p.

A directory of all U.S. organizations representing horse-related interests concerned with the health and welfare of horses and horse businesses. These include educational institutions; breeders; veterinarians; farriers; breed registries; horsemen's associations; race tracks; horse shows; commercial suppliers; and state horse councils. Continues: *Horse Industry Trade Press Directory*.   [D290]

Blood-Horse Directory of North American Racing and Breeding. 1989+. Lexington, Ky.; The Blood-Horse. 1991, 354p.

5,590 entries. An alphabetical listing of national and international equine facilities and services covering 76 categories. Continues: *List* (Blood-Horse, Inc.).

Thoroughbred Times, Inc. *Stallion Directory*. Annual. Lexington, Ky.; Thoroughbred Times, Inc. 1991, 319p.

An alphabetical listing of all stallions reported to be standing at stud in North America and Europe in 1991; state and stud fee index; sires of sires index; pedigree index; inbreeding index; new sires index; sires averages index; farm index and sire lists. Vol. for 1989 has title: *Stallion Directory for.* . . . Absorbed: *Sire Book*, 1989.

Dictionaries and Encyclopedias

Bongianni, Maurizio. *The Macdonald Encyclopedia of Horses*. English translation by Ardele Dejey. London; Macdonald Orbis, 1988. 255p.

Hope, Charles Evelyn Graham, and G. N. Jackson, eds. *The Encyclopedia of the Horse*. William Steinkraus, advisory ed.; Diane R. Tuke, picture ed. New York; Viking Press, 1973. 336p. (A Studio Book)

McBane, Susan. *Behaviour Problems in Horses*. North Pomfret, Vt.; David & Charles, 1987. 304p. Bibliography, p. 296.

Histories

Barclay, Harold B. *The Role of the Horse in Man's Culture*. London and New York; J. A. Allen, 1980. 398p. Bibliography, pp. 375–394.

Dossenbach, Monique, and Hans D. Dossenbach. *The Noble Horse*. Foreword by H. R. H. the Duke of Edinburgh. Boston; G. K. Hall, 1983. 448p. Bibliography, pp. 447–448.

Translation of: *Konig Pferd*.

Edwards, Elwyn Hartley. *Horses: Their Role in the History of Man*. London; Willow Books, 1987. 224p. Bibliography pp. 218–219.

Based on the original screenplay by Jan Damley-Smith.

Fraser, Andrew Ferguson. *The Days of the Gerron: The Story of the Highland Pony*. Loanhead; Macdonald, 1980. 102p.

Kust, Matthew J. *Man and Horse in History*. Alexandria, Va.; Plutarch Press; New York: Distributed by Advent Books, 1983. 158p.

Loch, Sylvia. *The Royal Horse of Europe: The Story of the Andalusian and Lusitano*. Foreword by Fernando d'Andrade. London; J. A. Allen, 1986. 256p. Bibliography, pp. 248–254.

Symanski, Richard. *Wild Horses and Sacred Cows*. Foreword by Edward Abbey. Flagstaff, Ariz.; Northland Press, 1985. 223p.

Thompson, F. M. L., ed. *Horses in European Economic History. A Preliminary Canter*. Reading; British Agricultural History Society, 1983. 206p.

Willett, Peter. *Makers of the Modern Thoroughbred*. Lexington, Ky.; University Press of Kentucky, 1986. 272p.

Worcester, Donald Emmet. *The Spanish Mustang: From the Plains of Andalusia to the Prairies of Texas*. El Paso; Texas Western Press, University of Texas at El Paso, 1986. 95p. Bibliography, pp. 87–91.

Breeds

Bongianni, Maurizio. *Simon and Schuster's Guide to Horses and Ponies of the World*. Translated by Ardele Dejey. New York; Simon & Schuster, 1988. 255p. (A Fireside Book) Bibliography, p. 253.

Translation of: *Cavalli*.

Churchill, Peter, ed. *The World Atlas of Horses and Ponies*. Maidenhead; Sampson Low, 1980. 160p.

Illustrates the types and varieties of animals found throughout the world.

Edwards, Elwyn Hartley, and Candida Geddes, eds. *The Complete Horse Book*. Revised ed. London; Ward Lock, 1987. 344p.

Previous ed., 1982, published as: *The Complete Book of the Horse*.

Edwards, Elwyn Hartley, general ed. *A Standard Guide to Horse and Pony Breeds*. New York; McGraw-Hill, 1980. 352p.

Foster, Carol. *The Athletic Horse: His Selection, Work, and Management*. New York; Howell Book House, 1986. 143p. Bibliography, p. 137.

Packer, Dianne E., and Talib M. Ali. *The Colours and Markings of Horses*. Ipswich, Suffolk, U.K.; Farming Press, 1985. 70p.

Realistic illustrations of coat colours and body, limb and head markings.

Patnet, Dorothy Hinshaw. *Quarter Horses*. Photographs by William Munoz and others. New York; Holiday House, 1985. 91p.

An introduction to the quarter horse, the most popular horse in the world.

Sponenberg, Dan Phillip, and Bonnie V. Beaver. *Horse Color*. College Station; Texas A&M University Press, 1983. 124p. Bibliography, pp. 117–119.

Husbandry

Biracree, Tom, and Wendy Insinger. *The Complete Book of Thoroughbred Horse Racing*. Garden City, N.Y.; Dolphin Books, 1982. 364p.

Breeding Management and Foal Development. [P.O. Box 9001, Tyler, TX 75711]; Equine Research, Inc., 1982. 700p. Bibliography, pp. 649–663.

Cassell, D. *The Horse and the Law*. Newton Abbot; David & Charles, 1987. 160p.

For the horse owner; covers all aspects of the law including a chapter on veterinary and other services.

Cunha, Tony Joseph. *Horse Feeding and Nutrition*. 2d ed. San Diego; Academic Press, 1991. 445p.

Ensminger, M. Eugene. *Horses and Tack*. Revised ed. Boston; Houghton, 1991. 499p. Bibliographical references, pp. 471–485.

Evans, J. Warren. *Horses, a Guide to Selection, Care, and Enjoyment*. 2d ed. New York; W. H. Freeman, 1989. 717p. Bibliography, pp. 683–706.

Evans, J. Warren, et al. *The Horse*. 2d ed. New York; W. H. Freeman, 1990. 844p.

A reference work for the specialist; covers various breeds in the U.S. and their use; normative biology of the horse; its nutrition and feeding; reproduction and genetics and its management. Extensive reference list: breed associations and registries; horse magazines and riding associations.   [D414]

Frape, David Lawrence. *Equine Nutrition and Feeding*. Harlow, Essex, U.K.; Longman Scientific & Technical; New York; Longman; New York; Churchill Livingstone, 1986. 373p. Bibliography, pp. 327–358.

Hardman, Ann Leighton. *Henry Wynmalen's Horse Breeding and Stud Management*. Revised and enlarged ed. London; J. A. Allen, 1989. 202p.

Revised ed., 1971, of: *Horse Breeding & Stud Management*.

Hawcroft, Tim. *The Complete Book of Horse Care*. New York; Howell Book House; Sydney, N.S.W.; Lansdowne Press, 1983. 208p.

Hewitt, Abram S. *The Great Breeders and Their Methods*. Lexington, Ky.; Thoroughbred Publishers, 1982 (1984 printing). 410p.

Companion volume to the author's: *Sire Lines* (1977).
"Some of the Material herein is reprinted by permission of the Thoroughbred Owners and Breeders Association."

Hickman, John, and M. Humphrey. *Hickman's Farriery: A Complete Illustrated Guide*. 2d ed. London; J. A. Allen, 1988. 245p.

Hickman, John, ed. *Horse Management*. 2d ed. London and Orlando, Fla.; Academic Press, 1987. 405p. Bibliography, pp. 239–241.

Hill, Cherry. *The Formative Years: Raising and Training the Young Horse from Birth to Two Years*. Millwood, N.Y.; Breakthrough Publications, 1988. 240p. Bibliography, pp. 233–234.

Kellon, E. M. *The Older Horse: A Complete Guide to Care and Conditioning for Horses 10 and Up*. [P.O. Box 594, Millwood, NY 10546]; Breakthrough Publications, 1988. 212p.

Lasley, John F. *Genetic Principles in Horse Breeding*. Rev. ed. Houston; Cordovan Press, 1981. 124p. Bibliography, pp. 122–124.

McBane, Susan. *The Horse in Winter: His Management and Work*. London; Methuen, 1988. 157p.

McCarthy, Gillian. *Pasture Management for Horses and Ponies*. London; Collins Professional Books, 1987. 259p. Bibliography, pp. 252–253.

National Research Council (U.S.). Subcommittee on Horse Nutrition, Board on Agriculture. *Nutrient Requirements of Horses*. 5th ed., rev. Washington, D.C.; National Academy Press, 1989. 100p. (Nutrient Requirements of Domestic Animals)

Pilliner, Sarah. *Getting Horses Fit: A Guide to Improving Performance*. Oxford and Boston; BSP Professional, 1988, c1986. 226p.

Sagittarius Bloodstock Association. *Bloodstock Breeders' Review: An Illustrated Worldwide Survey of the British Thoroughbred*. 1977 + . Annual. London; The Association. Vol. 70, 453p.

Continues: *Bloodstock Breeders' Annual Review*.   [D409]

Stud Manager's Handbook. Vols. 1–21, 1965–1988. Annual. Clovis, Calif.; Westview Press, 1988. 2 vols. 236p.   [D416]

Svendsen, Elisabeth D., compiler. *The Professional Handbook of the Donkey*. 2d ed. Sidmouth, Devon, U.K.; The Donkey Sanctuary, 1989. 284p. Bibliography, p. 264.

About a quarter of the book is concerned with the health of donkeys. The remainder covers nutrition, management, housing and the uses of donkeys.

Weir, Barbara J., et al., eds. *Equine Reproduction IV; Proceedings of the Fourth International Symposium on Equine Reproduction held at the University of Calgary, Aug. 1986*. Cambridge, U.K.; Journal of Reproduction and Fertility, 1987. 761p. (Journal of Reproduction and Fertility, Suppl. no. 35)

Willis, Larryann C. *The Horse-Breeding Farm*. 3d ed., rev. Millwood, N.Y.; Breakthrough Publications, 1985. 429p.

Wood, Kenneth A. *Law for the Horse Breeder: A Reference Book for Professionals, Equine Breeders of Show and Race Horses and Students of the Horse Business Covering the Legal and Tax Aspects of Breeding, Showing and Racing Horses*. 1982 + . Rancho Santa Fe, Calif.; Wood Publications. 1 vol., loose-leaf, 16 sections. Paging not continuous.

Covers U.S. laws and legislation.

Swine

Abstracts and Indexes

Index of Current Research on Pigs. Shinfield, U.K.; Published for the Agricultural Research Council, 1990. Vol. 36.

Annually revised index. Previous editions are obsolete. Provides information on scientists and institutions doing research on pigs, worldwide, from abnormalities and anatomy, to breeding, feeding, diseases, wounds, and zinc.   [D417]

Pig News and Information. 1980 + . Quarterly. Wallingford; CAB International.

Contains about 3,000 abstracts per year; each issue also contains news items, several review articles and a "country report" describing an aspect of pig production in a single territory.

Bibliographies

Larson, Jean A. *Biotechnology: Growth Hormone in the Pig, January 1979–December 1988: 70 Citations.* Beltsville, Md.; U.S. Dept. of Agriculture, National Agricultural Library, 1989. 7p. (Quick Bibliography Series no. 89-26)

Swanson, Janice C., and Jean Larson. *Stress in Swine, 1979–August 1990: 398 Citations from AGRICOLA.* Beltsville, Md.; U.S. Dept. of Agriculture, National Agricultural Library, 1990. 37p. (Quick Bibliography Series no. 91-16)

Swanson, Janice C.
Swine Housing and Facilities, January 1985–August 1990. Beltsville, Md.; U.S. Dept. of Agriculture, National Agricultural Library, 1990. 30p. 298 citations from AGRICOLA. (Quick Bibliography Series no. 91-15)

Welfare, Care and Husbandry of Swine, January 1979–August 1990. 20p. 227 Citations from AGRICOLA. (Quick Bibliography Series no. 91-14)

U.S. Dept. of Agriculture. Science and Education Administration. *Swine Publications and Visual Materials.* Washington, D.C.; For sale by the Supt. of Docs., U.S. Govt. Print. Off., 1980. 47p. (USDA Miscellaneous Publication no. 1397)

Histories

Wiseman, J. *History of the British Pig.* London; Duckworth, 1986. 118p.

Husbandry

AFRC Technical Committee on Responses to Nutrients. *Nutrient Requirements of Sows and Boars; An Advisory Booklet.* Derbyshire; HGM Publications, 1990. 31p.

Baxter, Seaton Hall. *Intensive Pig Production: Environmental Management and Design.* London and New York; Granada, 1984. 588p. Bibliography, pp. 547–584. CORE

Brent, G. *Housing the Pig.* Ipswich, Suffolk, U.K.; Farming Press, 1986. 248p. CORE

Brent, G. *The Pigman's Handbook.* 2d ed. Ipswich, Suffolk, U.K.; Farming Press, 1987. 244p.

Guide to the management of pig units with a discussion of health problems. Previous edition: 1982.

Drochner, W. *Aspects of Digestion in the Large Intestine of the Pig*. Berlin; Paul Parey, 1987. 84p. CORE

Ensminger, M. Eugene, and R. O. Parker. *Swine Science*. 5th ed. Danville, Ill.; Interstate Printers, 1984. 568p. (Ensminger, M. Eugene—Animal Agriculture Series) CORE

"How-to" manual for hog farmers and others interested in swine industry. The final chapter provides feed composition tables. [D421]

Krider, J. L., and W. E. Carroll. *Swine Production*. 5th ed. New York; McGraw-Hill, 1982. 679p. (McGraw-Hill Publications in the Agricultural Sciences) CORE [D422]

Mitchelmore, Peter. *The Pigkeeper's Guide*. Newton Abbot, U.K., and North Pomfret, Vt.; David & Charles, 1981. 128p.

National Research Council (U.S.). Subcommittee on Swine Nutrition, Board on Agriculture. *Nutrient Requirements of Swine*. 9th ed., rev. Washington, D.C.; National Academy Press, 1988. 93p. (Nutrient Requirements of Domestic Animals) Bibliography, pp. 63–90. CORE

Nutrient Requirements of Pigs: Technical Review by an Agricultural Research Council Working Party. 2d ed. Farnham Royal, U.K.; CAB International, 1981. 307p. CORE

Five chapters review in detail the energy, protein and amino acid, vitamin, mineral and water requirements. There is a glossary of terms.

Pig Health and Production Recording. Rev. ed. Alnwick; MAFF, 1983. 59p. (MAFF Booklet no. 2075)

A guide to the collection and farm data. Includes definitions of terms used to describe reproductive events in pig herds.

Pond, Wilson G., et al. *Pork Production Systems: Efficient Use of Swine and Feed Resources*. New York; Van Nostrand Reinhold, 1991. Paging unknown.

Pond, Wilson G., and J. H. Maner. *Swine Production and Nutrition*. Westport, Conn.; Avi Pub. Co., 1984. 731p. (Animal Science Textbook Series) CORE

Sainsbury, David W. B. *Pig Housing*. 5th ed., rev. Ipswich, U.K.; Farming Press, 1978. 222p.

Thornton, Keith. *Outdoor Pig Production*. Ipswich, U.K.; Farming Press; Alexandria Bay, N.Y.; Distributed in North America by Diamond Farm Enterprises, 1988. 206p.

Thornton, Keith. *Practical Pig Production*. 3d ed. Ipswich, U.K.; Farming Press, 1981. 234p. Bibliography, pp. 226–229. CORE

Sheep and Goats

Bibliographies

Davies, Alexander S., complier. *A Bibliography of Sheep and Goat Anatomy*. Palmerston North, New Zealand; Veterinary Continuing Education, Massey University, 1990. 167p. 509 citations. (Publication, Foundation for Continuing Education of the N.Z. Veterinary Association No.128)

Krausman, Paul R., John R. Morgart, and Mary Ellen Chilelli. *Annotated Bibliography of Desert Bighorn Sheep Literature. . . 1897–1983*. Phoenix, Ariz.; Southwest Natural History Association, 1984. 204p. "Nearly 600 citations." — Preface

Swanson, Janice C.
Sheep and Goat Housing and Facilities: January 1979–August 1990. Beltsville, Md.; National Agricultural Library, 1990. 18p. 226 Citations from AGRICOLA. (Quick Bibliography Series no. QB 91-22)

Stress in Sheep and Goats: January 1979–August 1990. 14p. 139 Citations from AGRICOLA. (Quick Bibliography Series no. QB 91-21)

Directories

Dairy Goat Breeders Directory. 1981 + . Calistoga, Calif.; Dairy Goat Breeders Directory. 1982, 103p.

Continues: *Dairy Goat Directory*.

King, J. W. B., ed. *Directory of Current Research on Sheep and Goats*. Wallingford, Oxon, U.K.; CAB International, 1988. 271p.

Lists current research projects together with details of publications arising from them. The basic organization is by the institute at which the work is being performed. Author and subject indexes.

Histories

Day, G., and J. Jessup, general eds.; K. Cameron et al., contributing eds. *The History of the Australian Merino*. Richmond, Vic.; W. Heinemann Australia, 1984. 180p. Bibliography, pp. 173–174.

Garran, John Cheyne, and L. White. *Merinos, Myths and Macarthurs: Australian Graziers and Their Sheep, 1788–1900*. Rushcutters Bay, N.S.W.; Australian National University Press, 1985. 288p. Bibliography, pp. 261–270.

Reinhardt, Mrs. Robert M., and Alice Hall. *Nubian History: America and Great Britain*. 2d ed. Sketches by Dorothy Schott. San Bernadino, Calif.; Hall Press, 1978. 119p. Bibliography, p. 124.

Rogers, Allan L. *Saanen Roots: A History of the Saanen Dairy Goat Breed in the United States*. Scottsdale, Ariz.; Dairy Goat Journal Pub. Co., 1981. 85p.

Ryder, Michael L. *Sheep and Man*. London; Duckworth, 1983. 846p. Bibliography, pp. 802–829.

Sands, Michael, and Robert E. McDowell. *A World Bibliography on Goats*. Ithaca, N.Y.; Dept. of Animal Science, New York State College of Agriculture and Life Sciences, Cornell University, 1979. 112p. (Cornell International Agriculture Mimeograph no. 70) Bibliography, p. 9. CORE

Breeds

Acharya, R. M. *Sheep and Goat Breeds of India*. Rome; Food and Agriculture Organization, 1982. 190p. (FAO Animal Production and Health Paper no. 30) CORE

Devendra, C., and Marcia Burns. *Goat Production in the Tropics*. 2d ed. Farnham Royal, U.K.; Commonwealth Agricultural Bureaux, 1983. 183p. CORE

Sourcebook on breeds and their comparative performance and management relative to meat and milk, hair and skin production, nutrition, and reproduction. Bibliography, pp. 152–176.   [D436]

Fitzhugh, H. A., and G. E. Bradford, eds. *Hair Sheep of Western Africa and the Americas: A Genetic Resource for the Tropics*. Boulder, Colo.; Westview Press, 1983. 319p. (A Winrock International Study)

Hall, Alice. *The Pygmy Goat in America*. Illustrated by Jamie Smith. San Bernadino, Calif.; Hall Press, 1982. 127p. Bibliography, p. 127.

Hasnain, H. U. *Sheep and Goats in Pakistan*. Rome; Food and Agriculture Organization, 1985. 135p. (FAO Animal Production and Health Paper no. 56) Bibliography, pp. 102–103.

Mason, Ian Lauder, with the assistance of the United Nations Environment Programme. *Prolific Tropical Sheep*. Rome; Food and Agriculture Organization, 1980. 124p. (FAO Animal Production and Health Paper no. 17) CORE

Ponting, Kenneth G. *Sheep of the World*. Poole, U.K., and New York; Blandford Press; Distributed by Sterling Pub. Co., 1980. 155p. Bibliography, p. 142. CORE

Gives a brief account of the early history of sheep and describes the breeds. Includes 52 color illustrations.

Sobral, Marcelino, et al. *Animal Genetic Resources: Indigenous Breeds: Sheeps and Goats*. Lisbon; Direccao-Geral da Pecuaria, 1987. 207p.

United Kingdom. National Sheep Association. *British Sheep*. 7th ed. Tring, Herts, U.K.; The Association, 1987. 242p.

Illustrated description of British breeds, sheep industry and sheep production, glossary of sheep terms and addresses of breed societies.   [D428]

Yalcin, B. G. *Sheep and Goats in Turkey*. Rome; Food and Agriculture Organization, 1986. 168p. (FAO Animal Production and Health Paper no. 60) Bibliography, pp. 127–153.

Husbandry

Botkin, M. P., Ray A. Field, and C. LeRoy Johnson. *Sheep and Wool: Science, Production, and Management*. Englewood Cliffs, N.J.; Prentice-Hall, 1988. 451p. CORE

Considine, Harvey, and George W. Trimberger. *Dairy Goat Judging Techniques*. 2d ed. Scottsdale, Ariz.; Dairy Goat Journal Pub. Co., 1985. 328p.

Coop, I. E., ed. *Sheep and Goat Production*. Amsterdam and New York; Elsevier Scientific Pub. Co., 1982. 492p. (World Animal Science, C. Production-System Approach no. 1) CORE

Devendra, C., and G. B. McLeroy. *Goat and Sheep Production in the Tropics*. London and New York; Longman Group, 1982. 271p. (Intermediate Tropical Agriculture Series) CORE

Downing, E. *Keeping Sheep*. 2d ed. London; Pelham Books, 1987. 144p. (Garden Farming Series)

A guide to small-scale sheep farming.

Dunn, P. *The Goatkeeper's Veterinary Book*. 2d ed. Ipswich, U.K.; Farming Press, 1987. 198p.

A popular reference work on the ailments of goats for both the goat-keeper and veterinary surgeon.

Ensminger, M. Eugene, and R. O. Parker. *Sheep and Goat Science*. 5th ed. Danville, Ill.; Interstate Printers & Publishers, 1986. 643p. (Animal Agriculture Series) CORE

A comprehensive work of particular relevance to those engaged in sheep and goat husbandry in the U.S. Revised ed. of: *Sheep and Wool Science*. 4th ed., 1970.   [D433]

Gall, C., ed. *Goat Production*. London and New York; Academic Press, 1981. 619p. CORE

Gatenby, Ruth M. *Sheep Production in the Tropics and Sub-Tropics*. London and New York; Longman, 1986. 351p. (Tropical Agriculture Series) Bibliography, pp. 293–335. CORE

Includes a directory of breeds of sheep in the tropics.

Haenlein, George F. W., and Donald L. Ace, eds. *Extension Goat Handbook: Management, Housing, Nutrition, Genetics, Reproduction, Milk, Anatomy, Health*. Washington, D.C.; Extension Service, U.S. Dept. of Agriculture, 1984. 1 vol. (various paging). Printed and distributed in cooperation with the Extension Service, USDA, Washington, D.C.

"To keep this Handbook updated, a committee of Extension specialists and goat industry leaders will be asked to review its contents annually and recommend fact sheets for development, revision and deletion." —Introduction.

Harrison, Virden L. *Sheep Production: Intensive Systems, Innovative Techniques Boost Yields*. Washington, D.C.; Dept. of Agriculture, Economics, Statistics, and Cooperatives Service; For sale by the Supt. of Docs., G.P.O., 1980. 42p. (USDA Agricultural Economic Report no. 452) Bibliography, pp. 38–42.

International Stockman's School. *Sheep and Goat Handbook*. Vol. 1, 1980–vol. 5, 1987. Annual. Sponsored by Agriservices Foundation. Clovis, Calif.; The Foundation.

Jaudas, Ulrich. *The New Goat Handbook: Housing, Care, Feeding, Sickness, and Breeding: With a Special Chapter on Using the Milk, Meat, and Hair*. Consulting ed., Matthew M. Vriends; translated from the German by Elizabeth D. Crawford; drawings by Fritz W. Kohler; color photographs by well-known animal photographers. New York; Barron's, 1989. 93p.

Translation of: *Ziegen*.

Juergenson, Elwood M. *Approved Practices in Sheep Production*. 4th ed. Danville, Ill.; Interstate Printers & Publishers, 1981. 455p. CORE

A practical guide to tried and tested methods currently in use in the husbandry of sheep in the U.S.

Kruesi, William K. *The Sheep Raiser's Manual*. Charlotte, Vt.; Williamson Pub., 1985. 288p.

Leach, Corl A. *Aids to Goatkeeping*. 9th ed. Scottsdale, Ariz.; Dairy Goat Journal Pub. Co., 1983. 268p.

Also incorporates: *Dairy Goat Husbandry and Disease Control*, by G. E. Leach.

Luttmann, Gail. *Raising Milk Goats Successfully*. Charlotte, Vt.; Williamson Pub., 1986. 172p. Bibliography, pp. 157–164.

Mackenzie, David. *Goat Husbandry*. Rev. and edited by Jean Laing. 4th ed. London and Boston; Faber & Faber, 1980. 375p. Bibliography, pp. 363–364. CORE

Technically written; covers all aspects of goat husbandry: breeding, feeding, dairy production, meat, leather and mohair, marketing, etc. One of the first scientific textbooks on the subject.   [D439]

Marai, I. Fayez M., and J. B. Owen., eds. *New Techniques in Sheep Production*. London and Boston; Butterworths, 1987. 292p. CORE

McCammon-Feldman, B., et al. *Feeding Strategy of the Goat*. Ithaca, N.Y.; Dept. of Animal Science, New York State College of Agriculture and Life Sciences, Cornell University, 1981. 37p. (Cornell International Agriculture Mimeograph no. 88) Bibliography, pp. 29–37.

Mills, Olivia. *Practical Sheep Dairying: The Care and Milking of the Dairy Ewe*. Fully revised and updated ed. Foreword by John MacGregor. Wellingborough, U.K.; Thorsons, 1989. 320p.

National Research Council (U.S.). Commission on Natural Resources, Board on Agriculture and Renewable Resources, Committee on Animal Nutrition, Subcommittee on Goat Nutrition. *Nutrient Requirements of Goats: Angora, Dairy, and Meat Goats in Temperate and Tropical Countries*. Washington, D.C.; National Academy Press, 1981. (Nutrient Requirements of Domestic Animals no. 15) Bibliography, pp. 73–91. CORE

National Research Council (U.S.). Committee on Animal Nutrition, Board on Agriculture, Subcommittee on Animal Nutrition. *Nutrient Requirements of Sheep*. 6th ed., rev. Washington, D.C.; National Academy Press, 1985. 99p. (Nutrient Requirements of Domestic Animals no. 5) Bibliography, pp. 79–92. CORE

Ott, Randall S., and Mushtaq A. Memon. *Sheep and Goat Manual*. Hastings, Nebr.; Society for Theriogenology, 1980. 50p. "Volume X." CORE

Salmon, Jill. *The Goatkeeper's Guide*. 3d ed. David & Charles, 1990. 200p.

Thear, Katie. *Goats and Goatkeeping*. London; Merehurst Press, 1988. 176p. CORE

Turner, M. *Goat Care: A Complete Handbook*. Jefferson, N.C.; McFarland, 1984. 186p. CORE

Wickham, G. A., and M. F. McDonald. *Sheep Production*. 1982 + . Wellington; R. Richards in association with the New Zealand Institute of Agricultural Science. Vol. 1, 1982, has 269p. Titled: *Breeding and Production*.

Wilkinson, J. M., and B. A. Stark. *Commercial Goat Production*. Oxford; Blackwell; Boston; BSP Professional Books, 1987. 159p. CORE

Winrock International. *Sheep and Goats in Developing Countries: Their Present and Potential Role*. Washington, D.C.; World Bank, 1983. 116p. (World Bank Technical Paper; ISSN: 0253-7494) Bibliography, pp. 109–116.

Rabbits

Bibliographies

Rafats, Jerry. *Rabbit Production for Food, Fur, and Fun, January 1979–December 1989*. Beltsville, Md.; National Agricultural Library, 1990. 25p. 273 Citations from AGRICOLA. (Quick Bibliography Series no. QB 90-36)

Breeds

Ambrose, T. J., revised by J. Barnes. *Dutch Rabbits.* Alton, U.K.; Nimrod, 1988. 80p. (The Rabbit Library)

American Rabbit Breeders Association. *Standard of Perfection; Standard Bred Rabbits and Cavies.* Pittsburgh; The Association, 1986. 206p. CORE   [D442]

Fisher, Judy, ed. *Angora Handbook.* Illustrated by Jennifer Cole. Calif.; Northern California Angora Guild, 1985. 117p.

Directories

American Rabbit Breeders Association. *Yearbook.* 1967/68 + . Annual. Chicago; The Association. 1989/90 ed., 304p.   [D442]

Husbandry

Cheeke, P. R. *Rabbit Feeding and Nutrition.* London; Academic Press, 1987. 376p. (Animal Feeding and Nutrition) CORE

Cheeke, P. R., et al. *Rabbit Production.* 6th ed. Danville, Ill.; Interstate Printers & Publishers, 1987. 472p. CORE

An established work on the husbandry of rabbits which contains a section on diseases; has color illustrations of the major breeds.

Lebas, F., et al. *The Rabbit: Husbandry, Health and Production.* Rome; Food and Agriculture Organization, 1986. 235p. (FAO Animal Production and Health Series no. 21) Bibliography, pp. 231–234. CORE

Leverett, B. *Keeping Rabbits: A Complete Manual.* London and New York; Blandford Press; Distributed in the U.S. by Sterling Pub. Co., 1987. 160p. (A Guide to Management) Bibliography, pp. 154.

Portsmouth, John. *Commercial Rabbit-Keeping.* 3d ed. 15 The Maltings, Turk St., Alton, Hants, GL134 IDL, U.K.; Nimrod Press, 1987. 142p.

Raising Rabbits 1: Learning about Rabbits, Building the Pens, Choosing Rabbits. Rome; Food and Agriculture Organization, 1988. 56p. (FAO Economic and Social Development Series no. 3/36; *Better Farming Series* no. 36)

Raising Rabbits 2: Feeding Rabbits, Raising Baby Rabbits, Further Improvements. Rome; Food and Agriculture Organization, 1988. 49p. (FAO Economic and Social Development Series no. 3/37; *Better Farming Series* no. 37)

Sandford, John Cecil. *The Domestic Rabbit.* 4th ed. London; Collins; Distributed in the U.S. by Sheridan House, 1986. 272p. CORE

Intended for rabbit farmers and covers every aspect of production, management and marketing.

Sandford, John Cecil. *Rabbits: A Guide to Management*. Ramsbury, Marlborough; Crowood Press, 1988. 128p. Bibliography, pp. 261–263.

Popular guide for small scale breeders.   [D445]

Vriends-Parent, Lucia; Matthew M. Vriends, consulting ed. *The New Rabbit Handbook: Everything about Purchase, Care, Nutrition, Breeding, and Behavior*. Color photographs by well-known photographers and drawings by Michelle Earle-Bridges. New York; Barron's, 1989. 133p. Bibliography, pp. 125–126.

Other Domesticated Species

Cheney, Sheldon. *Llamas and South American Camelids, January 1970–October 1988: 153 Citations from AGRICOLA*. Beltsville, Md.; U.S. Dept. of Agriculture; National Agricultural Library, 1989. January 1970–December 1978, 5p.; January 1979–February 1989, 10p. (Quick Bibliography Series no. QB 89-29)

Cockrill, W. Ross, ed. *The Camelid: An All-Purpose Animal*. Khartoum Workshop on Camels, 1979. Uppsala; Scandinavian Institute of African Studies, 1984–1985. 2 vols. CORE

Vol. 1: Thirty-two papers reviewing camelid species, breeds and status, diseases, feeding, reproduction, physiology, and meat and milk production; contains a useful review of the Camelidae of South America (pp. 112–143); most of the papers were first published in the *International Foundation for Science's Provisional Report no. 6: Camels (1979)*, 544p. Vol. 2: A companion bibliography; over 3,000 references.

Farid, Mohamed F. A. *Camelids Bibliography*. Damascus, Syria; Arab Centre for the Studies of Arid Zones and Dry Lands, 1981. 546p.

Contains 2,539 annotated references up to July 1981; has indexes to subjects and species and a geographical index. Updates. have appeared in the *Camel Newsletter* published by the Centre. A second edition of the bibliography is in preparation.

Hill, Desmond. *Cattle and Buffalo Meat Production in the Tropics*. Harlow, Essex, Eng; Longman Scientific & Technical, 1988. 210p. (Intermediate Tropical Agriculture Series) CORE

Joergensen, Gunnar, ed. *Mink Production*. English ed. Hilleroed, Denmark; SCIENTIFUR, 1985. 399p.

Danish ed., 1984, by the Danish Fur Breeders Association.

Lensch, Jurgen. *Problems and Prospects of Cattle and Buffalo Husbandry in India with Special Reference to the Concept of "Sacred Cow": Shaping and Controlling the Course of Future Development; Possibilities and Limitations*. Hamburg (P.O. Box 10, 2204 Krempe), Germany; Jurgen Lensch, 1987. 277p. Bibliography, pp. 271–276.

Mukasa-Mugerwa, E. *The Camel (Camelus Dromedarius): A Bibliographical Review*. Addis, Ababa, Ethiopia; International Livestock Centre for Africa, 1981. 147p. (ILCA Monograph no. 5) CORE

National Research Council (U.S.). Board on Agriculture and Renewable Resources, Committee on Animal Nutrition, Subcommittee on Furbearing Nutrition. *Nutrient Requirements of Minks and Foxes*. 2d ed., rev. Washington, D.C.; National Academy Press, 1982. 72p. (Nutrient Requirements of Domestic Animals no. 7) Bibliography, pp. 67–72. CORE

Ornas, Anders Hjort af, ed. *Camels in Development: Sustainable Production in African Drylands*. Uppsala, Sweden; Scandinavian Institute of African Studies, 1988. 165p.

The seminar, "The Case of African Drylands and Balanced Camel Production," was arranged as part of a research programme, Human Life in Arid Lands, held at Furudal, near Rattvik, Sweden, October 20–22, 1987.

Smith, Bruce William. *Nature's Jewels: A History of Mink Farming in the United States*. Brookfield, Wis.; National Board of Fur Farm Organizations, 1981. 100p.

Von Kerckerinck zur Borg, Josef. *Deer Farming in North America: The Conquest of a New Frontier*. Rhinebeck, N.Y.; Phanter Press, 1987. 225p. Bibliography, pp. 214–216.

Wilson, R. T. *The Camel*. London and New York; Longman, 1984. 223p. Bibliography, pp. 178–217. CORE

An excellent and comprehenive work on all aspects of the one-humped camel (Camelus Dromedarius); many figures and illustrations; a vast amount of numerical information is presented in over seventy tables; over 2,000 references are listed in the bibliography.

Statistics

Great Britain. Meat and Livestock Commission. *Performance Recorded Flocks*. Bletchley; M.L.C., 1983. 60p.

"Provides a list of the purebred flocks included in the MLC Individual-Ewe Recording Scheme whose owners have agreed to publication. Details of 366 flocks representing 49 breeds and about 42,000 ewes put to the ram in 1982 are included. The flocks are grouped by breed and arranged in alphabetical order of owners' names." —Foreword

Henson, Elizabeth, compiler. *AMBC 1985 North American Livestock Census*. Updated, March 1986. Pittsboro, N.C.; American Minor Breeds Conservancy, 1986, c1985. 34p. Bibliography, p. 32.

1948–1985 World Crop and Livestock Statistics: Area, Yield, and Production of Crops: Production of Livestock Products. Rome; Food and Agriculture Organization, 1987. 760p. (FAO Processed Statistics Series). Chiefly tables. Title also in French and Spanish.

Sarma, J. S., and Patrick Yeung. *Livestock Products in the Third World: Past Trends and Projections to 1990 and 2000*. Washington, D.C.; International Food Policy Research Institute, 1985. 87p. (Research Report no. 49) Bibliography, p. 87.

U.S. Department of Agriculture. Economics and Statistics Service, Crop Reporting Board. *Cattle*. 1973 + . Current frequency: semi-annual. Washington, D.C.; The Board.

With *Sheep and Goats,* continues: *Cattle, Sheep, and Goat Inventory*. Vols. for Feb. 4, 1987 + distributed to depository libraries in microfiche.

U.S. Department of Agriculture. Economics and Statistics Service, Crop Reporting Board. *Sheep and Goats*. 1973 + . Annual. Washington, D.C.; The Board.

With *Cattle*, continues: *Cattle, Sheep, and Goat Inventory*. Vols. for 1973–1981 issued by the Crop Reporting Board; 1990 + issued by the National Agricultural Statistics Service. Microfiche.

Animal Products

This section does not include works dealing with food hygiene and the inspection of animal products destined for human consumption.

Dairy Industry

Bibliographies

Dash, Suzanne L., and Judith Sommer. *Recent Dairy Policy Publications with Selected Annotations*. Washington, D.C.; U.S. Dept. of Agriculture; Economic Research Service; National Economics Division, 1984. 36p. (ERS Staff Report no. AGES 840417)

"Reproduced for limited distribution to the research community outside the U.S. Department of Agriculture." Distributed to depository libraries in microfiche.

Dictionaries

Dictionary of Dairy Terminology: In English, French, German, and Spanish. Compiled by International Dairy Federation. Amsterdam and New York; Elsevier Scientific Pub. Co., 1983. 328p. Bibliography, pp. vii–ix. CORE

Directories

Dryer, Jerry. *Dairy Foods 1988 Market Directory*. Chicago; Gorman Pub. Co., 1988. 284p.

Histories

Church, Gordon C. *An Unfailing Faith: A History of the Saskatchewan Dairy Industry*. Regina, Sask.; Canadian Plains Research Center, University of Regina, 1985. 308p. (Canadian Plains Studies no. 13) Bibliography, pp. 270–295.

Tauer, Janelle R., and Olan D. Forker. *Dairy Promotion in the United States, 1979–1986: The History and Structure of the National Milk and Dairy Product Promotion Program with Special Reference to New York*. Ithaca, N.Y.; Dept. of Agricultural Economics, Cornell University Agricultural Experiment Station, New York State College of Agriculture and Life Sciences, 1987. 314p.

General Works

National Commission on Dairy Policy (U.S.). *Report and Recommendations*. Submitted by the Subcommittee on Livestock, Dairy, and Poultry of the Committee on Agriculture, U.S. House of Representatives. Washington, D.C.; U.S. G.P.O., 1989. 111p.

Nelson, John A., and G. Malcolm Trout. *Judging Dairy Products*. 4th ed., rev. Westport, Conn.; Avi Pub. Co., 1981. 463p.   [D471]

Wong, Noble P., et al., eds. *Fundamentals of Dairy Chemistry*. 3d ed. New York; Van Nostrand Reinhold Co., 1988. 779p. CORE   [D472]

Animal and Plant Fibers and Textile Industry

Works listed below deal primarily with animal and plant fibers as textile raw materials, or cover these types of fibers along with other information about textiles and the textile industry.

Literature Guides

Vogel, J. Thomas, and Barbara W. Lowry. *The Textile Industry: An Information Sourcebook*. Phoenix, Ariz.; Oryx Press, 1989. 246p. (Oryx Sourcebook Series in Business and Management no. 19)

Abstracts, Indexes and Bibliographies

Arthur D. Jenkins Library. *Rug and Textile Arts: A Periodical Index, 1890–1982*. The Textile Museum, Arthur D. Jenkins Library. Boston; G. K. Hall, 1983. 472p.

Gordon, Beverly. *Domestic American Textiles: A Bibliographic Sourcebook*. Pittsburgh; Center for the History of American Needlework, 1978. 217p. 574 citations.

Also includes textile exhibits, magazines and periodicals.

Singh, I. B., and S. B. Singh, compilers. *Indian Textiles: A Select Bibliography.* Foreword by R. P. Rastogi. Varanasi; Bharat Kala Bhavan, Banaras Hindu University, 1986. 59p.

Encyclopedias and Dictionaries

Beech, S. R., ed. *Textile Terms and Definitions.* Compiled by the Textile Institute, Textile Terms and Definitions Committee. 8th ed., rev. and enlarged. Manchester; The Textile Institute, 1986. 297p.

Burnham, Dorothy. *Warp and Weft: A Dictionary of Textile Terms.* New York; Scribner, 1981. 216p. Bibliography, pp. 209–216.

Encyclopedia of Textiles. By the editors of *American Fabrics and Fashions Magazine.* 3d ed. Englewood Cliffs, N.J.; Prentice-Hall, 1980. 636p.

"Includes a comprehensive dictionary of textile terms."
2d ed. published as: *AF Encyclopedia of Textiles.*   [D478]

Grayson, Martin, ed. *Encyclopedia of Textiles, Fibers, and Nonwoven Fabrics.* New York; Wiley, 1984. 581p. (Encyclopedia Reprint Series)

Articles reprinted from 1978–1984 ed. of: *Kirk-Othmer Encyclopedia of Chemical Technology.*

Wingate, Isabel B., ed. *Fairchild's Dictionary of Textiles.* 6th ed. New York; Fairchild Publications, 1979. 691p.   [D479]

Handbooks and Reference Texts

Appleyard, H. M. *Guide to the Identification of Animal Fibres.* 2d ed. Leeds; Wire, 1978. 124p.

                                                                          [D482]
ASTM Standard Performance Specifications for Textile Fabrics. Philadelphia; American Society for Testing Materials, 1983. 167p.

Jurisdiction of ASTM Subcommittee D13.56.

Cook, James Gordon. *Handbook of Textile Fibres.* 5th ed. Durham, U.K.; Merrow Pub. Co., 1984. 2 vols.   [D485]

Needles, Howard L. *Handbook of Textile Fibers, Dyes, and Finishes.* New York; Garland STPM Press, 1981. 170p.

Directories

Davison's Textile Blue Book. 1st ed., 1988 + . Annual. Ridgewood, N.J.; Davison Pub. Co. 125th ed., 1991, 694p.   [D492]

Title and subtitle have varied. Most recently continues *Davison's Textile Blue Book; United States and Canada*. All listings are arranged by geographic location, first alphabetically by states in the U.S., then alphabetically by city within the state and then alphabetically within the city. Canadian listings follow the U.S. listings.

B. Poultry Husbandry, by Judith Levitt

Bibliographies and Lists of Periodicals

Clingerman, Karen J.
Stress in Poultry, January 1979–August 1990: 311 Citations from AGRICOLA. Beltsville, Md.; National Agricultural Library, 1990. 28p. (Quick Bibliography Series no. QB 91-01)

Poultry Housing and Facilities: January 1979–August 1990. Beltsville, Md.; National Agricultural Library, 1990. 36p. 417 Citations from AGRICOLA. (Quick Bibliography Series no. QB 91-02)

Welfare of Poultry: January 1979–August 1990. Beltsville, Md.; National Agricultural Library, 1990. 20p. 244 Citations from AGRICOLA. (Quick Bibliography Series no. QB 91-03)

Goldberg, David H. and Stanislaw J. Kosecki, compilers. *World List of Poultry Serials.* With a foreword by John L. Skinner. Beltsville, Md.; U.S. Dept. of Agriculture, National Agricultural Library, 1989. 182p. 1,641 citations. (USDA Bibliographies and Literature of Agriculture no. 76)

Maclean, Jayne T. *Poultry Wastes: Uses and Management, January 1979–January 1989: 226 Citations from AGRICOLA.* Beltsville, Md.; U.S. Dept. of Agriculture, National Agricultural Library, 1989. 23p. (Quick Bibliography Series no. QB 89-46)

Wiley, William H., compiler. *Bibliography on the Biology and Production of Turkeys.* Clemson, S.C.; Clemson University, 1977. 2 vols. Vol. 1, 574p.; vol. 2, 123p.

"The compiler reviewed 170 U.S. journals, bulletins from 38 State Experiment Stations, 93 non-U.S. journals and numerous textbooks. . . . This search covered the period 1919–1974 inclusive. It resulted in over 4,200 citations, almost all of which are annotated."   [D496]

Directories

American Poultry Association. *Yearbook.* Annual. Troy, N.Y.; The Association. 1990, 416p.

Continues: American Poultry Association. *What's What Yearbook.*

Association of Avian Veterinarians. *Membership Directory*. Annual. E. Northport, N.Y.; The Association. 1990, 107p.

Canada's Who's Who of the Poultry Industry. 1955 +. New Westminster, B.C.; Farm Papers. 1990 ed., 126p.

Published as a supplement to: *Canada Poultryman*.   [D498]

National Poultry Improvement Plan. *Directory of Participants Handling Egg-Type and Meat-Type Chickens and Turkeys*. Annual. Beltsville, Md.; Agricultural Research (Northeastern region), Science and Education Administration, U.S. Dept. of Agriculture, 1991. 46p. (National Poultry Improvement Plan Report No.1; *APHIS* 91)

Since 1984 distributed to depository libraries in microfiche.

National Poultry Improvement Plan. *Directory of Participants Handling Waterfowl, Exhibition Poultry, and Game Birds*. Annual. Beltsville, Md.; Agricultural Research (Northeastern region), Science and Education Administration, U.S. Dept. of Agriculture, 1991. 102p. (National Poultry Improvement Plan Reports; APHIS 91)

Since 1984 distributed to depository libraries in microfiche.

Who's Who in the Egg and Poultry Industries in the United States and Canada. 1987 +. Annual. Mt. Morris, Ill.; Watt Pub. Co. 1989 ed., 398p.

Continues: *Who's Who in the Egg and Poultry Industries* (1929–1986/87).
                    [D500]

Poultry Standards, Breeds, and Species

Batty, Joseph, assisted by other fanciers. *The Ancona Fowl*. Alton, U.K.; Nimrod, 1988. 53p. (Poultry Fanciers Library; Understanding Pure Breeds of Poultry)

Batty, Joseph. *Lewis Wright's Poultry*. Hindhead, Surrey; Triplegate; Liss, Hants, U.K.; Distributed by Nimrod Book Services, 1983. 130p.

80 pages of colored plates based on the plates taken from the *Illustrated Book of Poultry* by Lewis Wright.

Belshaw, R. H. Hastings. *Guinea Fowl of the World*. Liss, Hampshire, U.K.; Nimrod Book Services, 1985. 192p. (World of Ornithology) Bibliography, pp. 177–188.

Ducks and Geese. 6th ed. London; H.M.S.O., 1980. 85p. (MAFF Reference Book no. 70)

Frith, Harold James. *Pigeons and Doves of Australia*. Adelaide and New York; Rigby, 1982. 304p. Bibliography, pp. 292–298.

Goodwin, Derek. *Pigeons and Doves of the World*. 3d ed. Colour plates by Robert Gillmer. London; British Museum (Natural History); Ithaca, N.Y.; Comstock Pub. Associates, 1983. 363p. CORE

Nomenclature, adaptive behavior, plumage, feeding, and reproduction of typical pigeons, turtle doves, and other types of pigeons. Gives description, distribution, and habitat, feeding and general habits, nesting, voice, and display for each species.   [D503]

Hansell, Peter and Jean Hansell. *Doves and Dovecotes*. Bath, U.K.; Millstream Books, 1988. 248p. Bibliography, pp. 241–245.

Kemp, Rick. *Pure Breed Poultry Raising*. Kenthurst, Australia; Kangaroo Press, 1985. 80p.

Levi, Wendell Mitchell. *The Pigeon*. Sumter, S.C.; Levi Publishing, 1986, c1974. 667p. Reprint. Bibliography, pp. 616–641. CORE

Complete discussion of the breeds, biology and husbandry of this bird.   [D505]

May, C. G., ed. *British Poultry Standards: Complete Specifications and Judging Points of All Standardized Breeds and Varieties of Poultry as Compiled by the Specialist Breed Societies and Recognized by the Poultry Club of Great Britain*. 4th ed., rev. by David Hawksworth. London and Boston; Butterworth Scientific, 1982. 375p.

Handbook giving specifications and judging points of breeds of fowl, turkeys, ducks, and geese.   [D507]

Selected Annuals and Congresses

European Symposium of Poultry Nutrition. 1st, 1977 + . (2d, 1979; Troelstra Oord, Beekbergen, Netherlands.)

Nixey, C. and T. C. Grey, eds. *Recent Advances in Turkey Science; Papers From the 21st Poultry Sciences Symposium held at Harper Adams Agricultural College, Newport, Shropshire, September 8–11, 1987*. London and Boston; Butterworths, 1989. 373p. (Poultry Science Symposium No.21) CORE

Sorensen, L. Yding, ed. European Symposium on Poultry Welfare (1st; 1981; Koge, Denmark). *First European Symposium on Poultry Welfare; Report of Proceedings*. Denmark; W.P.S.A., Danish Branch, 1981. 240p.

Manuals and Handbooks

French, Kenneth M. *Practical Poultry Raising*. 1984 + . Edited by Larry Ritter; illustrated by Marilyn Kaufman. Washington, D.C.; Peace Corps Information Collection & Exchange, 1984. 1 vol., looseleaf. (Appropriate Technologies for Development, Manual no. M-11) Bibliography, pp. 207–210.

National Institute of Poultry Husbandry. *History of the National Institute of Poultry Husbandry: Incorporated by Harper Adams Agricultural College, Newport, Shropshire. . . .* Newport Salop; The Institute, 1986. 227p.

Prepared to celebrate the diamond jubilee of its foundation and as a memorial to the contributions of the late Dr. Harold Temperton.

North, Mack O. and Donald D. Bell. *Commercial Chicken Production Manual.* 4th ed. New York; Van Nostrand Reinhold, 1990. 913p. Includes bibliographical references, pp. 889–891.   [D554]

Reece, Floyd N. *Solar Heating for Brooding Chickens.* Prepared by Science and Education Administration. Washington, D.C.; The Administration, 1981. 12p. (USDA Farmers' Bulletin no. 2272)

Schwartz, L. Dwight. *Poultry Health Handbook.* 3d. ed. University Park, Pa.; College of Agriculture, Pennsylvania State University, 1988. 203p.

1st ed., 1972, published as: *Pennsylvania Poultry Handbook.*

Summers, John D. and Steven Leeson. *Poultry Nutrition Handbook.* Rev. ed. Guelph, Ontario; Dept. of Animal and Poultry Science, Ontario Agricultural College, University of Guelph, 1985. 230p.

U.S. Agricultural Marketing Services. *Egg-Grading Manual.* Rev., April 1983. Washington, D.C.; U.S. Department of Agriculture, 1983. 44p. (USDA Agriculture Handbook no. 75)   [D519]

U.S. Agricultural Marketing Service. *Poultry-Grading Manual.* Rev., June 1989. Washington, D.C.; U.S. Dept. of Agriculture, 1989. 28p. (USDA Agriculture Handbook no. 31)   [D518]

Reference Texts

Poultry Genetics

Crawford, R. D., ed. *Poultry Breeding and Genetics.* Amsterdam and New York; Elsevier, 1990. 1123p. (Developments in Animal and Veterinary Sciences no. 22)

An advanced level treatise on poultry breeding and genetics. Designed as a reference work and a comprehensive critical review of the field. Forty-two chapters written by 37 authors. Covers domestic fowl, turkey, Japanese quail, guineafowl, ring-necked pheasant, domestic duck, Muscovy duck and goose.

Hill, W. G., J. M. Manson and D. Hewitt, eds. *Poultry Genetics and Breeding; Proceedings of the 18th Poultry Science Symposium, 1983.* Harlow, Essex; British Poultry Science; Available from Longman Group, 1985. 178p. (Poultry Science Symposium no. 18)

Leclercq, B. and C. C. Whitehead, eds. *Leanness in Domestic Birds: Genetic, Metabolic, and Hormonal Aspects; Proceedings of a Symposium held in Tours,*

France, August 4–7, 1987. London and Boston; Published by arrangement with the Institut National de la Recherche Agronomique by Butterworths, 1988. 405p.

Eggs and Embryology

Butler, H. and B. H. J. Juurlink. *An Atlas for Staging Mammalian and Chick Embryos*. Boca Raton, Fla.; CRC Press, 1987. 218p. Bibliography, pp. 205–206.

Metcalfe, James, Michael K. Stock and Rolf L. Ingermann, eds. *Development of the Avian Embryo; International Union of Physiological Sciences Satellite Symposium, Lester B. Pearson College of the Pacific, Victoria, B.C., Canada, July 19–22, 1986*. New York; A. R. Liss, 1987. 376p.

Also issued as a supplement to the *Journal of Experimental Zoology,* 1987.

Anatomy and Histology

Koch, Tankred. *Anatomy of the Chicken and Domestic Birds*. Illustrated by Erwin Rossa. Edited and translated from the German manuscript by Bernard H. Skold and Louis DeVries. Ann Arbor, Mich.; Reprinted for the Iowa State University Press by University Microfilm International, 1978, c1973. 170p. Bibliography, p. 159. CORE   [D538]

Nickel, R., A. Schummer and E. Seiferle. *Anatomy of the Domestic Birds*. Translated by W. G. Siller and P. A. L. Wight. Berlin and Hamburg; Parey, 1977. 207p. Bibliography, pp. 164–194. CORE

Translation of: *Anatomie der Hausvogel*, which was originally published as vol. 5 of *Lehrbuch der Anatomie der Haustiere*.

Schwarze, Erich. *Kompendium der Geflugelanatomie*. 4th ed. Stuttgart; Fischer, 1985. 300p. Bibliography, pp. 267–284.

Physiology and Behavior

Abs, Michael, ed. *Physiology and Behavior of the Pigeon*. London and New York; Academic Press, 1983. 360p.

Bell, David James and B. M. Freeman, eds. *Physiology and Biochemistry of the Domestic Fowl*. London and New York; Academic Press, 1971–1984. 5 vols. CORE

Comprehensive multi-author work covering the functions of all body systems (digestive, respiratory, urinary, circulatory, nervous, reproductive and skeletal) and physiological chemistry that is important or regulated in poultry. Vols. 4–5, edited by B. M. Freeman, update the original work. An appendix in vol. 5 gives quantitative, biochemical and physiological data.   [D542]

Critical Reviews in Poultry Biology. Vol. 1, issue 1, 1987+. Quarterly journal. Boca Raton, Fla.; CRC Press.

Okawa, Takanori, ed. *The Brain and Behavior of the Fowl.* Tokyo; Japan Scientific Societies Press, 1983. 352p.

Sturkie, P. D., ed., with contributions by C. A. Benzo et al. *Avian Physiology.* 4th ed. New York; Springer-Verlag, 1986. 516p. CORE   [D544]

Zayan, Rene and Ian J. H. Duncan, eds. *Cognitive Aspects of Social Behaviour in the Domestic Fowl.* Amsterdam and New York; Elsevier, 1987. 492p. CORE

Poultry and Egg Production

Austic, Richard E. and Malden C. Nesheim. *Poultry Production.* Philadelphia; Lea & Febiger, 1990. 325p. CORE

An established text for students of poultry husbandry and a reference manual for the poultry farmer. Includes information on marketing and economics of the poultry industry in North America. Nesheim's name appears first on the previous ed.   [D553]

Clayton, G. A., et al. *Turkey Production: Breeding and Husbandry.* London; H.M.S.O., 1985. 122p. (Ministry of Agriculture, Fisheries and Food Reference Book [MAFF] no. 212) Bibliography, pp. 118–119. CORE

Covers housing, nutritional needs and ration formulation, and husbandry methods and equipment.

Ensminger, M. Eugene. *Poultry Science.* 2d ed. Danville, Ill.,; Interstate Printers & Publishers, 1980. 502p. (Animal Agriculture Series) CORE

Breeds and breeding, selection and culling, feeding and nutrition, housing, management, marketing, health, etc.   [D546]

Haynes, Cynthia. *Raising Turkeys, Ducks, Geese, Pigeons, and Guineas.* Blue Ridge Summit, Pa.; Tab Books, 1987. 354p.

Journal of Applied Poultry Research. Mar. 1992+. Quarterly. Athens, Ga.; Applied Poultry Science.

Manual of Poultry Production in the Tropics. English ed., translated by R. R. Say. Wallingford, Oxon, U.K.; CAB International, 1987. 119p. CORE

A basic introductory text. Translation of: *Manuel d'Aviculture en Zone Tropicale* (IEMVT, 1983).

Moreng, R. E. and J. S. Avens. *Poultry Science and Production.* Reston, Va.; Reston Pub. Co., 1985. 438p. CORE

Comprehensive guide to the production of chickens, turkeys, ducks and geese written for agricultural students and poultry farmers.

Oluyami, J. A. and F. A. Roberts. *Poultry Production in Warm Wet Climates.* London; Macmillan, 1979. 197p. (Macmillan Tropical Agriculture, Horticulture and Applied Ecology Series) CORE

Sainsbury, David. *Poultry Health and Management.* 2d ed. London and New York; Granada, 1984. 186p. Bibliography, pp. 181–182. CORE

Concise review of poultry production in temperate and hot climates; includes a chapter on welfare and alternative production systems.

Stadelman, William J. and Owen J. Cotterill, eds. *Egg Science and Technology.* 3d ed. Westport, Conn.; Avi Pub. Co., 1986. 449p. CORE

Egg production practices, quality of eggs, microbiology, nutritive value, industrial processing and utilization.   [D557]

Thear, Katie. *Keeping Quail: A Guide to Domestic and Commercial Management.* Saffron Walden; Broad Leys Publishing, 1987. 96p.

Walters, John and Michael Parker. *Keeping Chickens.* 2d ed. London; Pelham Books, 1982. 126p. (Garden Farming Series) Bibliography, p. 117.

Feeds and Nutrition

Balloun, Stanley L. *Soybean Meal in Poultry Nutrition* . . . edited by Kenneth C. Lepley. St. Louis, Mo.; American Soybean Association, 1980. 122p. Bibliography, pp. 111–122.

Cole, D. J. A. and W. Haresign, eds. *Recent Developments in Poultry Nutrition.* London and Boston; Butterworths, 1989. 344p.

Feltwell, Ray and Syd Fox. *Practical Poultry Farming.* London and Boston; Faber & Faber, 1978. 302p. Bibliography, p. 289.

Fisher, C. and K. N. Boorman, eds. *Nutrient Requirements of Poultry and Nutritional Research; Proceedings of the 19th Poultry Science Symposium, held in Edinburgh, September 1984.* London and Boston; Butterworths, 1986. 224p. (Poultry Science Symposium no. 19) CORE

National Research Council (U.S.). Subcommittee on Poultry Nutrition, Committee on Animal Nutrition. *Nutrient Requirements of Poultry.* 8th ed., rev. Washington, D.C.; National Academy Press, 1984. 71p. (Nutrient Requirements of Domestic Animals no. 1) Bibliography, pp. 49–65. CORE

Data were prepared from all available literature. Requirements for energy, protein, minerals, vitamins, choline and essential fatty acids, and water are shown.   [D559]

Patrick, Homer and Philip J. Schaible. *Poultry, Feeds and Nutrition.* 2d ed. Westport, Conn.; Avi Pub. Co., 1980. 668p. Bibliography, pp. 637–660. CORE

Treatise on feeds, feed additives, and feeding of poultry in health and disease, written for the nutritionist, veterinarian, teacher, and student of nutrition and feed technology, and for the general poultryman. Appendix, glossary.   [D560]

Scott, Milton, Malden C. Nesheim and Robert J. Young. *Nutrition of the Chicken*. 3d ed. Ithaca, N.Y.; M. L. Scott, 1982. 562p. CORE

Text and ready reference for students and researchers in poultry nutrition, with chapters on energetics, nutrients, nutritional requirements, feedstuffs, feed formulation and measurement of nutritive quality.   [D561]

Statistics

Baker, Allen J. and Eunice Armstrong. *Poultry and Egg Statistics, 1960–85*. Washington, D.C.; U.S. Dept. of Agriculture, Economic Research Service, 1986. 84p. (USDA Statistical Bulletin no. 747)

Hatchery Production. Eggs, Chickens and Turkeys. 1983 + . Annual. Washington, D.C.; Crop Reporting Board; U.S. Dept. of Agriculture; Distributed by Supt. of Docs., U.S. G.P.O. Title varies.

Lasley, Floyd Alvin, William L. Henson and Harold B. Jones, Jr. *The U.S. Turkey Industry*. Washington, D.C.; U.S. Dept. of Agriculture, Economic Research Service, 1985. 64p. (USDA Agricultural Economic Report no. 525) Bibliography, pp. 55–58.

Distributed to depository libraries in microfiche.

U.S. Department of Agriculture. Economic Research Service. *Livestock and Poultry Update*. 1988 + . Monthly. Washington, D.C.; The Service.

Supplement to: *Situation and Outlook Report. Livestock and Poultry*.

U.S. Dept. of Agriculture. Economic Research Service. *Situation and Outlook Report. Livestock and Poultry*. 1986 + . Bimonthly. Washington, D.C.; The Service.

Title varies. Has supplement: *Livestock and Poultry Update*.
Absorbed: *Poultry and Egg Situation*.   [D563]

Weimar, Mark R. and Shauna Cromer. *U.S. Egg and Poultry Statistical Series, 1960–87*. Washington, D.C.; U.S. Dept. of Agriculture, Economic Research Service, 1989. 198p. (USDA Statistical Bulletin no. 775). Chiefly tables.

C. Veterinary Medicine, by Jo Anne Boorkman

Literature Guides and Lists of Periodicals

Darling, Louise, ed. *Handbook of Medical Library Practice*. 4th ed. Chicago; Medical Library Association, 1982–1988. 3 vols.   [D001]

Gibbs, Mike. *Keyguide to Information Sources in Veterinary Medicine*. London and New York; Mansell Pub., 1990. 459p.

Part I presents a narrative survey of the literature; Part II provides an annotated bibliography of key references; and Part III provides an international directory of veterinary associations, societies, selected libraries, online systems, online databases and publishers.

Schwabe, Calvin W. *Veterinary Medicine and Human Health*. 3d ed. Baltimore, Md.; Williams & Wilkins, 1984. 680p.

"A Key to the Literature" is found at the conclusion of each chapter, following chapter references and suggestions for further readings.   [D004]

Veterinary Serials: A Union List of Serials Held in Veterinary Collections in Canada, Europe and the U.S.A. Sponsored by the Veterinary Medical Libraries Section of the Medical Library Association. Produced by the Union List Committee. 2d ed. Chicago; Veterinary Medical Libraries Section, Medical Library Association, 1987–1988. 2 vols.

Abstracts and Major Indexes

Animal Disease Occurrence = Incidence des Maladies Animales. 1980 + . Annual. Farnham Royal, U.K.; Commonwealth Agricultural Bureaux.

Provides abstracts and convenient tabular indexes for identifying disease occurrence by disease, species and geographical location. Was semi-annual 1980–1989.

Mastitis Research Index. Feb. 1984 + . Annual. Brussels, Belgium; International Dairy Federation.

Resulting from a questionnaire. Section I, Projects organized by country and institution conducting research; Section II, Worker index; Section III, Subject index.

Wildlife Disease Review. 1983 + . Monthly. Fort Collins, Colo.; Wildlife Disease Review.

A taxonomic guide to the literature of diseases in captive and free-ranging wildlife. Looseleaf binder with tabular arrangement (Mammals, Birds, Fish and Reptiles, including Amphibians). Arranged by order with citation numbers listed numerically by family. Subject, taxonomic, geographic and author indexes. Entries provide bibliographic citation, abstract and first author's address.

Veterinary Update: Clinical Abstract Service. Large Animal ed. Vol. 27, no. 6, June 1986 + . Monthly. Santa Barbara, Calif.; American Veterinary Publications.

Continues: *Veterinary Reference Service Update*, vol. 16, no.1, Jan. 1975–vol. 27, no. 4, Apr. 1986. Published in two editions: Equine and Food Animal (cattle, swine, goats and sheep), each published on alternate months: Food Animal

Abstracts published in January, March, May, July, September and November; Equine Abstracts published in February, April, June, August, October and December. Volume numbering changes to vol. 2, no. 1, January-February 1987. Small Animal ed. continues numbering of *Veterinary Reference Service Update*.
[D018]

Bibliographies and Catalogs

Bebee, Charles N., compiler and ed. *Protection of Farm Animals 1979–April 1989; Citations from AGRICOLA Concerning Diseases and Other Environmental Considerations*. Beltsville, Md.; U.S. Dept. of Agriculture, National Agricultural Library; Washington, D.C.; U.S. Environmental Protection Agency, Office of Pesticide Programs, 1989. 456p. (Bibliographies and Literature of Agriculture no. 88)

Foot and Mouth Disease Bibliography. USDA, APHIS, Emergency Programs, Veterinary Services. Hyattsville, Md.; USDA-APHIS, Veterinary Services, Emergency Programs, 1980. 443p.

"Part of the Emergency Programs Foreign Animal Disease Data Bank." [D042]

Gluckstein, Fritz P. *Zoonoses: January 1985 through September 1986*. Bethesda, Md.; U.S. Dept. of Health and Human Services, Public Health Service, National Institutes of Health, National Library of Medicine, 1986. 22p. (Literature Search no. 86–12) 277 citations from the MEDLARS database. [D044]

Gray, D. E. *Bibliographical References in Veterinary Scientific Publications*. Ministry of Agriculture, Fisheries and Food, Agricultural Development and Advisory Service, 1982. 34p. Classified list of books and serials. Includes index.

Hoogstraal, Harry. *Bibliography of Ticks and Tickborne Diseases from Homer (about 800 B.C.) to 19-- +*. Cairo, Egypt, U.A.R., U.S. Naval Medical Research Unit no. 3, 1970–1982. (Public Health Service Publication no. 229, Suppl. no. 1; U.S. Navy Special Publication. Naval Medical Research Unit no. 3) Vol. 1 lists serial publications, pp. 1–173. [D045]

Mathias-Mundy, Evelyn and Constance M. McCorkle. *Ethnoveterinary Medicine: An Annotated Bibliography*. Ames, Iowa; Orders may be placed with the Technology and Social Change Program, 1989. 199p. (Bibliographies in Technology and Social Change Series no. 6)

Ryu, E. *Chronological Reference of Zoonoses: Leptospires and Leptospirosis*. 2d ed. Taipei, Taiwan; International Laboratory for Zoonoses, 1978 +. 2 vols.

Ryu, E. *Chronological Reference of Zoonoses: Toxoplasma and Toxoplasmosis*. Taipei, Taiwan; International Laboratory for Zoonoses, 1978 +. 2 vols.

Smith, Lynn M. and Edward M. Addison. *A Bibliography of Parasites and Diseases of Ontario Wildlife*. Ontario Ministry of Natural Resources, 1982. 267p. (Wildlife Research Report no. 99) Includes indexes; bibliography, pp. 201–259.

World Catalogue of Veterinary Films/Video Tapes and Films/Video Tapes of Veterinary Interest, 1983. 3d ed. Geneva; World Veterinary Association, 1983. 114p.
[D157]

Dictionaries

Akzhigitov, G. N., et al. *Anglo-Russkii Meditsinskii Slovar': Okolo 70,000 Terminov.* Moscow; "Russkii Iazyk", 1988. 602p.

English-Russian medical dictionary.

Black's Medical Dictionary. 35th ed. Edited by C. W. H. Havard. Totowa, N.J.; Barnes & Noble, 1987. 750p.

British counterpart to *Dorland's* or *Stedman's* dictionaries, providing British spelling and usage of medical terminology.   [D066]

Black's Veterinary Dictionary. Edited by Geoffrey P. West. 16th ed. Totowa, N.J.; Barnes & Noble, 1988. 703p.   [D097]

Blood, D. C. and Virginia P. Studdert. *Bailliere's Comprehensive Veterinary Dictionary.* Anatomical tables by John Grandage; consultants, John H. Arundel et al. Edited by Robert C. J. Carling. London and Philadelphia; Bailliere Tindall, 1988. 1123p.

Comprehensive dictionary "intended to include every word which the typical practising veterinarian or veterinary student might encounter . . ."—Preface. Terms were selected from a survey of the literatures of veterinary and allied sciences. Includes many cross references. Miscellaneous appendixes.

Brown, Christopher M., D. A. Hogg and D. F. Kelly, consulting eds. *Concise Veterinary Dictionary.* Oxford and New York; Oxford University Press, 1988. 890p.

Bunges, Werner E. *Medical and Pharmaceutical Dictionary: English-German.* 4th ed. with a suppl. comprising more than 17,000 new entries. Stuttgart and New York; G. Thieme, 1991. 556p., 140p.

Dorland, W. A. Newman. *Dorland's Illustrated Medical Dictionary.* 27th ed. Philadelphia; Saunders, 1988. 1888p.   [D069]

Mack, Roy. *Dictionary for Veterinary Science and Biosciences: German-English/ English-German; with trilingual appendix, Latin terms- Worterbuch fur Veterinarmedizin und. . . .* Berlin; Paul Parey, 1988. 321p.

Stedman, Thomas Lathrop. *Stedman's Medical Dictionary.* 25th ed. Baltimore, Md.; Williams & Wilkins, 1990. 1784p.   [D076]

Worterbuch der Veterinarmedizin. Herausgegeben von Ekkehard Wiesner, Regine Ribbeck. Bearbeitet von 72 Fachwissenschaftelern. 2d new ed. Stuttgart and New York; G. Fischer, 1983. 2 vols. (1362 p.)   [D089]

Nomenclature

Animal Disease Thesaurus. 12th revision, June 1986. Hyattsville, Md.; Animal Health Information, Program Planning and Development, Veterinary Services, Animal and Plant Health Inspection Service, U.S. Dept. of Agriculture, 1986. 111p.

CAB Thesaurus. Wallingford, U.K.; CAB International. 1990 ed. 2 vols.

Used to index bibliographic records for the CAB Abstracts and AGRICOLA databases. Used to formulate bibliographic searches of these databases. Supersedes *Controlled Vocabulary 1985; For Subject Indexing in Veterinary Bulletin, Index Veterinarius, Animal Disease Occurrence and Small Animal Abstracts.* Weybridge, U.K.; Commonwealth Bureau of Animal Health, 1985. 110p. Used in 1985–1989; provides cross references to terms used prior to 1985.

Palotay, James L. and David J. Rothwell, eds. *SNOVET, Systematized Nomenclature of Medicine: Microglossary for Veterinary Medicine.* Schaumberg, Ill.; American Veterinary Medical Association, 1984. 200p. Includes indexes.

Directories

Three types of directories are identifiable in the veterinary field: 1) General, which serve more than a single purpose; 2) Veterinary Education; and 3) Veterinary Regulatory and Specialty Groups, which include government regulatory directories, as well as membership listings of special groups, bylaws, information about meetings, governing bodies, etc.

General

American Veterinary Medical Association. Division of Membership and Field Services. *AVMA Directory*. Annual. Schaumburg, Ill.; Division of Membership and Field Services. American Veterinary Medical Association. 33d ed., 1984.

Continues: American Veterinary Medical Association, *Directory*, which was biennial 1974–1983. Arranged in three sections: Alphabetical Section listing name, city, state, province, or country of each veterinarian and the member status code; Geographic Section by state and town (or country), veterinarian's name, spouse's name, full address, telephone number, school and year of graduation, professional activity, type of employment and employment function; and Reference Section, which contains AVMA organization and history, names and addresses of other veterinary and related associations, federal and state government agencies, and veterinary colleges.   [D108]

Diagnosis of Animal Health in the Americas. Washington, D.C.; Pan American Health Organization, Pan American Sanitary Bureau, Regional Office of the World Health Organization, 1983. 278p. (WHO Scientific Publication no. 452)

Thirty-five countries in the Americas were surveyed. Directory information includes: Chap. V, Directory of Animal Facilities; Chap. VI, Veterinary Diagnostic Laboratories in the Americas; Annex II, Directory of Animal Quarantine Stations in the Americas; Annex III, Directory of Animal Facilities in the Americas; Annex IV, Directory of Diagnostic Veterinary Laboratories in the Americas; Annex V, Directory of Schools of Veterinary Medicine in the Americas; Annex VI, Directory of Professional Veterinary Associations; Annex VII, Directory of Livestock Farmer's Associations.

Health Organizations of the United States, Canada, and the World; A Directory of Voluntary Associations, Professional Societies, and Other Groups Concerned with Health and Related Fields. Paul Wasserman, managing editor; Marek Kaszubski, associate editor. 5th ed. Detroit, Mich.; Gale Research Co., 1981. 411p. 4th ed., 1977. [D109]

International Animal Health Directory. Animal Pharm. Richmond, U.K.; V & O Publications, 1983. 181p.

International Directory of Animal Health and Disease Data Banks. Compiled by Herner & Co. for the National Agricultural Library. Beltsville, Md.; National Agricultural Library, U.S. Dept. of Agriculture, 1982. 93p. (USDA Miscellaneous Publication no. 1423)

Who's Who in Veterinary Science and Medicine. 1st ed., 1987–1988. Van Nuys, Calif.; Crown Publications, 1987. 315p.

World Veterinary Association. *List of Members of the World Veterinary Association: National Members, Associate Members, Affiliated Members, Honorary Members, and Organizations with Observer Status.* Madrid; World Veterinary Association, 1989. 17p.

Zeitak, G. and F. Berman, compilers and eds. *Directory of International and National Medical and Related Societies.* 2d ed., completely revised. Rehovot, Israel; PBZ Informatics; Elmsford, N.Y.; Pergamon Press, 1990. 340p.

Veterinary Education

Directory of Internship and Residencies Matching Programs for. . . . Prepared by the American Association of Veterinary Clinicians. Annual. St. Louis, Mo.; Ralston Purina Co., 1986–1987.

Currently distributed by the American Association of Veterinary Clinicians, the directory serves as a means of disseminating internship and residency information to the profession to stimulate the interest of senior students and recent graduates in these programs. Participation in the listing is strictly voluntary and does not construe accreditation. [D111]

Giammattei, Victor M. and Jamie G. Anderson. *Training Programs and Careers in Animal Health Technology and Veterinary Nursing in North America.* 1st ed. Napa, Calif.; Dillon-Tyler, 1985. 164p.

Peterson's Guide to Graduate Programs in the Biological and Agricultural Sciences. 23d ed. Princeton, N.J.; Peterson's Guides, 1988 + . (Peterson's Annual Guides, Graduate Study; Book 3) Annual.

Continues: *Peterson's Annual Guides/Graduate Study. Book 3, Graduate Programs in the Biological, Agricultural, and Health Sciences.*   [D113]

Peterson's Guide to Graduate Programs in Business, Education, Health and Law. 23d ed. Princeton, N.J.; Peterson's Guides, 1988 + . (Peterson's Annual Guides, Graduate Study; Book 6) Annual.

Academic and Professional Programs in Health-Care Professions includes Section 15: Veterinary Medicine and Sciences.   [D113]

Training Programs in Pathology and Clinical Pathology in North American Colleges and Schools of Veterinary Medicine, 1988–89. Prepared by the Association of Veterinary Pathology Chairpersons; Sponsored by UAREP and the Armed Forces Institute of Pathology, 1988. 62p.   [D112]

Veterinary Regulatory and Specialty Groups

Adressbuch der Deutschen Tierarzteschaft. Stand 1. January 1986: Nach den offiziellen Unterlagen der Tierarztekammerm. Hannover; Schlutersche Verlagsanstalt, 1986. 586p.   [D116]

AAHA Directory of Membership 19-- + . Annual. South Bend, Ind.; American Animal Hospital Association.   [D117]

American Association of Zoo Veterinarians. *Membership Directory.* 1991. Irregular. AAZV.   [D120]

Directory of Animal Disease Diagnostic Laboratories. U.S. Dept. of Agriculture, Animal and Plant Health Inspection Service, Veterinary Service. Irregular. Ames, Iowa; The Veterinary Service; Washington, D.C.; For sale by the Supt. of Docs., U.S. Govt. Print. Off. 1989, latest ed.   [D124]

Meat and Poultry Inspection Directory. Irregular. Washington, D.C.; U.S. Dept. of Agriculture, Meat and Poultry Inspection Program, Dec. 1991. 694p.   [D125]

Royal College of Veterinary Surgeons. *Registers and Directory.* London; The College. 1989, latest ed. Supplements issued between editions.   [D122]

Veterinary Biological Products: Licensees and Permittees. Prepared by Veterinary Services, Animal and Plant Health Inspection Service, U.S. Dept. of Agriculture. Hyattsville, Md.; The Service, Jan. 1992. Semiannual.   [D126]

Veterinary Congresses, Conferences, and Symposia

Blanchard and Farrell listed the congresses of four national and four international veterinary groups. Below is a selective listing of congresses of interest to large animal, wildlife and zoo veterinarians which have appeared since 1980.

American Association of Zoo Veterinarians. *Proceedings, Joint Conference of the American Association of Zoo Veterinarians and American Association of Wildlife Veterinarians, November 1988, Sheraton Centre, Toronto, Ontario*, 1988. 204p.

Animal Health and Economics. Paris; Office International des Eppizooties, 1983. 381p. (OIE Technical Series no. 3)

Economics of Animal Diseases; Proceedings of a Conference held at Michigan State University, June 1986. Sponsored by the W. K. Kellogg Foundation. Edited by Edward C. Mather and John B. Kaneene. East Lansing; Michigan State University, 1987. 354p.

Interamerican Commission on Animal Health. *1st Meeting of the Interamerican Commission on Animal Health*. Mexico City; IICA, 1983. 531p.

International Conference on Veterinary Preventive Medicine and Animal Production; Proceedings . . . University of Melbourne, Australia, November 1985. Victoria; Australian Veterinary Association, 1985. 151p.

International Conference on Zoological and Avian Medicine, 1st, September 1987, Turtle Bay Hilton and Country Club, Oahu, Hawaii; Proceedings. . . . Sponsored by Association of Avian Veterinarians and American Association of Zoo Veterinarians. Madison, Wis.; Omnipress, 1987. 586p.

International Workshop on Enzyme Immuno Assay Techniques in Animal Reproduction and Health, 1st, April 1983, Zeist, Netherlands; Syllabus. . . . Compiled by D. F. M. van de Wiel. Zeist; Research Institute for Animal Production "Schoonoord," 1983. 220p.

Karstad, Lars, Barry Nestel and Michael Graham, eds. *Wildlife Disease Research and Economic Development; Proceedings of a Workshop . . . Habete, Kenya, September 1980*. Ottawa; International Development Research Centre, 1981. 80p.

Symposium '88 on Veterinary Epidemiology, Zoonoses, and Economics, 1st, September 1988, Ramada Inn, Bethesda, Maryland; Proceedings. . . . Washington, D.C.; U.S. Dept. of Agriculture, Animal and Plant Health Inspection Service, 1989. 109 leaves.

Woodbine, Malcolm, ed. International Symposium on Antibiotics in Agriculture: Benefits and Malefits, 4th. *Antimicrobials and Agriculture; Proceedings. . . .* London and Boston; Butterworths, 1984. 583p.

Literature and Course Reviews

Foundation for Continuing Education of the New Zealand Veterinary Association. *Publications*. Palmerston North, New Zealand; Massey University Centre for Veterinary Continuing Education. Irregular.

Recent titles include: Dairy Cattle Medicine, 101; The Veterinary Handbook (of diseases affecting animals in New Zealand), 102; Clinical Immunology, 104;

Goat Husbandry and Medicine, 106; Ectoparasites of Sheep in New Zealand and Their Control, 107; Clinical Neurology of Farm Animals, 108; Zoonoses in New Zealand, 112; Equine Reproduction, 114; Goat Seminar 1987, 115; Equine Seminar 1988, 117; Slaughter of Stock, 118; Avian Veterinary Handbook, 120.

Office International des Epizooties. *Technical Series*. Paris, France; L'Office, 1981 + . Irregular.

Includes the following reviews to date: no. 1, Rift Valley Fever (1981); no. 2, Infectious Laryngotracheitis (1982); no. 3, Animal Health and Economics (1983); no. 4, Diseases Transmissible by Semen and Embryo Transfer Techniques (1985); no. 5, Cryptosporidiosis: A Cosmopolitan Disease in Animals and in Man, 2d ed. (1988); no. 6, Brucellosis in Cattle, Sheep and Goats (1987); no. 7, Enzyme Immunoassay Techniques, ELISHA, in Animal and Plant Diseases, 2d ed. (1987); no. 8, Update on Avian Diseases (1988).

Progress in Veterinary Microbiology and Immunology. Basel and New York; Karger, 1985 + . Annual.

Refresher Course for Veterinarians; Proceedings. . . . Sydney; University of Sydney, Post-Graduate Committee in Veterinary Science. Irregular.

Since 1980, includes such topics as: no. 60, Advances in Veterinary Virology (1982); no. 65, Equine Practice—Diagnosis and Therapy (1983); no. 66, Disease Prevention and Control in Poultry Production (1983); no. 67, Sheep: Production and Preventive Medicine (1983); no. 68, Beef Cattle Production (1984); no. 70, Embryo Transfer (1984); no. 71, Clinical Pharmacology and Therapeutics (1984); no. 72, Deer Refresher Course (1984); No.73, Goats (1984); no. 74, Equine Gastroenterology (1985); no. 78, Dairy Cattle Production (1985); no. 82, Equine Exercise Physiology Seminar (1985); no. 83, Equine Surgery (1986); no. 92, Poultry Health (1986); no. 93, Clinical Pathology (1986); no. 95, Pig Production, 2 vols. (1987); no. 96, Artificial Breeding in Sheep and Goats (1987); no. 103, Veterinary Clinical Toxicology (1987); no. 104, Australian Wildlife (1988); no. 106, Fish Diseases (1988); no. 110, Sheep Health and Production (1988).

Veterinary Clinics of North America. Equine Practice. Philadelphia; Saunders. Vol. 1 + , April 1985 + . Three nos. a year.

Continues in part: *Veterinary Clinics of North America. Large Animal Practice*.
[D150]

Veterinary Clinics of North America. Food Animal Practice. Philadelphia; Saunders. Vol. 1 + , March 1985 + . Three nos. a year.

Continues in part: *Veterinary Clinics of North America. Large Animal Practice*.
[D150]

Veterinary Clinics of North America. Large Animal Practice. Philadelphia; Saunders. Vols. 1–6, May 1979–Nov. 1984. Two to three a year.

Histories

Representative veterinary histories published since 1980.

Barker, C. A. V. and T. A. Crowley. *One Voice; A History of the Canadian Veterinary Medical Association*. Ottawa; Canadian Veterinary Medical Association = Association Canadienne des Veterinaires, 1989. 260p. Includes bibliographical references.

Karasszon, Denes. *A Concise History of Veterinary Medicine*. Translated by E. Farkas; translation revised by Iringo K. Kecskes. Budapest; Akademiai Kiado, 1988. 458p. Includes indexes; bibliography, pp. 430–438.

Pattison, Iain. *The British Veterinary Profession 1791–1948*. London; J. A. Allen, 1983. 207p. Includes index; bibliography, pp. 198–201.

Manuals and Handbooks

Veterinary Practice, General

Callis, Jerry J., et al. *Illustrated Manual for the Recognition and Diagnosis of Certain Animal Diseases*. Greenport, N.Y.; Plum Island Animal Disease Center; Mexico-U.S. Commission for the Prevention of Foot and Mouth Disease, 1982. 68p.

Faulkner, D. E., compiler. *Manual for Animal Health Auxiliary Personnel*. Rome; Food and Agriculture Organization, 1983. 400p.

Fenner, William R., ed. *Quick Reference to Veterinary Medicine*. Philadelphia; Lippincott, 1982. 592p. Includes index and bibliographies.

A Guide for Accredited Veterinarians. Hyattsville, Md.; U.S. Dept. of Agriculture, Animal and Plant Health Inspection Service, Veterinary Services, 1981. 79p. (APHIS 91–18)

Kirk, Robert W., Stephen I. Bistner and Richard B. Ford. *Handbook of Veterinary Procedures and Emergency Treatment*. 5th ed. Philadelphia; Saunders, 1990. 1008p.   [D179]

Manketelow, B. W. *The Veterinary Handbook*. 1st ed. Palmerston, North; New Zealand Veterinary Association Foundation for Continuing Education, 1984. 269p.

Successor to: *Diseases of Domestic Animals in New Zealand*. New Zealand Veterinary Assoc., Technical Committee. 3d ed., rev. Includes index.

The Merck Veterinary Manual: A Handbook of Diagnosis, Therapy, and Disease Prevention and Control for the Veterinarian. Editorial Board, Clarence M. Fraser, editor; Asa Mays, associate editor; Harold E. Amstuts et al. 7th ed. Rahway, N.J.; Merck, 1991. 1832p.   [D180]

Veterinary Values; The Pocket Compendium of Veterinary Knowledge. Compiled by Ag. Resources, Inc. 2d ed. Wyman Guin, 1985. 296p.

Veterinary Practice, Special

American Association of Zoo Keepers, Inc. *Diet Notebook*. Project Coordinator, Susan Bunn. Topeka, Kans.; American Association of Zoo Keepers, in cooperation with Assiniboine Park Zoo AAZK Chapter, 1988+. Loose-leaf.

American Assocation of Zoo Veterinarians. Veterinary Standards Committee. *Guidelines for Zoo Veterinary Medical Programs and Veterinary Hospitals*. Prepared by Janis Ott et al. 1981. 14p. Includes bibliography, p. 14.

Klos, Heinz-Georg and Ernst M. Lang. *Handbook of Zoo Medicine; Diseases and Treatment of Wild Animals in Zoos, Game Parks, Circuses, and Private Collections*. Contributors, H.-P. Brandt et al.; English editors, Reinhard Goltenboth, Dietmar Jarofke; English text, Gunter Speckmann; translation by G. Speckmann. New York; Van Nostrand Reinhold, 1982. 453p. Includes indexes; bibliography, pp. 388–420.

Laboratory Training Manual on Radioimmunoassay in Animal Reproduction; A Joint Undertaking by the Food and Agriculture Organization and the International Atomic Energy Agency. Vienna; International Atomic Energy Agency; New York; UNIPUB, distributor, 1984. 269p. (IAEA Technical Reports Series no. 233)

Monnig, Hermann O. and F. J. Veldman. *Handbook on Stock Diseases*. 3d rev. ed. Cape Town; Tafelberg, 1982. 392p. Includes index.

Poppensiek, George C. *Foreign Animal Diseases, 1987*. Edited by Paul G. Rudenberg. Ithaca, N.Y.; Dept. of Microbiology, College of Veterinary Medicine, Cornell University, 1987. 375p. Includes index; bibliography, pp. 336–352.

Reibel, Jaime Isaac. *Caring for Livestock: A Veterinary Handbook*. New York; Arco Pub., 1984. 296p. Includes index.

Schmidt, Robert E. and Gene B. Hubbard. *Atlas of Zoo Animal Pathology*. Boca Ratan, Fla.; CRC Press, 1987. 2 vols.

Contents: Vol. 1, Mammals; Vol. 2, Avian, Reptile, and Miscellaneous Species. Includes bibliography and indexes.

Stockner, Priscilla K. *A Practice Management Manual for Veterinarians*. Ocean Shores, Wash.; Stockner & Associates, 1984. 1 vol. Includes bibliographies. (P.O. Box 962, Ocean Shores, WA 95869; Loose-leaf for updating)

United States Animal Health Association. Committee on Foreign Animal Diseases. *Foreign Animal Diseases: Their Prevention, Diagnosis, and Control*. Rev. 4th ed., 1984. Richmond, Va.; The Committee, 1984. 381p. Includes bibliographies. (Suite 205, 6924 Lakeside Avenue, Richmond, VA 23228)

Whiteman, C. E. and A. A. Bickford. *Avian Disease Manual*. 3d ed. Dubuque, Iowa; Kendall/Hunt; Kennett Square, Pa.; American Association of Avian Pathologists, 1989. 242p. Includes bibliographical references. (283 W. Street Rd., Kennnett Square, PA 19348)

Veterinary, Pharmaceutical

Animal Drug Analytical Manual. Prepared and edited by the Center for Veterinary Medicine, Food and Drug Administration, and Association of Official Analytical Chemists; co-editors, John R. Markus and Joshep Sherma. Arlington, Va.; AOAC, 1985. 1 vol. (various paging). Includes bibliographies.

Animal Drugs, Feeds and Related Products, March 1936–March 1978. Washington, D.C.; U.S. Dept. of Health and Human Services, Public Health Service, Food and Drug Administration; for sale by the Supt. of Docs., U.S. Govt. Print. Off., 1981. 886p.

"Containing a redesignation table for parts 500–599"—Cover.
"All narrative preambles have been compiled from published Federal Register Documents." Includes bibliographical references.

Arzneimittel-Verzeichnis. Im Auftr. d. Ministeriums fuer Gesundheitswesen d. DDR hrsg. vom Inst. fur Arzneimittelwesen d. DDR; zsgest. u. bearb. von K. Gerecke. Ausg. 1977, 1. Aufl. Berlin; Verlag Volk und Gesundheit. (1977).

List of veterinary drugs and biologicals used in East Germany.   [D192]

Blodinger, Jack, ed. *Formulation of Veterinary Dosage Forms*. New York; M. Dekker, 1983. 316p. Includes bibliographies and indexes. (Drugs and the Pharmaceutical Sciences; Vol. 17)

Brander, George C. *Chemicals for Animal Health Control*. London and Philadelphia; Taylor & Francis, 1986. 170p. Includes index; bibliography, pp. 161–164.

The Bristol Veterinary Handbook of Antimicrobial Therapy. Edited by Dudley E. Johnston. 2d ed. Syracuse, N.Y.; Veterinary Learning Systems Co., 1987. 296p. Includes bibliographies.

British Pharmacopoeia Commission. *British Pharmacopoeia (Veterinary), 1985*. London; H.M.S.O., 1985. 213p. Includes index.   [D183]

Center for Veterinary Medicine (U.S.). *Importing Veterinary Products into the United States*. Rockville, Md.; U.S. Dept. of Health and Human Services, Public Health Service, Food and Drug Administration, Center for Veterinary Medicine, 1986. 17p. (HHS Publication; FDA 86–6044)

The Henston Veterinary Vade Mecum. Large Animals. London; Henston, 1984–1985 + . Annual.

Issued in parts to be updated separately. Continues in part: *Henston Veterinary Vade Mecum*. 1982.

IVS; Index of Veterinary Specialties. Epsom, Surrey, U.K.; A. E. Morgan Publications, Ltd., 1961 + . 6 issues a year.

"A service to veterinary surgeons listing ethical veterinary preparations including a new preparations section when applicable and a guide to pharmaceutical companies and services. A completely revised issue is published each alternate month."   [D186]

Lewis, Benjamin P. and Leon O. Wilken. *Veterinary Drug Index*. Philadelphia; Saunders, 1982. 327p.

List of Approved Animal Drugs. U.S. Department of Health and Human Services, Public Health Services, Food and Drug Administration, Bureau of Veterinary Medicine. Rev. ed. Washington, D.C.; The Bureau, 1984. 216p.

The Merck Index: An Encyclopedia of Chemicals, Drugs, and Biologicals. Edited by Susan Budavari; associate editor, Maryadele J. O'Neil. 11th ed., centennial ed. Rahway, N.J.; Merck, 1989. 1 vol. (various paging).

Authoritative, comprehensive, computer produced and maintained listing of compounds useful to biologists, practitioners of health professions, and pharmacologists. For each compound, it provides condensed information on properties, principal pharmacological action, use, and toxicity.   [D188]

Sittig, Marshall. *Veterinary Drug Manufacturing Encyclopedia*. Park Ridge, N.J.; Noyes Publications, 1981. 507p. Includes bibliographies and index.

Veterinarians' Product and Therapeutic Reference: A Guide to Pharmaceuticals and Biologicals. 5th ed. Caldwell, N.J.; Therapeutic Communications, 1979. 534p.   [D193]

Veterinary Drug Formulary. Cornell Research Foundation, Inc. Baltimore; Williams & Wilkins, 1985. 168p.

"Combined effort of the pharmacy staff, the Pharmacy and Therapeutics Committee, and the clinical staff of the New York State College of Veterinary Medicine, Cornell University."—Introduction. Bibliography, p. 9.

Veterinary Practitioner's Guide to Approved New Animal Drugs: A Practical Guide to New Animal Drugs Approved for Use in the United States of America. 1988 ed. Dallas, Tex.; Shotwell & Carr, 1988. 169p.

Reference Texts

Sciences Basic to Veterinary Medicine

Anatomy

Loeffler, Klaus. *Anatomy and Physiology of Domestic Animals*. Edited by Andre Darbre. 4th ed. New York; Harper & Row, 1986. 383p. Translation of *Anatomie und Physiologie de Haustiere*. Includes index; bibliography, pp. 367–371.

Pasquini, Chris and Tom Spurgeon. *Anatomy of Domestic Animals: Systemic and Regional Approach*. Contributors, Susan Pasquini et al. 4th ed. La Porte, Colo.; Sudz Pub., 1989. 582p. Includes index.

Physiology

Dukes, H. H. *Dukes' Physiology of Domestic Animals*. Edited by Melvin J. Swenson. 10th ed. Ithaca, N.Y.; Comstock Pub. Associates, 1984. 1463p. Includes bibliographies.   [D198]

Pharmacology

Booth, Nicholas H. and Leslie E. McDonald, eds. *Veterinary Pharmacology and Therapeutics*. 6th ed. Ames; Iowa State University Press, 1988. 1227p. Includes bibliographies and index.

Toxicology

Humphreys, D. J. *Veterinary Toxicology*. 3d ed. London and New York; Bailliere Tindall, 1988. 356p. Includes bibliographies and index.   [D200]

Osweiler, Gary D., et al. *Clinical and Diagnostic Veterinary Toxicology*. 3d ed. Dubuque, Iowa; Kendall/Hunt Pub. Co., 1985. 494p. Includes bibliographies and index.   [D201]

Microbiology

Linton, Alan H., ed., with contributions by Mary P. English et al. *Microbes, Man, and Animals: The Natural History of Microbial Interactions*. Chichester, Sussex, U.K., and New York; Wiley, 1982. 342p. Includes bibliographies and index.

Veterinary Microbiology: Molecular and Clinical Perspectives. Volume editor, R. Pandey. Basel and New York; Karger, 1986. 220p. (Progress in Veterinary Microbiology and Immunology; Vol. 2) Includes bibliographies and index.

Parasitology

Soulsby, E. J. L. *Helminths, Arthropods and Protozoa of Domesticated Animals*. 7th ed. Philadelphia; Lea & Febiger, 1982. 809p.

"First published 1934 as *Veterinary Helminthology and Entomology* by H. O. Monnig"—Verso t.p. Includes bibliographies and index.   [D204]

Pathology

Jubb, K. V. F., Peter C. Kennedy and Nigel Palmer. *Pathology of Domestic Animals*. 3d ed. Orlando, Fla.; Academic Press, 1985. 3 vols. Includes bibliographies and indexes.   [D205]

Clinical Biochemistry

Kaneko, Jiryo J., ed. *Clinical Biochemistry of Domestic Animals.* 4th ed. San Diego, Calif.; Academic Press, 1989. 932p. Includes bibliographies and index.
[D206]

Clinical Veterinary Medicine

Large Animals

Amstutz, H. E., ed. *Bovine Medicine and Surgery.* 2d ed. Santa Barbara, Calif.; American Veterinary Publications, 1980. 2 vols. 1269p. Includes bibliographies and indexes.
[D208]

Blood, D. C. and O. M. Radostits. *Veterinary Medicine: A Textbook of the Diseases of Cattle, Sheep, Pigs, Goats and Horses.* Contributions by J. H. Arundel and C. C. Gay. 7th ed. London and Philadelphia; Bailliere Tindall, 1989. 1502p. Includes bibliographies and index.
[D207]

Colahan, Patrick T., et al., eds. *Equine Medicine and Surgery.* 4th ed. Goleta, Calif.; American Veterinary Publications, 1991. 2 vols.
[D210]

Hall, Harold T. B. *Diseases and Parasites of Livestock in the Tropics.* 2d ed. London and New York; Longman, 1985. 328p. Includes bibliographies and index.

Jensen, Rue. *Jensen and Swift's Diseases of Sheep.* 3d ed. By Cleon V. Kimberling. Philadelphia; Lea & Febiger, 1988. 394p. (Rev. ed. of *Diseases of Sheep.* 2d ed., 1982.)
[D212]

Kirkbride, Clyde A. *Control of Livestock Diseases.* Springfield, Ill.; Thomas, 1986. 152p. Includes index.

Leman, A. D., et al., eds.; with 99 authorized contributors selected for their recognized leadership in this field. *Diseases of Swine.* 6th ed. Ames; Iowa State University Press, 1986. 930p. Includes bibliographies and indexes.
[D209]

Oehme, Frederick W., ed. *Textbook of Large Animal Surgery.* 2d ed. Baltimore, Md.; Williams & Wilkins, 1988. 714p. Includes bibliographies and index.
[D213]

Birds, Poultry

Coutts, G. S. *Poultry Diseases under Modern Management.* 3d ed. Alton, U.K.; Nimrod, 1987. 245p. Includes 8 pages of plates.

Calnek, B. W., et al. *Diseases of Poultry.* 9th ed. Ames; Iowa State University Press, 1991. 929p. Includes bibliographies and index.
[D221]

Jordan, F. T. W. *Poultry Diseases.* 3d ed. Philadelphia; Saunders, 1990. 497p.

Lofts, Norah. *Poultry Diseases: Short Notes Containing Stragegic Information for Veterinary Students.* By Peter Curtis. 2d ed. Liverpool; Liverpool University Press, 1987. 64p.

Previous ed., Liverpool; Department of Veterinary Clinical Science, University of Liverpool, 1986. Includes index.

Randall, C. J. *Color Atlas of Diseases of the Domestic Fowl and Turkey.* Ames; Iowa State University Press, 1985. 116p. Includes index; bibliography, p. 111.

Schrag, Ludwig. *Healthy Pigeons: Recognition, Prevention and Treatment of the Major Pigeon Diseases.* Trans. by Winifried Mehlig in cooperation with Cyril J. Morley. 19th ed.; 5th English ed., completely rev. ed. Hengersberg, Germany; Schober Verlags-GMBH, 1985. 108p. (Translation of *Gesunde Tauben.*) Includes index.

Veterinary Specialties

Barber, Don L. *Guidelines for Radiology Service in Veterinary Medicine.* Compiled by Don L. Barber and R. E. Lewis on behalf of the American College of Veterinary Radiology Committee to Formulate Standards for Radiology. . . . Chicago; American Veterinary Medical Association, 1982. 25p.

"Approved by the Council on Veterinary Service, AVMA, March 1, 1982." Bibliography, pp. 24–25.

Lumb, William V. and E. Wynn Jones. *Veterinary Anesthesia.* 2d ed. Philadelphia; Lea & Febiger, 1984. 693p. Includes bibliographies and index.   [D224]

Roberts, Stephen J. *Veterinary Obstetrics and Genital Diseases (Theriogenology).* 3d ed. Woodstock, Vt.; The Author; North Pomfred, Vt.; Distributed by David & Charles Inc., 1986. 981p. Includes bibliographies and index.   [D225]

Schalm, O. W. *Schalm's Veterinary Hematology.* 4th ed. By Nemi C. Jain. Philadelphia; Lea & Febiger, 1986. 1221p. Includes 25 pages of plates. Errata slip inserted. Includes bibliographies and index.   [D226]

Short, Charles E., ed. *Principles and Practice of Veterinary Anesthesia.* Baltimore, Md.; Williams & Wilkins, 1987. 609p. Includes bibliographies and index.

Thielen, Gordon H. and Bruce R. Madewell, eds. *Veterinary Cancer Medicine.* 2d ed. Philadelphia; Lea & Febiger, 1987. 676p. Includes bibliography and index.

Zoo and Wildlife Diseases

Fowler, Murray E., ed. *Zoo and Wild Animal Medicine.* 2d ed. Philadelphia; Saunders, 1986. 1127p.

"Sponsored by Morris Animal Foundation, Denver, Colorado." Includes bibliographies and index.   [D228]

Frye, Fredric L. *Biomedical and Surgical Aspects of Captive Reptile Husbandry.* 2d ed., enl. Malabar, Fla.; Krieger Pub. Co., 1991. 2 vols. 637p.

Heavily illustrated with color photographs. Includes bibliographical references and indexes.

Griner, Lynn A. *Pathology of Zoo Animals: A Review of Necropsies Conducted over a Fourteen-Year Period at the San Diego Zoo and San Diego Wild Animal Park.* San Diego, Calif.; Zoological Society of San Diego, 1983. 608p. Includes index.

Hoff, Gerald L. and John W. Davis, eds. *Noninfectious Diseases of Wildlife.* 1st ed. Ames; Iowa State University Press, 1982. 174p. Includes bibliographies and index.

Jacobson, Elliott R. and George V. Kollias, Jr., eds. *Exotic Animals.* New York; Churchill Livingstone, 1988. 328p. (Contemporary Issues in Small Animal Practice, Vol. 9) Includes bibliographies and index.

Zoonoses and Communicable Diseases

Hagan, William A. *Hagan and Bruner's Microbiology and Infectious Diseases of Domestic Animals; With Reference to Etiology, Epizootiology, Pathogenesis, Immunity, Diagnosis, and Antimicrobial Susceptibility.* 8th ed. By John F. Timoney et al. Ithaca, N.Y.; Comstock Pub. Associates, 1988. 951p.

Laws and Disease Reporting

AAZP Manual of Federal Wildlife Regulations. Wheeling, W.Va.; American Association of Zoological Parks and Aquariums, 1985 + .

Animals and Their Legal Rights: A Survey of American Laws from 1641 to 1990. With chapters by the Animal and Plant Health Inspection Service of the U.S. Dept. of Agriculture et al. 4th ed. Washington, D.C.; Animal Welfare Institute, 1990. 441p. (P.O. Box 3650, Washington, DC 20007)

Revised ed. of *Animals and Their Legals Rights.* By Emily Stewart Leavitt. 3d ed., 1978. Includes bibliographical references, pp. 440–441.   [D265]

Beal, Victor C., Jr. *Regulatory Statistics.* 6th ed. Hyattsville, Md.; U.S. Dept. of Agriculture, Animal and Plant Health Inspection Service, Veterinary Services, 1983 + .

Blackman, D. E., P. N. Humphreys and P. Todd, eds. *Animal Welfare and the Law.* Cambridge, U.K., and New York; Cambridge University Press, 1989. 283p. Includes bibliographical references and index.

Blood, D. C. *Veterinary Law: Ethics, Etiquette, and Convention.* North Ryde, New South Wales; Law Book Co., 1985. 368p. Includes index. Bibliography, p. xvii.

Clingermann, Karen J., Sean Gleason and Janice Swanson. *Animal Welfare Legislation: Bills and Public Laws 1989*. Beltsville, Md.; Animal Welfare Information Center, National Agricultural Library, 1990. 15p. (AWIC Series no. 2) Updates earlier ed. covering 1980–October 1988.

Crofts, Wendy. *A Summary of the Statute Law Relating to the Welfare of Animals in England and Wales*. Revised, Aug. 1989. Potters Bar, Hertfordshire; Universities Federation for Animal Welfare, 1989. 227p. Bibliography, p. 227.

Favre, David S. and Murray Loring. *Animal Law*. Westport, Conn.; Quorum Books, 1983. 253p. Includes bibliographical references and index.

Model Code of Practice for the Welfare of Animals. Canberra; Australian Bureau of Animal Health, 1983 + . 5 vols. in 1.

"This Model Code . . . has been prepared by the Sub-Committee on Animal Welfare (SCAW) of the Animal Health Committee within the Australian Agricultural Council (AAC) System." Vol. 1, The Pig; Vol. 2, The Domestic Fowl; Vol. 3, Road Transport of Livestock; Vol. 4, Rail Transport of Livestock; Vol. 5, Air Transport of Livestock; Annex C, Intensive Husbandry of Rabbits.

Rumore, James J. *Veterinary Medical Records and the Law*. Baton Rouge, La.; Claitor's Pub. Division, 1980. 32 leaves. Bibliography, pp. 30–31.

Soave, Orland A. and Lester M. Crawford. *Veterinary Medicine and the Law*. Baltimore, Md.; Williams & Wilkins, 1981. 146p. Includes bibliographical references and index.

Standards for the Preparation and Carriage of Cattle by Sea. Australian Bureau of Animal Health. Canberra; Australian Government Pub. Service, 1984. 10p.

Veterinary and Plant Health Controls; Veterinary Control, Plant Health Control. Luxembourg; Office for Official Publications of the European Communities, 1990. 149p. (Completing the Internal Market)

Wilson, James F. *Law and Ethics of the Veterinary Profession*. Bernard E. Rollin and Jo Anne L. Garbe, contributing authors. Yardley, Pa.; Priority Press Ltd., 1988. 513p. Includes bibliographies and index.

D. Wildlife and Its Management, by Jo Anne Boorkman

Literature Guides

Loubou, Robert. *Wildlife Rehabilitation: A Guide to the Literature*. Wilmington, Del.; Tri-State Bird Rescue and Research, 1984. 49p. (P.O. Box 1713, Wilmington, DE 19899)

In four sections: Publications of primary interest to rehabilitators; Publications of secondary interest to rehabilitators; Selected periodicals of interest to rehabilitators; and Selected works on animal rights and animal welfare.

Miller, Melanie Ann. *Birds: A Guide to the Literature*. New York; Garland Pub., 1986. 887p. (Garland Reference Library of the Humanities, Vol. 680)

Moore, Julie L. "Wildlife Management Literature." In: *Wildlife Management Techniques Manual*. 4th ed., rev. Edited by Sanford D. Schemnitz; illustrated by Larry Toschik. Washington, D.C.; Wildlife Society, 1980. (Chapter 2, pp. 7–38.)

Revision of the 1969 chapter by Robert W. Burns; provides a succinct overview of the literature. Includes information on print and electronic sources. Also, a section on organization and preparation of a research paper.   [D564]

Indexes and Abstracts

No new indexing or abstracting services have begun since 1980; however, the following index of *Contaminant Hazard Reviews* is of note.

Eisler, Ronald and Joyce Haber Corley. *Index to Common and Scientific Names of Species Listed in Contaminant Hazard Reviews 1 through 15*. Laurel, Md.; Fish and Wildlife Service, U.S. Department of the Interior, 1989. 44p. Bibliography, pp. 43–44.

Bibliographies

Wildlife Management and Conservation

Bebee, Charles N., compiler and ed. *The Protection of Wildlife, January 1979–April 1989: Citations from AGRICOLA Concerning Diseases and Other Environmental Considerations*. Beltsville, Md.; U.S. Dept. of Agriculture, National Agricultural Library; Washington, D.C.; U.S. Environmental Protection Agency, Office of Pesticide Programs, 1989. 199p. (Bibliographies and Literature of Agriculture no. 86)

Boyle, Stephen A. and Fred B. Samson. *Nonconsumptive Outdoor Recreation: An Annotated Bibliography of Human-Wildlife Interactions*. Washington, D.C.; U.S. Dept. of the Interior, Fish and Wildlife Service, 1983. 113p. (Special Scientific Report—Wildlife no. 252)

Hall, Christine and Philip Dearden. *The Impact of "Non-Consumptive" Recreation on Wildlife: An Annotated Bibliography*. Monticello, Ill.; Vance Bibliographies, 1984. 45p. (Public Administration Series, Bibliography P-1458)

Shank, Christopher C. and Fred L. Bunnell. *The Effects of Snow on Wildlife; An Annotated Bibliography*. Victoria, B.C.; Research Branch, Ministry of Forests: Fish and Wildlife Branch, Ministry of Environment, 1982. 58p. (Integrated Wildlife Intensive Forestry Research, IWIFR- 1; Ministry of Forests, Research Branch, EP 934; Ministry of Environment, Fish and Wildlife Bulletin B-25)

Smeltzer, John F. *Wildlife Law Enforcement; An Annotated Bibliography*. Fort Collins; Colorado Division of Wildlife, 1985. 139p. (Colorado Division of Wildlife; Division Report no. 13)

Wood, Don A. *Endangered Species: Concepts, Principles, and Programs: A Bibliography*. Tallahassee; Florida Game and Fresh Water Fish Commission, 1981. 228p.

Zoology

General

Melville, R. V. and J. D. D. Smith, eds. *Official Lists and Indexes of Names and Works in Zoology*. London; International Trust for Zoological Nomenclature on behalf of the International Commission on Zoological Nomenclature, 1987. 366p.

Includes "Bibliographic references to directions and opinions", pp. 357–366.

Sims, Reginald W., Paul Freeman and David L. Hawksworth, eds. *Key Works to the Fauna and Flora of the British Isles and North-Western Europe*. 5th ed. Oxford; Published for the Systematics Association by the Clarendon Press, 1988. 312p. (Systematics Association Special Volume no. 33)

Mammals

Worthen, Gary L. *An Annotated Computerized Bibliography of the Use of Karyotypic Analysis in the Subspecific Taxonomy of Mammals*. Utah State University, Logan, Utah. La Jolla, Calif.; National Oceanic and Atmospheric Administration, National Marine Fisheries Service, Southwest Fisheries Center, 1981. 154p. (NOAA Technical Memorandum NMFS-SWFC no. 9)

Birds

Larson, Jean A. *Raising Quail, Partridge, Pheasant, Bobwhites, and Ostriches, January 1979–May 1989: 103 Citations*. Beltsville, Md.; U.S. Dept. of Agriculture, National Agricultural LIbrary, 1989. 10p. (Quick Bibliography Series; NAL-BIBL. QB 89–95)

Scott, Thomas G. *Bobwhite Thesaurus*. Edgefield, S.C.; International Quail Foundation, 1985. 306p.

Amphibians and Reptiles

Ratermann, Mary M. and John M. Brode. *Annotated Bibliography of Amphibian and Reptile Field Study Methods*. Sacramento; California Dept. of Fish and Game, 1983. 45p. (Inland Fisheries Administration Report no. 83–3)

Villa, Jaime, Larry D. Wilson and Jerry D. Johnson. *Middle American Herpetology: A Bibliographic Checklist*. Columbia; University of Missouri Press, 1988. 131p.

In English and Spanish. Includes index; bibliography, pp. 91–113.

Welch, Kenneth R. G. *Herpetology of Africa: A Checklist and Bibliography of the Orders Amphisbaenia, Sauria, and Serpentes.* Malabar, Fla.; R. E. Krieger Pub. Co., 1982. 293p. Includes indexes; bibliography, pp. 211–272.

Welch, Kenneth R. G. *Herpetology of Europe and Southwest Asia: A Checklist and Bibliography of the Orders Amphisbaenia, Sauria and Serpentes.* Malabar, Fla.; R. E. Krieger Pub. Co., 1983. 135p. Includes indexes; bibliography, pp. 92–126.

Dictionaries, Encyclopedias, and Field Guides

Campbell, Bruce and Elizabeth Lack, eds. *A Dictionary of Birds.* Vermillion, S.Dak.; Published for the British Ornithologists' Union by Buteo Books, 1985. 670p. Includes bibliography.

Choate, Ernest A., ed. *The Dictionary of American Bird Names.* Revised by Raymond A. Paynter, Jr. Boston; Harvard Common Press, 1985. 226p.

Ferlin, Guy. *Elsevier's Dictionary of the World's Game and Wildlife; in English, Latin, French, German, Dutch, and Spanish with equivalents in Afrikaans and Kiswahili, with thirteen original drawings by the author.* Amsterdam and New York; Elsevier, 1989. 426p. Includes bibliographical references.

Headstrom, Richard. *Identifying Animal Tracks: Mammals, Birds, and Other Animals of the Eastern United States.* New York; Dover Publications, 1983. 141p.

Originally published as: *Whose Track Is It?* 1971. Includes index.

Lincoln, Roger J. and G. A. Boxshall. *The Cambridge Illustrated Dictionary of Natural History.* Illustrations by Roberta Smith. Cambridge and New York; Cambridge University Press, 1987. 413p.

Wood, Gerald L. *The Guinness Book of Animal Facts and Feats.* 3d ed. Enfield, Middlesex, U.K.; Guinness Superlatives, 1982. 252p. Includes index; bibliography, pp. 223–239.   [D599]

Directories

1985 United Nations List of National Parks and Protected Areas. Prepared by the IUCN Conservation Monitoring Centre and IUCN's Commission on National Parks and Protected Areas. Gland, Switzerland; IUCN, 1985. 171p. In English and French.   [D606]

The Animal Finders' Directory. Prairie Creek, Ind.; AFD Publications, 1985. 40p.

"A classified directory of the exotic wildlife field."

Hudson, Kenneth and Ann Nicholls. *The Directory of Museums and Living Displays.* 3d ed. New York; Stockton Press, 1985. 1047p.

Lowe, David W., managing ed; John R. Matthews and Charles Moseley, eds. *The Official World Wildlife Fund Guide to Endangered Species of North America.* Washington, D.C.; Beacham Pub., 1990. 2 vols. 1180p.

Includes bibliographical references and indexes. Contents: Vol. 1, Plants, Mammals; Vol. 2, Birds, Reptiles, Amphibians, Fishes, Mussels, Crustaceans, Snails, Insects and Arachnids.

Moseley, Charles and David Lowe, researchers and eds. *Endangered Species Photo Locator.* Washington, D.C.; Beacham Pub., 1990. 73p.

List of sources of photographs and directory of photographers published in *The Official World Wildlife Fund Guide to Endangered Species of North America.* Includes indexes.

Reece, Kathleen A., compiler and ed. *Animal Organizations and Services Directory 1985.* Huntington Beach, Calif.; Animal Stories, 1985. 170p. Includes index; periodicals, pp. 145–170.

U.S. Fish and Wildlife Service. *Directory, Pacific States Region National Wildlife Refuge and Fish Hatcheries.* Washington, D.C.; Dept. of the Interior, U.S. Fish and Wildlife Service, 1980. 32p.   [D607]

Zucker, Barbara Fleisher. *Children's Museums, Zoos, and Discovery Rooms: An International Reference Guide.* New York; Greenwood Press, 1987. Includes index; bibliography, pp. 241–260.

Histories

Allen, Thomas B. *Guardian of the Wild: The Story of the National Wildlife Federation, 1936–1986.* Bloomington; Indiana University Press, 1987. 212p.

Published in association with the National Wildlife Federation. Includes index; bibliography, p. 203.

Belanger, Dian Olson. *Managing American Wildlife: A History of the International Association of Fish and Wildlife Agencies.* Amherst; University of Massachusetts Press, 1988. 247p. Includes index; bibliography, pp. 227–236.

Day, David. *The Doomsday Book of Animals: A Unique Natural History of Three Hundred Vanished Species.* Foreword by the Duke of Edinburgh; illustrated by Tim Bramfitt et al. London; Ebury Press, 1981. Includes index; bibliography, pp. 282–284.

Dunlap, Thomas R. *Saving America's Wildlife.* Princeton, N.J.; Princeton University Press, 1988. 222p. Includes index; bibliography, pp. 177–214.

Matthiessen, Peter. *Wildlife in America.* Drawings by Bob Hines. Rev., updated ed. New York; Viking, 1987. 332p. Includes index; bibliography, pp. 315–320.

Restoring America's Wildlife, 1937–1987: The First 50 Years of the Federal Aid in Wildlife Restoration (Pittman-Robertson) Act. Prepared in cooperation with the wildlife agencies of the states and territories; Harmon Kallman, chief editor et al. Washington, D.C.; U.S. Dept. of the Interior, U.S. Fish and Wildlife Service; Superintendent of Documents, U.S. Govt. Print. Off., 1987. 394p. Includes index.

Handbooks, Manuals, and Texts

Wildlife Management and Conservation

Average Physiological Values. International Species Inventory System and American Association of Zoo Veterinarians. Apple Valley, Minn.; ISIS, 1987. 190p.

Also called *ISIS Average Laboratory Data.* Chiefly tables. Includes index.

Brownie, Cecil, et al. *Statistical Inference from Band Recovery Data: A Handbook.* 2d ed. Washington, D.C.; U.S. Dept. of the Interior, Fish and Wildlife Service, 1985. 305p. (U.S. Fish and Wildlife Resource Publication no. 156)   [D621]

Byrd, Nathan A., compiler. *A Forester's Guide to Observing Wildlife Use of Forest Habitat in the South.* Atlanta, Ga.; U.S. Dept. of Agriculture, Forest Service, Southern Region, 1985. 36p. (Forestry Report RB, i.e. R8–FR; 5) Includes bibliographies.

Cornfield, Timothy. *The Wilderness Guardian.* Nairobi, Kenya; David Sheldrick Wildlife Appeal; Nairobi Space Publications, 1984. 621p.

On cover: African Wildlife Foundation. Includes index; bibliography, pp. 619–621.

Ffolliott, Peter and Sonia Gallina, eds. *Deer Biology, Habitat Requirements, and Management in Western North America.* Mexico, D.F.; Instituto de Ecologia, 1981. 238p. (Publication, Instituto de Ecologia, A.C. no. 9)

"A binational Mexico-United States Man and Biosphere (MAB) Program investigation."
"Bibliography of deer biology, habitat requirements, and management, by Linda M. Ffolliott", pp. 213–238.

Giles, Robert H., Jr. *Wildlife Management.* San Francisco; W. H. Freeman, 1978. 416p. Includes bibliographies and index.

IUCN and Natural Resources Amphibia-Reptilia Red Data Book. Compiled by Brian Groombridge; assisted by Lissie Wright, with the help and advice of the Species Survival Commission of the International Union for Conservation of Nature and other experts throughout the world. 4th ed., fully rev. and expanded. Gland, Switzerland; IUCN, 1982. 1 vol.

Revision and expansion of *Amphibia and Reptilia.* By Rene E. Honegger, 1979. Includes bibliographical references and index.   [D632]

IUCN and Natural Resources Mammal Red Data Book. Compiled by Jane Thornback and Martin Jenkins, with the help and advice of the Species Survival Commission of International Union for the Conservation of Nature and other experts throughout the world. Gland, Switzerland; IUCN, 1982. 1 vol.

Contents: Pt. 1, Threatened Mammalian Taxa of the Americas and the Australasian Zoogeographic Region (excluding Cetacea). Includes bibliographies and index.   [D632]

Leopold, Aldo. *Game Management*. With a new foreword by Laurence R. Jahn; drawings by Allan Brooks. Madison; University of Wisconsin Press, 1986. 481p. Originally published, New York; Scribner, 1933.

A classic. Includes index; bibliography, pp. 427–449.   [D633]

Robinson, William L. and Eric G. Bolen. *Wildlife Ecology and Management*. 2d ed. New York; Macmillan; London; Collier Macmillan, 1989. 574p. Includes index; bibliography, pp. 497–547.

Rue, Leonard Lee, III. *The Deer of North America*. 2d ed., updated and expanded. Danbury, Conn.; Grolier Book Clubs, 1989. 544p. Includes index; bibliography, pp. 509–525.

Sanderson, Glen C., ed. *Management of Migratory Shore and Upland Game Birds in North America*. 1st Bison Book Print. Lincoln; University of Nebraska Press, 1980. 358p.

Originally produced through the cooperation of the International Association of Fish and Wildlife Agencies, and the U.S. Fish and Wildlife Service. Reprint of the 1977 ed. published by the International Association of Fish and Wildlife Agencies, Washington, D.C. Includes bibliographies and index.

Standards for the Development of Habitat Suitability Index Models. Division of Ecological Services, U.S. Fish and Wildlife Service, Dept. of the Interior. Washington, D.C.; The Division, 1981. 1 vol. (various pagings).

Performing organization: Western Energy and Land Use Team, U.S. Fish and Wildlife Service. Cover title: *Standards for the Development of Habitat Suitability Index Models for Use with the Habitat Evaluation Procedures*. Includes bibliographies.

Wakeley, James S., ed. *Wildlife Population Ecology*. University Park; Pennsylvania State University Press, 1982. 385p. Bibliography, pp. 381–385.

Wallmo, Olof C., compiler and ed. *Mule and Black-Tailed Deer of North America*. Illustrated by Dean Rocky Barrick; technical eds., Richard E. McCabe and Laurence R. Jahn. Lincoln; University of Nebraska Press, 1981. 605p. (A Wildlife Management Institute Book) Includes index; bibliography, pp. 556–598.

Wildlife and Fisheries Habitat Improvement Handbook. Neil F. Payne and Frederick Copes, technical editors. Washington, D.C.; U.S. Dept of Agriculture, Forest Service, Wildlife and Fisheries, 1990. 1 vol. (various pagings).

"Replaces FSH 2609, *Wildlife and Fish Habitat Improvement Handbook* . . . published in 1969." Includes bibliographical references, pp. LC-1—LC-33.
                                                                              [D642]

Young, E., ed. *The Capture and Care of Wild Animals: The Work of Eighteen Veterinary, Medical, and Wildlife Experts*. 1st U.S. ed. Hollywood, Fla.; Curtis Books, 1975. 224p.

"This publication was compiled by the Wildlife Group of the South African Veterinary Association and the Southern African Wildlife Management Association." Includes bibliographies.

Zoology

General

Banks, Richard C., Roy W. McDiarmid and Alfred L. Gardner, eds. *Checklist of Vertebrates of the United States, the U.S. Territories, and Canada*. Washington, D.C.; U.S. Dept. of the Interior, Fish and Wildlife Service, 1987. 79p. (U.S. Fish and Wildlife Service Resource Publication no. 166)

International Commission on Zoological Nomenclature. *International Code of Zoological Nomenclature*. Adopted by the XX General Assembly of the International Union of Biological Sciences; editorial committee, W. D. L. Ride et al. 3d ed. London; International Trust for Zoological Nomenclature, in association with British Museum (Natural History); Berkeley; University of California Press, 1985. 338p.

Includes bibliographical references and indexes. Later taxonomic changes are published in the *Bulletin of Zoological Nomenclature*.   [D649]

Mayr, Ernst and Peter D. Ashlock. *Principles of Systematic Zoology*. 2d ed. New York; McGraw-Hill, 1991. Includes index; bibliography, pp. 434–463.   [D650]

Mammals

Anderson, Sydney and J. Knox Jones, Jr., eds. *Orders and Families of Recent Mammals of the World*. New York; Wiley, 1984. 686p. Sponsored by the American Society of Mammalogists. Includes index; bibliography, pp. 589–657.
    [D653]

Booth, Ernest S. *How to Know the Mammals*. 4th ed. Dubuque, Iowa; W. C. Brown Co., 1982. 198p. Includes index; bibliography, pp. 9–11.   [D654]

Chapman, Joseph A. and George A. Feldhamer, eds. *Wild Mammals of North America: Biology, Management, and Economics*. Baltimore; Johns Hopkins University Press, 1982. 1147p. Includes bibliographies and index.

Clark, Michael. *Mammal Watching*. Drawings by the author. London; Severn House, 1981. 175p. Includes index; bibliography, pp. 170–173.

Dawson, Terence J. *Monotremes and Marsupials: The Other Mammals*. London; E. Arnold, 1983. 87p. (Institute of Biology's Studies in Biology no. 150) Includes index; bibliography, pp. 84–87.

Green, Richard. *Wild Cat Species of the World*. Plymouth, U.K.; Basset Pub., 1991. 163p.

Identifies 39 species of cats using Helmut Hemmer's 1978 classification. Provides general description, distribution, status, habitat, behavior, reproduction and taxonomy of each species.

Hall, E. Raymond. *The Mammals of North America*. 2d ed. New York; Wiley, 1981. 2 vols. Includes indexes; bibliography, vol. 2, pp. 1138–1175.   [D662]

International Conference on Bear Research and Management, 5th, 1980, Madison, Wis. *Bears, Their Biology and Management; A Selection of Papers from a Conference* . . . . Edited by E. Charles Meslow. West Glacier, Mont.; International Association for Bear Research and Management; Available from Clifford J. Martinka, Glacier National Park, 1983. 328p. Sponsored by the Bear Biology Association (BBA). Includes bibliographical references.   [D664]

Kelsey-Wood, Dennis. *The Atlas of Cats of the World; Domesticated and Wild*. Neptune City, N.J.; T. F. H. Publications, 1989. 384p. Includes bibliographical references and index.

Partridge, John, ed. *Management Guidelines for Exotic Cats*. Eastvale, U.K.; Association of British Wild Animal Keepers, 1991. 153p.

Describes 35 species. Concentrates on the captive management of cats. Bibliography, p. 150.

Sea Mammals. New York; Torstar Books, 1985. 158p. Includes index; bibliography, p. 152.

Stirling, Ian. *The Polar Bear*. London; Blanford, 1992. 232p.

Covers aspects of polar bear biology and interactions between bears and man. Illustrated with 163 color photos and extensive reference to scientific literature.

Vaughn, Terry A. *Mammalogy*. 3d ed. Philadelphia; Saunders College Pub., 1986. 576p. Includes index; bibliography, pp. 527–561.

Walker's Mammals of the World. 4th ed. Edited by Ronald M. Nowak and John L. Paradiso. Baltimore, Md.; Johns Hopkins University Press, 1983 + . Includes index.   [D668]

Birds

Brown, Leslie, Emil K. Urban and Kenneth Newman. *The Birds of Africa*. Illustrated by Martin Woodcock and Peter Hayman. London and New York; Academic Press, 1982–1988. 3 vols.

Includes indexes. Vols. 2–3 edited by Emil K. Urban, C. Hilary Fry and Stuart Keith. Bibliography, vol. 1, pp. 479–507.

Check-List of Birds of the World. Cambridge; Harvard University Press, 1931–1987. 16 vols.

Cover title: *Birds of the World*. Recognized authoritative work with literature citations to newer literature. Volumes have different editors. Vols. 8 and 11 unpublished. Comprehensive index by Raymond A. Paynter, Jr.   [D682]

Check-List of North American Birds: The Species of Birds of North America from the Arctic through Panama, Including the West Indies and Hawaiian Islands. Prepared by the Committee on Classification and Nomenclature of the American Ornithologists' Union. 6th ed. Washington, D.C.; The Union, 1983. 877p.

Spine title: *A. O. U. Check-List of North American Birds*. Maps on lining papers. Includes index.   [D670]

Clements, James F. *Birds of the World, a Checklist*. 3d ed. New York; Facts on File, 1981. 562p. Maps on lining paper. Includes indexes; bibliography, pp. 527–531.   [D674]

Edwards, Ernest Preston. *Birds of the World*. Sweet Briar, Va.; E. P. Edwards, 1989. 1 computer file: 31/2 in. + guide. 2p.

"These files do not contain family, order, or subfamily headings, or any of the taxonomic notes, maps or introductory material or indexes from the *Coded Workbook*."

"The accompanying 720k disk contains a sample portion of *A Coded List of Birds of the World: Non-Passerines and Passerines*. Any IBM PS/2 or compatible should be able to read this disk. These are not databases or programs. These are text files (ASCII files) . . ."

Edwards, Ernest Preston. *A Coded Workbook of Birds of the World*. 2d ed. Sweet Briar, Va.; E. P. Edwards, 1982–1986. 2 vols.

"A revision and enlargement of the passerine portion of Edition A of *A Coded List of Birds of the World*."—Vol. 2. Includes bibliographies and indexes.

[D677]

Farner, Donald S. and James R. King, eds. *Avian Biology*. Taxonomic editor, Kenneth C. Parkes; contributors, N. Philip Ashmore et al. New York; Academic Press, 1971–1985. 8 vols. Includes bibliographies and indexes.   [D678]

Gensbol, Benny. *Collins Guide to the Birds of Prey of Britain and Europe, North Africa and the Middle East*. Illustrated by Bjarne Bertel; trans. by Gwynne Vevers; adapted for the English language edition by C. J. Mead. English language ed. London; Collins, 1984. 384p. Includes maps, index; bibliography, pp. 380–383.

Howard, Richard and Alick Moore. *A Complete Checklist of the Birds of the World*. With a foreword by Leslie Brown; revised by Alick Moore. Rev. ed. London; Macmillan, 1984. 732p. Includes indexes; bibliography, pp. 8–47.

[D679]

Madge, Steve and Hilary Burns. *Waterfowl: An Identification Guide to the Ducks, Geese, and Swans of the World*. Boston; Houghton Mifflin, 1988. 298p. Includes index; bibliography, pp. 292–294.

Palmer, Ralph S. *Handbook of North American Birds*. New Haven; Yale University Press, 1962 + . Vols. 1–3 and 5.

"Sponsored by the American Ornithologists' Union and New York State Museum and Sciences Services." Vol. 5 sponsored by the Smithsonian Institution. Includes bibliographies. Contents: Vol. 1, Loons through Flamingos; Vols. 2–3, Waterfowl; Vol. 5, Family Accipitridae (concluded); Family Falconidae. [D681]

Pendleton, Beth A. Giron et al., eds. *Raptor Management Techniques Manual*. Foreword by John J. Craighead; editorial assistant, Kathleen M. Walsh. Washington, D.C.; Institute for Wildlife Research, National Wildlife Federation, 1987. 420p. (National Wildlife Federation Scientific and Technical Series no. 10) Includes bibliographies and index.

Pennychuick, C. J. *Bird Flight Performance: A Practical Calculation Manual*. With photographs by the author. Oxford and New York; Oxford University Press, 1989. 153p. + 1 computer disk (51/4 in.)

Includes index; bibliography, pp. 146–148.
System requirements for computer disk (Version 1.0): IBM compatible computers; 360K; MS-DOS; BASIC Interpreter (preferably Microsoft BASIC; printer.

Smith, Loren M., Roger L. Pederson and Richard M. Kaminski, eds. *Habitat Management for Migrating and Wintering Waterfowl in North America*. Lubbock; Texas Tech University Press, 1989. 560p. Includes bibliographical references.

Reptiles and Amphibians

Gans, Carl, ed. *Biology of the Reptilia*. London and New York; Academic Press, 1969–1988. 16 vols. Includes bibliographies and indexes.   [D689]

Halliday, Tim R. and Kraig Adler, eds. *The Encyclopedia of Reptiles and Amphibians*. New York; Facts on File, 1986. 143p. Includes index; bibliography, pp. viii-ix.

Harding, Keith A. and Kenneth R. G. Welch. *Venomous Snakes of the World: A Checklist*. 1st ed. Oxford and New York; Pergamon Press, 1980. 188p. (Supplement no. 1 (1980) to the journal *Toxicon*.) Includes indexes; bibliography, pp. 149–153.

Stebbins, Robert C. *A Field Guide to Western Reptiles and Amphibians; Field Marks of All Species in Western North America, Including Baja California*. Illustrations by the author. 2d ed., rev. Boston; Houghton Mifflin, 1985. 336p. (The Peterson Field Guide Series no. 16)

Sponsored by the National Audubon Society and the National Wildlife Federation. Illustrations on lining papers. Includes index; bibliography, pp. 278–781.

Zoogeography

Andrewartha, H. G. and L. C. Birch. *The Ecological Web; More on the Distribution and Abundance of Animals*. Chicago; University of Chicago Press, 1984. 506p. Includes indexes; bibliography, pp. 563–495.

Banarescu, Petru. *Zoogeography of Fresh Waters*. Wiesbaden; AULA-Verlag, 1990 + . 3 vols.

Contents: Vol. 1, General Distribution and Dispersal of Freshwater Animals; Vol. 2, Distribution and Dispersal of Freshwater Animals in North America and Eurasia; Vol. 3, Distribution and Dispersal of Freshwater Animals in Africa, Pacific Areas and South America.

Lean, Geoffrey, Don Hinrichsen and Adam Markham. *Atlas of the Environment*. London; Hutchinson, 1990.

Sponsored by the World Wildlife Fund. "The most up-to-date report on the state of the world."—Dust jacket. Bibliography, pp. 187–192.

Lidiker, William Z., Jr. and Roy L. Caldwell, eds. *Dispersal and Migration*. Stroudsburg, Pa.; Hutchinson Ross Pub. Co.; New York; Distributed world-wide by Van Nostrand Reinhold Co., 1982. 311p. (Benchmark Papers in Ecology no. 11) Includes bibliographies and indexes.

Trense, Werner. *The Big Game of the World*. Hamburg; Paul Parey, 1989. 413p.

With supplements by A. B. Bubenik, V. Geist and Sigrid Schwenk. Illustrated by Clare Abbott et al. Includes indexes; bibliography, pp. 394–398.

Wildlife Legislation

AAZPA Manual of Federal Wildlife Regulations. Wheeling, W. Va.; American Association of Zoological Parks and Aquariums, 1985 + . 2 vols., loose-leaf.

Includes index. Contents: Vol. 1, Protected Species, compiled by Alan H. Shoemaker; Vol. 2, Laws and Regulations, compiled by Kristin L. Vehrs.

African Wildlife Laws. By the IUCN Environmental Law Centre, with the assistance of Cyrille de Klemm and Barbara Lausche. Gland, Switzerland; International Union for Conservation of Nature and Natural Resources, 1987. 1712p. (IUCN Environmental Policy & Law Occasional Paper no. 3)

The Animal Rights Movement in the United States; Its Composition, Funding Sources, Goals, Strategies and Potential Impact on Research. Prepared by the Harvard University's Office of Government and Community Affairs, based on research by Phillip W. D. Martin. Clarks Summit, Pa.; Society for Animal Rights, 1982. 12p.

Bean, Michael J. *The Evolution of National Wildlife Law*. Rev. & expanded ed. New York; Praeger, 1983. 449p.

Revision of earlier edition prepared for the Council on Environmental Quality by the Environmental Law Institute, 1977. Includes index; bibliography, pp. 430–436.

Burton, Edward C. *Enforcement of Natural Resources Legislation: A Handbook.* Agincourt, Ontario; Carswell, 1984. 154p.

Spine title: *Natural Resource Handbook.* Includes index.

Du Saussay, Christian. *Legislation on Wildlife and Protected Areas in Africa.* For Legislation Branch, Legal Office. Rome; Food and Agriculture Organization, 1984. 158p. (Legislative Study no. 25) Includes bibliographical references.

Endangered Species Act of 1973, as Amended through the 100th Congress, December 15, 1988. Washington, D.C.; U.S. Govt. Print. Off., 1988. 45p. (Serial no. 100–C)

Estes, Carroll Lynn and Keith W. Sessions. *Controlled Wildlife: A Three-Volume Guide to U.S. Wildlife Laws and Permit Procedures.* Lawrence, Kans.; Association of Systematics Collections, 1983– 1985. 3 vols.

Includes indexes. Contents: Vol. 1, Federal Permit Procedures; Vol. 2, Federally Controlled Species; Vol. 3, State Wildlife Regulations, compiled by Steven T. King and John R. Schrock.

Facts about Federal Wildlife Laws. Washington, D.C.; Dept. of the Interior, U.S. Fish and Wildlife Service, 1982. 13p.

Favre, David S. *Wildlife: Cases, Laws, and Policy.* Tarrytown, N.Y.; Associated Faculty Press, 1983. 277p. Includes bibliographical references.

Fuller, Kathryn S. and Brian Swift. *Latin American Wildlife Trade Laws.* 2d ed. Revisors for 2d ed., Kathryn S. Fuller, Amanda Jorgenson and Amie Brautigam. Washington, D.C.; World Wildlife Fund, 1985. 354p.

In English and Spanish. In loose-leaf.

Lyster, Simon. *International Wildlife Law: An Analysis of International Treaties Concerned with the Conservation of Wildlife.* Cambridge; Grotius, 1985. 470p.

"A publication of the Research Centre for International Law, University of Cambridge in association with the International Union for Conservation of Nature and Natural Resources." Includes texts of treaties. Includes bibliographical references and index.

Marashi, Sadat. *Compendium of National Legislation on the Conservation of Marine Mammals.* Rome; Food and Agriculture Organization, 1986 + .

At head of title: Food and Agriculture Organization of the United Nations: United Nations Environment Programme. "FAO/UNEP Project no. 0501–78/02". Includes bibliographical references.

Wildlife Economics: Useful and Noxious Wildlife

Gasaway, William C., et al. *Interrelationships of Wolves, Prey, and Man in Interior Alaska*. Washington, D.C.; Wildlife Society, 1983. 50p. (Wildlife Monographs no. 84)

The study of wolves, moose, caribou, and man was conducted during the 1970s in a 17,000 km^2 area in east-central Alaska near Fairbanks. "Literature cited", pp. 46–49.
Supplement to the *Journal of Wildlife Management*, vol. 47, no. 3, July 1983.

Halstead, Bruce W. *Poisonous and Venomous Marine Animals of the World*. 2d rev. ed. Princeton, N.J.; Darwin Press, 1989. 1168p. Includes bibliographies and indexes.   [D716]

Jerry, Danielle. *Selkirk Mountain Caribou: A Cooperative Management Plan*. Portland; U.S. Fish and Wildlife Service, 1985. 118p.

In cooperation with British Columbia Fish and Wildlife Branch et al.
Bibliography, pp. 115–118.

Klauber, Laurence M. *Rattlesnakes, Their Habitats, Life Histories, and Influence on Mankind*. Abridged by Karen Harvey McClung. Berkeley; University of California Press, 1982. 350p. Includes index; bibliography, pp. 337–339.   [D719]

Kyle, Russell. *A Feast in the Wild*. Kidlington; KUDU, 1987. 203p. Includes index; bibliography, pp. 185–200.

Marais, Johan. *Snake Versus Man: A Guide to Dangerous and Common Harmless Snakes of Southern Africa*. 1st ed. Braamfontein, Johannesburg; Macmillan South Africa, 1985. 102p. Includes index; bibliography, pp. 94–95.

Meredith, Thomas C. and Ludger Muller-Wille. *Man and Caribou: The Economics of Naskapi Hunting in Northeastern Quebec*. Montreal, Quebec; Centre for Northern Studies and Research, McGill University, 1982. 54p. (McGill Subarctic Research Paper no. 36)

Includes summary in French, Naskapi and Cree; abstract in English and French.
Bibliography, pp. 47–49.

Moore, Granville, M., ed. *Poisonous Snakes of the World*. Turnbridge Wells, Kent; Castle House, 1980. 212p. Includes index; bibliography, pp. 184–185.

Skjenneberg, Sven and Lars Slagsvold. *Reindeer Husbandry and Its Ecological Principles*. Edited by Candy M. Anderson and Jack R. Luick; translated by Tone Treider Deehr. Juneau, Alaska; U.S. Dept. of the Interior, Bureau of Indian Affairs, 1979. 395p.

"Translated from Norwegian." Originally published, Oslo; Universitetsforlaget, 1968. Includes bibliographies.

United States. Bureau of Sport Fisheries and Wildlife. *Birds in Our Lives*. Edited by Alfred Stefferud. Arnold L. Nelson, managing editor. Bob Hines, artist. New York; Arco, 1970. 447p.   [D726]

Waterfowl Production; Proceedings of the International Symposium on Waterfowl Production, the Satellite Conference for the XVIII World's Poultry Congress, September 1988, Beijing, China. Sponsored and organized by China Association of Animal Science and Veterinary Medicine. 1st ed. Beijing, People's Republic of China; International Academic Publishers; Oxford and New York; Pergamon Press, 1989. 441p. Includes bibliographical references.

Wildlife in Zoos and Captivity

Barzdo, Jon, ed. *Management of Canids and Mustelids.* Dunstable, U.K.; Association of British Wild Animal Keepers, 1981. 58p. (Proceedings of a Symposium . . . Association of British Wild Animal Keepers, 5th.)

Cover title: "The Fifth Specialist Symposium of the Association of British Wild Animal Keepers was held at the Zoological Society of London on March 8, 1980."—p.i. Includes bibliographical references.

Bendiner, Robert. *The Fall of the Wild, the Rise of the Zoo.* 1st ed. New York; Dutton, 1981. 196p. Includes index; bibliography, pp. 152–153.

Cherfas, Jeremy. *Zoo 2000: A Look beyond the Bars.* London; British Broadcasting Corp., 1984. 244p. Includes index; bibliography, p. 240.

Deere, Derek, ed. *Animal Transport by Sea.* A Collection of Papers prepared for the Anitrans Conference. London; Marine Publications International, 1983. 82p.

Sponsored by Universities Federation for Animal Welfare and World Society for the Protection of Animals. Conference not held.

Huxley, Elspeth J. G. *Whipsnade: Captive Breeding for Survival.* London; Collins, 1981. 159p. Includes index; bibliography, pp. 153–154.

Markowitz, Hal. *Behavioral Enrichment in the Zoo.* New York; Van Nostrand Reinhold, 1982. 210p. Includes indexes; bibliography, pp. 200–203.

McKenna, Virginia, Will Travers and Jonathan Wray, eds. *Beyond the Bars: The Zoo Dilemma.* Wellingborough, Northamptonshire and Rochester, Vt.; Thorsons Pub. Group, 1987. 208p. Includes index.

Mullan, Bob and Gerry Marvin. *Zoo Culture.* London; Weidenfeld & Nicolson, 1987. 171p. Includes bibliographical references.

Polakowski, Kenneth J. *Zoo Design: The Reality of Wild Illusions.* Ann Arbor; University of Michigan, School of Natural Resources, 1987. 193p. Includes index; bibliography, pp. 181–184.

Why Zoos? Herts, U.K.; Universities Federation for Animal Welfare, 1988. 58p. (UFAW Courier no. 24) Includes bibliographical references.

E. Commercial Fishing, Fisheries and Aquaculture, by Jo Anne Boorkman

Abstracts and Indexes

Compact Cambridge Aquatic Sciences and Fisheries Abstracts. Bethesda, Md.; Cambridge Scientific Abstracts, 1987+. Quarterly compact disks with cumulations.

Covers 1982/86+. Computer laser optical disks; 43/4 in., 2 program disks and user's manual. Issued also in printed form and on computer tape reels.   [D735]

Fisheries Review. Fort Collins, Colo.; Dept. of the Interior, U.S. Fish and Wildlife Service, Vol. 31+, 1986+. Four nos. a year.

Absorbed: *Fish Health News.* Continues: *Sport Fishery Abstracts.* (Vol. 1–30, 1955–1985).   [D743]

Wildlife and Fish Worldwide. Baltimore, Md.; National Information Services Corporation, Vol. 1+, 1989+. Quarterly compact disk service.

Computer laser optical disks; 43/4 in. plus documentation. "CD Answer (tm) retrieval software by Dataware Technologies, Inc." To be used with the latest of NISC Disc's access and retrieval software. Vol. 1 includes 1971–March 1990. Issued in print form as *Wildlife Review* [D568] and *Fisheries Review* [D743].

Bibliographies

Aquaculture and Related Publications of the School of Forestry and Wildlife Management, Agricultural Extension Station, Louisiana State University. Baton Rouge; Louisiana State University, 1983. 27p. Around 300 references.

Breisch, Linda L. and Victor S. Kennedy. *A Selected Bibliography of Worldwide Oyster Literature.* College Park, Md.; Sea Grant Program, University of Maryland, 1980? 309p.

3,781 references primarily from 1971–1980. 2,837 references from the primary literature; 810 reports and 130 theses. Each section arranged alphabetically with separate subject indexes.

Coche, A. G., compiler. *Lists of Serials, Newsletters, Bibliographies and Meeting Proceedings Related to Aquaculture.* Rome; Food and Agriculture Organization, 1983. 65p. (FAO Fisheries Circular no. 758) Includes index.

Dahm, E. *Bibliography of Existing Literature on Selectivity of Inland Water Fishing Gear Published by European Authors.* Rome; Food and Agriculture Organization, 1987. 46p. (EIFAC Occasional Paper no. 18) 55 references with detailed abstracts. Author and subject indexes.

Forbes, John B. and C. N. Bebee. *Literature for United States Aquaculture 1970–1982.* Beltsville, Md.; U.S. Dept. of Agriculture, National Agricultural Library,

1983. 228p. (Bibliographies and Literature of Agriculture no. 28) Contains 3,600 references.

Foster, Michelle E. and Deborah T. Hanfman. *Aquaculture Journals of the National Agricultural Library*. Beltsville, Md.; U.S. Dept. of Agriculture, National Agricultural Library, Aquaculture Information Center, 1988. 29p.

Hanfman, Deborah T., et al. *Aquaculture in the Caribbean Basin: A Bibliography, 1970–1988*. Washington, D.C.; U.S. Dept. of Agriculture, National Agricultural Library, 1988. 71p. (Bibliographies and Literature of Agriculture no. 71)

151 references with subject index, compiled for the Symposium on the *Status and Potential of Aquaculture in the Caribbean* at the Annual Meeting of the Gulf and Caribbean Fisheries Institute.

Hanfman, Deborah T., et al. *Aquaculture in the Northeast Pacific: A Bibliography*. Beltsville, Md.; U.S. Dept. of Agriculture, National Agricultural Library, 1990. 76p. (Bibliographies and Literature of Agriculture no. 93) 180 annotated references covering 1974–1989, with author and subject indexes.

Hanfman, Deborah T., Steven Tibbitt and Carol Watts. *The Potentials of Aquaculture: An Overview and Bibliography*. Beltsville, Md.; U.S. Dept. of Agriculture, National Agricultural Library, 1989. 73p. (Bibliographies and Literature of Agriculture no. 90) 128 annotated references with author and subject indexes.

McVey, Eileen, et al. *Practical Aquaculture Literature II: A Bibliography*. Beltsville, Md.; U.S. Dept. of Agriculture, National Agricultural Library, 1989. 175p. (Bibliography and Literature of Agriculture no. 75)

In cooperation with Joint Subcommittee on Aquaculture Information Task Force. Updates Bibliographies and Literature of Agriculture no. 35. Selected "how to" publications covering the literature from 1970 to 1989. In five parts: Part I, Species; Part II, Subjects; Part III, Other types of publications; Part IV, Contacts in aquaculture; Part V, Addresses for publications.

Mann, Joyce A., et al. *Fish Culture: An Annotated Bibliography of Publications of the National Fisheries Center, Leetown, 1972–1980*. Kearneysville, W.Va.; U.S. Fish and Wildlife Service, National Fisheries Center, Leetown, 1982. 124p.

1,975 references with brief annotations; arranged by subject with an author index.
"Publications from these components prior to 1972 are documented in U.S. Bureau of Sport Fisheries and Wildlife, *Resource Publication 120: Bibliography of Research Publications of the U.S. Bureau of Sport Fisheries and Wildlife, 1928–1972*."— Preliminary page.

Martin, Cynthia S., et al. *Fishery Publication Index, 1980–85; and Technical Memorandum Index, 1972– 85*. Seattle, Wash.; U.S. Dept. of Commerce, National Oceanic and Atmospheric Administration, National Marine Fisheries Service, 1987. 149p. (NOAA Technical Report NMFS no. 62; Suppl. to earlier

NMFS Circulars no. 400, 296 & 36) Indexes of publications of the Scientific Publ. Office, National Marine Fisheries Service.

Munro, J. L. and W. J. Nash. *A Bibliography of the Giant Clams (Bivalvia: Tridacnidae)*. Manila, Philippines; International Center for Living Aquatic Resources Management, 1985. 36p. (Bibliographies/ICLARM no. 5)

In two parts: Part 1, Alphabetical list of references; Part 2, Subject index.

Redout, L. M., compiler. *Aquaculture and Fish III*. Farnham Royal, Slough, U.K.; Commonwealth Agriculture Bureaux, 1983. 397p. (Annotated Bibliography no. F34) 1,490 annotated references from the CAB database, 1980–1982, arranged under broad headings with author and species indexes.

Ruff, Robert L. *A Bibliography of Cooperative Extension Service Literature on Wildlife, Fish and Forest Resources*. Madison, Wis.; Dept. of Wildlife Ecology, Cooperative Extension Program, University of Wisconsin, 1982. 42p. 105 aquaculture and fish citations.

Serial Holdings of the U.K. Marine and Freshwater Sciences Libraries, 1980. Wormley, Surrey; Distributed by Library, Institute of Oceanographic Sciences, 1980. 200p.   [D807]

Serials Monitored for the ASFIS Bibliographic Database. Aquatic Sciences and Fisheries Information System, Fishery Information, Data and Statistics Service, Fisheries Department. Rome; Food and Agriculture Organization, 1988. 153p. (ASFIS Reference Series no. 1, rev. 2)   [D806]

Shoenen, Peter. *A Bibliography of Important Tilapias (Pisces—Cichlidae) for Aquaculture*. Manila, Philippines; International Center for Living Aquatic Resources Management, 1982. 336p. (Bibliographies/ICLARM no. 3); Manila, Philippines; International Center for Living Aquatic Resources Management, 1985. 99p. (Bibliographies/ICLARM no. 6)

Arranged by species name. Each section has a separate bibliography with subject and geographic index.

Turnbull, Deborah A. *Keyguide to Information Sources in Aquaculture*. London and New York; Mansell Pub., 1989. 137p. Includes index; also contains directories.

Venema, S. C., compiler. *A Selected Bibliography of Acoustics in Fisheries Research and Related Fields*. Rome; Food and Agriculture Organization, 1985. 142p. (FAO Fisheries Circular no. 748, rev. 1)

"A preliminary version of this report was prepared as an FAO contribution to the ICES/FAO Symposium on Fisheries Acoustics held from 21–24 June, 1982, at Bergen, Norway as FAO Fisheries Circular no. 748."—p. i. Contains 1,791 references.

Ward, John. *Bureau of Commercial Fisheries, Economic Working Papers Series: Annotated Bibliography*. Miami, Fla.; U.S. Dept. of Commerce, National Oceanic and Atmospheric Administration, National Marine Fisheries Service, Southeast Fisheries Center, 1982. 37p. (NOAA Technical Memorandum NMFS SEFC no. 86) Abstracts of 122 working papers from U.S. Bureau of Commercial Fisheries on fisheries economics from 1969–1973.

World List of Aquatic Sciences and Fisheries Serial Titles: Preliminary ed. Compiled by Fishery Information, Data and Statistics Service; prepared by Gillian Dore-Medichini. Rome; Food and Agriculture Organization, 1975 + . (FAO Fisheries Technical Paper no. 147) Supplement 3, 1978, 148p.; supplement 4, 1980, 120p.; supplement 5, 1981, 96p.   [D808]

Zamora, Ma. Divina V., William P. Gabuelo and Amelia T. Arisola, compilers. *Grouper Abstracts.* Tigbauan, Iloilo, Philippines; Brackishwater Aquaculture Information System, SEAFDEC Aquaculture Dept., 1987. (Bibliography Series no. 8) 179 references with author, title, biological (subject), taxonomic and geographical indexes.

Dictionaries and Encyclopedias

Depestre Catony, Leonardo and Eladio Blanco Cabrera. *Diccionario Multilingue de Especies Marines: Espanol, Ingles, Frances, Aleman, Portugues.* La Habana, Cuba; Editorial Cientifico-Tecnica, 1987. 80p. (Coleccion Diccionario) Includes bibliographical references.

Groves, Donald G. and Lee M. Hunt. *Ocean World Encyclopedia.* New York; McGraw-Hill, 1980. 443p. Includes index.

Jean, Yves, Alex E. Peden and Don E. McAllister. *English, French, and Scientific Names of Pacific Fish of Canada = Noms Francais, Anglais et Scientifiques des Poissons de la Cote du Pacifique du Canada.* Victoria; British Columbia Provincial Museum, 1981. 51p. (Heritage Record no. 13) Includes index and bibliography.

Multilingual Dictionary of Fish and Fish Products = Dictionnaire Multilingue des Poissons et Produits de la Peche. Prepared by the Organisation for Economic Co-operation and Development. 2d ed. Farnham, U.K.; Fishing News, 1984. 430p.

"Reprinted with corrections, 1984."   [D775]

Negedly, Robert, compiler. *Elsevier's Dictionary of Fishery, Processing, Fish, and Shellfish Names of the World in Five Languages, English, French, Spanish, German, and Latin.* Amsterdam and New York; Elsevier, 1990. Includes indexes.

North, Jeannette P., compiler. *Annotated Acronyms and Abbreviations of Marine Science Related Activities.* 3d ed. Washington, D.C.; U.S. Dept. of Commerce, National Oceanic and Atmospheric Administration, Environmental Data and Information Service, National Oceanographic Data Center, 1981. 349p. Revision of 2d ed., 1976. Revised by Charlotte M. Ashby and Alan R. Flesh. Includes indexes.   [D778]

Selected Terms in Fish Culture = Choix de Termes de Pisciculture. Rome; Food and Agriculture Organization, 1981. 151p. (FAO Terminology Bulletin; Bulletin de Terminologie/Organization des Nations Unies pour l'Alimentation et l'Agriculture no. 19) In Arabic, English, French and Spanish. Bibliography, pp. 148–149.   [D782]

Directories

American Fisheries Society. Fish Culture Section. *The Fish Culturist Registry*. Bozeman, Mont.; Fish Culture Section of the American Fisheries Society, 1987. 175p. (Rt. 2, Box 333, Bozeman, MT 59715)

Aquaculture Research: A Directory of USDA and State Projects in CRIS. Beltsville, Md.; U.S. Dept. of Agriculture, National Agricultural Library and Cooperative State Research Service, 1983. 357p. (USDA Miscellaneous Publication no. 1432)

Compiled by Current Research Information System (CRIS), Cooperative State Research Service for National Agricultural Library, U.S. Dept. of Agriculture. Includes bibliographical references and indexes.

Ayers, James W., compiler. *National Aquaculture Directory*. Little Rock, Ark.; U.S. National Marine Fisheries Service, 1986. 222p.

Available from National Technical Information Service (PB87–110268).

Brackishwater Aquaculture Information System. *Directory of Brackishwater Aquaculture Institutions*. Tigbauan, Iloilo, Philippines; Brackishwater Aquaculture Information System, Aquaculture Dept., Southeast Asian Fisheries Development Center, 1988. 89p.

Carigma, Mari Assunta A. and Regina G. Morales, compilers. *Directory of Educational and Training Opportunities in Fisheries and Aquaculture*. Rome; Fisheries Dept., Food and Agriculture Organization; Manila, Philippines; International Center for Living Aquatic Resources Management, 1989. 46p. (ICLARM Contribution no. 528)

Digest of Fishery Assistance Offices. Washington, D.C.; U.S. Dept. of the Interior, Fish and Wildlife Service, Division of Program Operations—Fisheries, 1986. 39 leaves. Includes indexes.

Food and Agriculture Organization. *Directory of Fishing Technology Institutions and Services = Repertoire des Institutions et Services de Technologie de la Peche = Guia de Instituciones y Servicios de Tecnologia Pesquera*. Rome; FAO, 1980. (FAO Fisheries Technical Paper no. 205) Compiled by Fisheries Technology Service, Fisheries Dept. Text in English, French and Spanish.

Food and Agriculture Organization. *International Directory of Fish Inspection and Quality Control Institutes = Repertoire International des Institutions/Organismes Responsables du Controle de la Qualite et de l'Inspection du Poisson = Lista*

Internacional de Institutos de Inspeccion y Control de Calidad del Pescado. Rome; FAO, 1984. 139p. (FAO Fisheries Technical Paper no. 244)

Prepared by Fish Utilization and Marketing Services, Fishery Industries Division, Fisheries Dept.

Food and Agriculture Organization. *International Directory of Fish Technology Institutes.* New and enl. 2d ed. Rome; FAO, 1980. 106p. (FAO Fisheries Technical Paper no. 152, rev. 1)

Prepared by Fish Utilization and Marketing Service, Fishery Industries Division, Fisheries Dept. 1st ed. published as: *A Directory of University-Level Training Programmes in the Aquatic Sciences with Emphasis on Fisheries.* FAO, Fishery Resources and Environment Division, Research Information Unit, 1976.

Frimodt, Claus. *The European Fishing Handbook: Directory of the European Fish Trade.* 1st ed. Denmark; Scandinavian Fishing Year Book, 1988. 449p.

International Directory of Marine Scientists: A Product of the Joint FAO/IOC/UN (OETB) Aquatic Sciences and Fisheries Information System (ASFIS), with support from UNESCO. 3d ed. Paris; UNESCO; Rome; FAO, 1983. 488, 87, 173p. Includes indexes.   [D787]

Joncheere, H. L. Aspeslagh and S. Boni, compilers. *International Aquaculture Trade Directory.* Bredene, Belgium; European Aquaculture Society, 1989. 254p. Text in English, French, German, Norwegian and Spanish.

Major Aquaculture Associations, Education and Research Resources in the United States. Beltsville, Md.; U.S. Dept. of Agriculture, National Agricultural Library and Dept. of Fisheries and Allied Aquaculture, Auburn University, 1983. (Bibliographies and Literature of Agriculture no. 26) Includes index.

Martin, James W., ed. and publisher. *The American Fisheries Directory and Reference Book.* 2d ed. Camden, Maine; National Fisherman, 1991. 750, 100p.

Appendix: Statistics from Fisheries of the United States, 1980. Bibliography, pp. 535–547.   [D784]

McAleer, Beth A., ed. *Directory of North American Fisheries Scientists.* Bethesda, Md.; American Fisheries Society, 1987. 363p.

Over 10,000 entries to fisheries and aquatic scientists, not limited to AFS members. In three sections: Section I, Alphabetical listing of individuals with addresses and brief biographical information; Section II, Listing of individuals by geographic area; Section III, Listing of individuals by professional activities and primary fields of expertise.

National Agricultural Library. *Bibliography of Aquaculture Information Resources.* Beltsville, Md.; U.S. Dept. of Agriculture, 1982? 53p. (Bibliographies and Literature of Agriculture no. 25)

U.S. Joint Subcommittee on Aquaculture. *Aquaculture: A Guide to Federal Government Programs* . . . prepared in cooperation with the National Agricultural

Library. Beltsville, Md; U.S. Department of Agriculture, National Agricultural Library, 1991. 38p.

U.S. Ocean Scientists and Engineers . . . Directory. Washington, D.C.; American Geophysical Union, (1986+). Latest ed., 1987.

Continues: *U.S. Directory of Marine Scientists*, 1975–1982.   [D792]

Varley, Allen and Stella E. L. Wheeler, eds. *Ocean Research Index: A Guide to Ocean and Freshwater Research Including Fisheries Research.* 2d ed. Guernsey, Channel Islands; F. Godgson, 1976. 637p.

Lists research organizations alphabetically by country. Includes indexes. Bibliography, pp. 503– 548.   [D789]

Who Hazzit?: A Guide to West Coast Seafood Products. 2d ed. Portland, Oreg.; West Coast Fisheries Development Foundation, 1982? 155p. Includes indexes.

Lists of Fishes

FAO Species Catalogue. Rome; United Nations Development Programme [and] Agriculture Organization of the United Nations, 1980+. (FAO Fisheries Synopsis no. 125)

"FAO series of worldwide annotated and illustrated catalogues of major marine groups of organisms that enter marine fisheries. . . Designed specifically for the use of fishery workers, laying emphasis on field identification of species available to non-taxonomists, as well as fisheries information . . ."—p. iii, vol. 8, 1988. Includes indexes and bibliography. 11 vols. to date, all by different authors.

International Committee for the Check-List of the Fishes of the North-Eastern Atlantic and Mediterranean. *Check-List of the Fishes of the North-Eastern Atlantic and of the Mediterranean, Clofnam = Catalogue des Poissons de l'Atlantique du Nord-Est et de la Mediterranee.* Edited by J. C. Hureau and Th. Monod. 2d impression, with suppl. Paris; United Nations Educational, Scientific and Cultural Organization, 1979. 2 vols. Text in English and French. Includes indexes and bibliographies.   [D799]

Nelson, Joseph S. *Fishes of the World.* 2d ed. New York; Wiley, 1984. 523p. Includes index. Bibliography, pp. 425–474.   [D803]

Page, Lawrence M. and Brooks M. Burr. *A Field Guide to Freshwater Fishes: North America North of Mexico.* Boston; Houghton Mifflin, 1991. 432p.

Sponsored by the National Audubon Society, the National Wildlife Federation, and the Roger Tory Peterson Institute, this is the first and only guide to all 790 freshwater fishes found north of Mexico. Using the Peterson Identification System, volume identifies fish size, range, habitat, and behavior. Also lists those fish on the federal endangered species list.

Wheeler, Alwyne C. *The World Encyclopedia of Fishes*. London; Macdonald, 1985. 368p. Line drawings by Annabel Milne and Peter Stebbing; photographs supplied by Photo Aquatics.   [D805]

Handbooks, Texts, and Statistics

Atlas of the Living Resources of the Sea = Atlas des Resources Biologiques des Mers = Atlas de los Recursos Vivos del Mar. Prepared by the FAO Department of Fisheries. 4th ed. Rome; Food and Agriculture Organization; New York; UNIPUB, sales agent, 1981. 23p. (FAO Fisheries Series no. 15)

Parallel text in English, French and Spanish. Maps on lining papers. Bibliography, p. 12.   [D809]

Brandt, Andres von. *Fish Catching Methods of the World*. 3d ed., rev. and enl. Farnham, Surrey, U.K.; Fishing News Books; New York; Distributed in the USA by W. S. Heinman, 1984. 419p. Includes indexes. Bibliography, pp. 394–406.   [D812]

Browning, Robert J., et al. *Fisheries of the North Pacific: History, Species, Gear and Processes*. Rev. ed. Edmonds, Wash.; Alaska Northwest Pub. Co., 1980. 423p. Includes bibliographical references and index.   [D814]

Bryan, C. F., ed. *Warmwater Streams Techniques Manual: Fishes*. Baton Rouge; Louisiana State University Printing Office, 1984. 1 vol., loose-leaf.

"Contributions from the Warmwater Streams Committee, Southern Division, American Fisheries Society." Includes bibliographies.

Coche, A. G. *Soil and Freshwater Fish Culture*. Graphic design and layout, T. Laughlin. Rome; Food and Agriculture Organization, 1985. 174p. (FAO Training Series no. 6) Simple methods for aquaculture. Bibliography, p. 165.

Food and Agriculture Organization. Fishery Information, Data and Statistics Service, Fisheries Dept. *Aquaculture Production (1984–1987) = Production de l'Aquaculture (1984–1987)/Prepare par Service de l'Information, des Donnees et des Statistiques sur la Peche, Department des Peches, FAO = Produccion de Acuicultura (1984–1987)/Preparada por Servicio Pesca, FAO*. Rome; FAO, 1989. 130p. (FAO Fisheries Circular no. 815, rev. 1)

Gulland, J. A., ed. *Fish Population Dynamics: The Implications for Management*. 2d ed. Chichester and New York; Wiley, 1988. 422p. Includes bibliographies and indexes.   [D817]

Kennish, Michael J., ed. *Practical Handbook of Marine Science*. Boca Raton, Fla.; CRC Press, 1989. 710p. Includes index. Bibliography, pp. 680–689.

Mangone, Gerald J. *Mangone's Concise Marine Almanac*. 2d ed., rev. and expanded. New York; Taylor & Francis, 1991. 199p. Includes bibliographical references and index.

McGoodwin, James Russell. *Crisis in the World's Fisheries: People, Problems, and Politics*. Stanford, Calif.; Stanford University Press, 1990. 235p.

Broad coverage of international and domestic fisheries, and the economics of current fisheries management.

Robinson, M. A. *Trends and Prospects in World Fisheries*. Rome; Food and Agriculture Organization, 1984. 25p. (FAO Fisheries Circular no. 772) Includes bibliographical references.

Ross, Lindsay G. and Barbara Ross. *Anaesthetic and Sedative Techniques for Fish*. 1st ed. Stirling, Scotland; Institute of Aquaculture, University of Sterling, 1984. 35p. Bibliography, pp. 30–32.

Saila, Saul B., Conrad W. Recksiek and Michael H. Prager. *Basic Fishery Science Programs: A Compendium of Microcomputer Programs and Manual of Operation*. Amsterdam and New York; Elsevier, 1988. 230p. (Developments in Aquaculture and Fisheries Science no. 18) Includes bibliographical references and index.

U.S. Peace Corps. *Aquaculture Training Manual*. Washington, D.C.; Peace Corps, Office of Training and Program Support, 1990. 350p. (Training Manual no. T0057) Includes bibliographical references, pp. 337–343.

U.S. Peace Corps. *Small-Scale Marine Fisheries: An Extension Training Manual*. Washington, D.C.; Peace Corps, Office of Program Development, 1983 + . 1 vol. (loose-leaf). (TR-30) "Produced for the Peace Corps by the Technos Corporation." Includes bibliographical references.

Index of References, Chapter 7

Authors and titles referenced in Chapter 7 are included in this index. Subject indexing is only to the broad subject categories of the Chapter; there is no subject indexing of titles or the contents of notations.

8. Primary Historical Literature, 1860–1949

HENRY T. MURPHY

DOROTHY W. WRIGHT

Mann Library, Cornell University

The objective of this phase of the study has been to identify a body of the agricultural literature which, by various measures, has been deemed worthy of preservation for posterity. The need for preservation results from the fact that about the time of the U.S. Civil War, the technology of paper-making changed from relying on a high rag content to depending on ground wood pulp. This new process, a revolutionary development creating cheaper paper to meet the increased demands from newspaper, book and magazine publishers, was based on a chemical technique for the digestion of the wood to pulp which resulted in an acidic paper that over time self-destructs. The yellowing, brittle paper of older books tears easily, entire pages break away from the binding, and the paper is soon pulverized to dust. This is all too familiar in books published after the Civil War. Older books, those printed in the eighteenth century on paper with a high rag content, have pages which are still white and pliable with little evidence of the yellowing and brittleness of later publications. Therefore, this effort to identify the primary historical or heritage literature that should be preserved concentrates on those publications which appeared between 1860 and 1949. The importance of permanent records in agriculture is well established, but our objective is to help ensure that these records are indeed permanent.

In order to address the problem of this massive deterioration in agricultural libraries, this phase of the study has been undertaken to identify those publications within the subject parameters which appeared between 1860 and 1949 and would be most valuable to future generations. While a few books published prior to 1860 have been included here because of their special significance, in general it is assumed that because of their age, rarity, and historical value, all monographs published before 1860 should have high priority for preservation.

The decade of the 1860s was significant in U.S. agriculture. In 1862 Lincoln signed the bill that established the U.S. Department of Agriculture (USDA). The Homestead Act, which also passed in 1862, opened half the continent to agricultural development. In that same year, Senator Justin Morrill of Vermont introduced a bill providing for the sale of federally owned land, the proceeds of which would be used for the perpetual endowment in each state of at least one college "to teach such branches of learning related to agriculture and the mechanic arts." The Morrill Act as enacted by Congress became the foundation of the sixty-eight colleges and universities of the land-grant system in the United States. A later related development was the passage of the Hatch Act in 1887, which provided for the establishment in all states of agricultural experiment stations which were generally associated with the state land-grant college.

Many other changes were occurring during the nineteenth century which had an impact on American agriculture. Transportation was being transformed with the expansion of canals, rail lines, and steamship service. The industrial revolution was under way, which resulted in increased urban population and market centers. Westward expansion beyond the Alleghenies and western wheat and cattle development contributed to the growth of the nation beyond the Mississippi River. New farm implements and machinery aided in increasing production. Farms were undergoing a change from family subsistence and general agriculture to more commercial and specialized agriculture.

The tremendous changes of nineteenth century farming are reflected in the growth and development of the published agricultural literature in the United States. With the publication of the first agricultural experiment station bulletins in 1888, followed by the U.S. Department of Agriculture's *Farmers Bulletins* in 1889, a new medium of publication for the results of expanding agricultural research was made available. For the next sixty or seventy years the publications of the agricultural experiment stations and USDA would represent a significant percentage of the agricultural research literature. In fact, these publications formed the foundation for the development of many libraries within the land-grant system. They were generally available free to agricultural scientists and therefore widely distributed throughout the land-grant colleges. Many researchers compiled extensive personal libraries of these experiment station and USDA bulletins which they made available to their students.

Agricultural societies proliferated in the 1800s. In 1858, 912 state and county agricultural societies were listed by the U.S. Commissioner of Patents. Most were mainly concerned with the operation of local agricultural fairs, but some periodically published results of scientific, agricultural experiments in their Memoirs or Transactions. The Columbian Agricultural Society's *Agricultural Museum* (Georgetown, District of Columbia), beginning publication in 1810, was the first agricultural journal in the United States. Although it lasted less than two years, its editor, the Reverend David Wiley, broke ground for a new specialty in journalism.

Almanacs were a valuable publication for the nineteenth-century farmer and frequently the only one available to him. Intended primarily to record astronomical data, they became a source of a variety of miscellaneous rural information. The farmer, being totally dependent on the climate and weather conditions, needed the information provided by the almanac to schedule his work in order to keep pace with the seasons. No doubt many early nineteenth-century farm homes had only the almanac and the family Bible for reading material.

At the time of the American Revolution nearly 90% of the American people were farmers. The importance of agriculture to the nation was recognized by our founding fathers and the importance of agricultural literature to them is evidenced by an examination of the catalogs of the libraries of George Washington and Thomas Jefferson. Washington had over fifty agricultural volumes in his library and Jefferson had 133, impressive numbers considering the difficulty of obtaining books in America in the 1700s. Both men were farmers interested in the results of agricultural experimentation and both had in their collections the publications of the outstanding British agriculturists of the day such as Arthur Young, the forerunner of modern agricultural authors, with whom Washington corresponded on several occasions about agricultural husbandry.

The first book on farming printed in England was Anthony Fitzherbert's *Boke of Husbondrye* published in 1523. This had been preceded by Latin classics and handwritten manuscripts. The first printed English book devoted to a particular aspect of animal husbandry was Leonard Mascall's *The Husbandrie, Ordering and Government of Poultrie* published in 1581. For most of the next three centuries North Americans were primarily dependent on English publishers for their books and journals in the fields of science including agriculture.

However, printing presses in the American colonies were not idle. The first agricultural book published in the United States was Jared Eliot's *Essays upon Field-Husbandry in New England*, which appeared in Boston in 1760. George Culley's *Observations on Live Stock: Containing Hints for Choosing and Improving the Best Breeds of the Most Useful Kinds of Domestic Animals*, published in New York in 1804, was one of the earliest American books devoted entirely to animal husbandry. The last half of the nineteenth century marked the beginning of the publication of significant numbers of American books in specific fields of agriculture.

Poultry was an early area of specialization in the agricultural literature. Poultry was not only a part of the rural scene; many nineteenth-century city dwellers had a chicken coop or hen house in the backyard with a few birds adequate to keep the family supplied with eggs and the occasional Sunday dinner. In the latter part of the century there was great interest in the specialty breeds of poultry. Poultry books and journals provided a wealth of information to the rural poultry farmer and the backyard chicken keeper. The first modern book on poultry by an English author was Bonington Moubray's *Treatise on Domestic Poultry* . . . published in London in 1815, followed by an American edition in 1832. Micajah Cock's (pseudonym for Caleb N. Bement) *American Poultry Yard*, the first poultry book by an American author, appeared in 1843. This was followed a year later by his *American Poulterer's Companion*. The first poultry magazine published in the United States was *The Poultry Bulletin*, founded in 1870. The *American Poultry Journal*, one of the oldest and most prominent poultry publications, first appeared in 1874. The early success of poultry journals led to an unprecedented proliferation in their numbers. In the thirty years from 1870 to 1900 more than 200 new ones had been established although many had very brief lives. While many were very regional or parochial in their coverage, a review of their content provides an intimate view of the life and economy of the era. A footnote on nineteenth-century poultry literature relates to the author of *The Hamburgs, a Brief Treatise upon the Mating, Rearing, and Management of the Varieties of Hamburgs*, published in Hartford, Conn., in 1886. The author, Frank L. Baum, later achieved fame with the publication of his children's books, most notably his *Wonderful Wizard of Oz*, published in 1900.

The literature of beekeeping is extensive and dates back to the time of the Greeks and Romans. Modern American beekeeping dates from 1853 with the publication of the Reverend Lorenzo L. Langstroth's *Langstroth on the Hive and the Honey Bee* and his invention of the movable frame hive. Beekeepers of the nineteenth century were enthusiasts, and their enthusiasm prompted them to record their ideas in numerous books and periodicals. Early specialty journals in this field were the *American Bee Journal* (Chicago, 1861 +) and *Gleanings in Bee Culture* (Medina, Ohio, 1873 +). Both of these pioneering journals are still being published. A. I. Root, the publisher of *Gleanings*, wrote not only about beekeeping but also about the activities of the Anti-Saloon League and warned about the use of tobacco. His column "Our Home" in the March 1, 1904, issue refers to the flight of two local brothers, Wilbur and Orville Wright, at Kitty Hawk, N.C., in a "flying machine constructed without the use of a balloon," one of the early published accounts of their historic accomplishment. These early specialty journals not only furnish information about the agricultural specialty itself but also afford a valuable insight into rural life and people, their values and their interests.

Sericulture or silk culture was another early area of agricultural specialization. Although it never developed into a profitable enterprise in the United States, an avid interest in silk culture began in the 1830s and persisted into the early twentieth century. The arrival of the now detested gypsy moth in New England from Europe in 1868 was the result of an entrepreneur importing it with the expectation that the insect would be the foundation of an American silk industry. The American Silk Society established a monthly journal in 1839 and others followed.

The introduction of scientific journals and monographs in animal science began around 1870 in the United States, although there are a few important works prior to this date. This nearly coincides with the introduction of poor quality paper. Therefore, most of the scholarly and general animal science publications from the United States fall in the period where historical preservation is critical.

Mann Library, Cornell University, set about identifying and evaluating this literature covering the period of 1860 until 1950. This was done as an adjunct to the current core literature from the 1950–1990 period which is presented earlier in this book. Distinct types of publications important to animal science and health in the United States have been identified in the sections following: (1) monographs; (2) popular periodicals; and (3) scholarly journals.

A. Identifying the Monographs

The aim of this historical investigation has been to identify those monographs important in academic and research literature in the field of animal science and beekeeping for approximately the one hundred years prior to 1950. These scholarly publications were identified by two methods: (1) citation analysis of key historical literature, and (2) recommendations made by scholars who reviewed lists.

The citation analysis methods used are the same as those described in Chapter 5 for the identification and weighting of the 1950–1990 publications. Titles and counts were kept each time a journal, journal article, book or chapter of a book was cited. Landmark and historically significant monographs were chosen for analysis covering the various subject fields such as animal breeding, and nutrition, beef cattle, beekeeping, dairy science, horses, poultry, sheep, swine, etc. The landmark volumes used for citation analysis are listed here.

Landmark Animal Science and Health Literature
Used for Citation Analysis

Anderson, Arthur L. *Introductory Animal Husbandry*. Rev. ed. New York; Macmillan, 1951. 679p.

Bailey, Liberty H., ed. *Cyclopedia of American Agriculture*. Vol. 3-Animals. New York and London; Macmillan Co., 1908. 708p.

Bartsch, Otto. *Auchtungs- und Vererbungslehre fur Geflugelzuchter*. 2d ed. Berlin; F. Pfenningstorff, 1954–1956. 2 pts. in 1 vol.

Becker, Raymond B. *Dairy Cattle Breeds; Origin and Development*. Gainesville; University of Florida Press, 1973. 554p.

Bundy, Clarence E., and Ronald V. Diggins. *Swine Production*. Englewood Cliffs, N.J.; Prentice-Hall, 1956. 337p.

Cole, Harold H., and Magnar Ronning, eds. *Animal Agriculture, the Biology of Domestic Animals and Their Use by Man*. San Francisco; Freeman, 1974. 788p.

Cole, Harold H., ed. *Introduction to Livestock Production, Including Dairy and Poultry*. San Francisco and London; W. H. Freeman & Co., 1962. 789p.

Crew, F. A. E. *Animal Genetics: An Introduction to the Science of Animal Breeding*. Edinburgh and London; Oliver & Boyd, 1925. 420p.

Davidson, H. R. *The Production and Marketing of Pigs*. 2d ed. London, New York and Toronto; Longmans, Green & Co. 1953. 537p.

Fraser, Allan. *Beef Cattle Husbandry*. London; Crosby Lockwood & Son, 1953. 244p.

Hagedoorn, A. L. *Animal Breeding*. 5th ed. London; Crosby Lockwood & Son, 1954. 355p.

Hammond, John. *Farm Animals; Their Breeding, Growth, and Inheritance*. 2d ed. London; Edward Arnold & Co., 1952. 266p.

Hammond, John, Ivar Johansson, and Fritz Haring, eds. *Handbuch der Tierzuchtung; Unter Mitwirkung von zahlreichen Mitarbeitern*. Hamburg; Parey, 1958–1961. 3 vols. in 4.

Henderson, H. O., and Paul M. Reaves. *Dairy Cattle Feeding and Management*. 4th ed. New York; J. Wiley & Sons; London; Chapman & Hall, 1954. 614p. (1st ed., 1917.)

Hutt, F. B. *Genetics of the Fowl*. 1st ed. New York, Toronto and London; McGraw-Hill Book Co., 1949. 590p.

Jull, Morley A. *Poultry Husbandry*. 3d ed. New York; McGraw-Hill Book Co., 1951. 511p.

Lerner, I. Michael, and H. P. Donald. *Modern Developments in Animal Breeding*. London; Academic Press, 1966. 271p.

Lush, Jay L. *Animal Breeding Plans*. Ames; Iowa State College Press, 1945. 443p.

Manley, R. O. B. *Bee-Keeping in Britain*. London; Faber & Faber, 1948. 439p.

Mason, I. L. *A World Dictionary of Breeds, Types, and Varieties of Livestock*. Slough, U.K.; Commonwealth Agricultural Bureaux, 1951. 272p. (Technical Communication no. 8 of the Commonwealth Bureau of Animal Breeding & Genetics)

Maynard, Leonard A. *Animal Nutrition*. 3d ed. New York; McGraw-Hill Book Co., 1951. 443p.

Mehner, Alfred. *Lehrbuch der Geflugelzucht; Zuchtung, Futterung und Haltung von Huhnern und Puten*. Hamburg; Parey, 1962. 531p.

Mellen, Ida M. *The Natural History of the Pig*. New York; Exposition Press, 1952. 157p.

Morse, Roger A. *Bees and Beekeeping*. Ithaca, N.Y.; Cornell University Press, 1975. 283p.

National Agricultural Library, Dictionary Catalog, 1862–1965. New York; Rowman & Littlefield, 1969. Vol. 50, pp. 62–69 (under heading: Poultry breeding).

Pellett, Frank C. *History of American Beekeeping*. Ames, Iowa; Collegiate Press, 1938. 213p.

Peters, Walter H., and Robert H. Grummer. *Livestock Production*. 2d ed. New York; McGraw-Hill Book Co., 1954. 409p.

Peterson, W. E. *Dairy Science: Its Principles and Practice*. 2d ed. Chicago; J. B. Lippincott Co., 1950. 695p. (1st ed., 1939.)

Plumb, Charles S. *Types and Breeds of Farm Animals*. Boston; Ginn & Company, 1906. 555p.

Porter, A. R., J. A. Sims, and C. F. Foreman. *Dairy Cattle in American Agriculture*. Ames; Iowa State University Press, 1965. 328p.

Rice, Victor A. *Breeding and Improvement of Farm Animals*. 3d ed. New York; McGraw-Hill Book Co., 1942. 750p.

Rouse, John E. *World Cattle III: Cattle of North America*. Norman; University of Oklahoma Press, 1973. 650p.

Sampson, Arthur W. *Livestock Husbandry on Range and Pasture*. New York; J. Wiley & Sons, 1928. 405p.

Towne, Charles W., and Edward N. Wentworth. *Cattle & Men*. Norman; University of Oklahoma Press, 1955. 341p.

Towne, Charles W., and Edward N. Wentworth. *Pigs: From Cave to Corn Belt*. Norman; University of Oklahoma Press, 1950. 295p.

Wentworth, Edward N. *America's Sheep Trails, History, Personalities*. Ames; Iowa State College Press, 1948. 627p.

Winter, A. R., and E. M. Funk. *Poultry; Science and Practice*, edited by R. W. Gregory. 3d ed. Chicago, Philadelphia and New York; J. B. Lippincott Co., 1951. 662p.

Yapp, William W., and William B. Nevens. *Dairy Cattle; Selection, Feeding and Management*. New York; J. Wiley & Sons; London; Chapman & Hall, 1941. 456p. (1st ed., 1926.)

Citation analysis of these source publications provided a count of the number of times each publication was cited.

Emphasis is on North American monographs but includes primary European works in English as well. Shorter monographs under fifty pages were excluded unless there was evidence of their historical significance. Also, all federal documents and land-grant agricultural publications in series were excluded since these have already been preserved on microfilm or plans to do so are under way.

Lists generated by this method were then evaluated by subject specialists in select fields, usually faculty members of land-grant agricultural colleges or U.S. Department of Agriculture scholars with long research and teaching experience.

Historical Monograph Reviewers

Randall K. Cole
  Cornell University
John K. Loosli
  Cornell University
T. Wayne Perry
  Purdue University
John L. Skinner
  University of Wisconsin

Clair E. Terrill
  USDA, Agricultural Research Service
George W. Trimberger
  Cornell University
George H. Wellington
  Cornell University

Reviewers were asked to rank the titles with any of these criteria in mind:

(1) The work has had an important influence in the subject field; this could be because the author was important, the work has been frequently referred to by later authors, the work was a major compilation or compendium of the time, or it was a foundation book on which later efforts were built.
(2) The work is the first of its kind published or records major advances in the field.
(3) The work embodies an historical record of daily or yearly transactions or changes in the field.
(4) The title is valuable because it is a superior work of a leader in the animal or agricultural sciences.
(5) The work includes unusual or valuable etchings, prints, or illustrations.
(6) The title has survived in a very limited number of copies.

Reviewers also made suggestions of worthy titles for inclusion in the list, in addition to those generated by citation analysis. Although these were few, they were incorporated in the list and evaluated. We are most grateful for the reviewers' willingness to share their time and expertise in this project. Most felt that the efforts toward literature preservation should not be delayed.

Reviewers were asked to rank each title under one of the following:

Category 1. A very important historical title worthy of preservation.
Category 2. Worthy of preservation but of secondary importance.
Category 3. A title of marginal historical value.

A total score was obtained for each title by adding the number of times that title appeared in the references in the various source documents, referred to as citation hits, plus the rankings of all reviewers. Category 1 rankings by reviewers were weighted by a factor of 3; Category 2 rankings, by a factor of 2; and Category 3 rankings by a factor of 1.

$$\text{Final ranking} = (1 \times \#\text{ hits}) + (3 \times \#1 \text{ category ranking})$$
$$+ (2 \times \#2) + (1 \times \#3)$$

Thus those receiving the highest scores derived from this formula were rated first rank; those scoring in the mid-range ranked second; and those with the lowest scores ranked third. Those titles in the first rank should be given top priority by book conservators for preservation while those in the second and third ranking should be of lower priority. The 612 titles appearing on the list were divided as follows:

First rank	108	17.6%
Second rank	362	59.2
Third rank	142	23.2
Total	612	100.0%

Special attention must be paid to the herdbooks which in the past twenty years have become a specialized format unto themselves. Many of the records are proprietary today and must be searched via specific negotiated arrangements. Much of the data is computerized and specific searches can be made for a fee. This has resulted in very little being published with general public access. Because of this situation, the herdbooks were not sought extensively nor incorporated in the evaluation.

Items designated with a dagger(†) in the following list are historically important poultry books designated by the American Poultry History Association in its *American Poultry History, 1823–1973,* ed. by Oscar August Hanke, John L. Skinner, and James Harold Florea (Madison, Wis.: 1974). The brief listing is on pp. 743–744. The books were considered "significant due to their influence on the industry because they were first, exclusives, unique, or received especially wide distribution."

Historically Important Monographs in Animal Science and Health, 1860–1949

Ranking

A

Second   Aikman, Charles M. Milk, Its Nature and Composition; A Handbook on the Chemistry and Bacteriology of Milk, Butter, and Cheese. London; A. & C. Black, 1895. 180p.

Second   Alexander, Alexander S. Udder Diseases of the Cow and Related Subjects. Boston; R. G. Badger, 1928. 213p.

Ranking

Third	Allee, Warder C., et al. Principles of Animal Ecology. Philadelphia; Saunders, 1949. 837p.
Second	Allen, Edgar, ed. Sex and Internal Secretions; A Survey of Recent Research. Baltimore; Williams & Wilkins Co., 1932. 951p. (3d ed., edited by William C. Young, 1961. 2 vols. 1609p.)
Third	Allen, George E. Angora Goats; The Wealth of the Wilderness. Wellsboro, Pa.; H. A. Field Co., 1900. 32p.
First	Allen, Lewis F. American Cattle: Their History, Breeding and Management. New York; Taintor Brothers & Co., 1868. 528p. (Later ed., New York; Orange Judd Co., 1883.)
First	Allen, Lewis F. History of the Short-Horn Cattle: Their Origin, Progress and Present Condition. Buffalo, N.Y.; The author, 1872. 266p. (2d ed., 1883. 280p.)
First	Allen, Richard L. Domestic Animals. History and Description of the Horse, Mule, Cattle, Sheep, Swine, Poultry, and Farm Dogs with Directions for Their Management, Breeding, Crossing, Rearing, Feeding, and Preparation for a Profitable Market; Also Their Diseases, and Remedies, Together with Full Directions for the Management of the Dairy. New York; C. M. Saxton, 1848. 227p.
Third	Altenburg, Edgar. Genetics. New York; Holt, 1945. 452p. (Rev. ed., 1957. 496p.)
Second	American Association for the Advancement of Science. The Chemistry and Physiology of Hormones, edited by Forest Ray Moulton. Washington, D.C.; American Association for the Advancement of Science, 1944. 243p.
Third	American Meat Institute. Reference Book of the Meat Industry. Chicago; American Meat Institute, Dept. of Public Relations, 1941. 64p.
First	†American Poultry Association. The American Standard of Perfection . . . Containing a Complete Description of All the Recognized Varieties of Fowls, edited by Harmon S. Babcock. Buffalo, N.Y.; American Poultry Association, 1888. 244p. (1985 ed. as American Standard of Perfection 1985. Troy, N.Y. 336p.)
Third	Anderson, Arthur L. Introductory Animal Husbandry. New York; Macmillan, 1943. 742p. (3d ed., 1958.)
Third	Anderson, Arthur L. Swine Management, Including Feeding and Breeding, edited by R. W. Gregory. Philadelphia; Lippincott, 1950. 531p. (2d ed., Chicago; Lippincott, 1957.)
Second	Anderson, James. The Semen of Animals and Its Use for Artificial Insemination. Edinburgh; Printed by Oliver & Boyd, 1945. 151p.
Second	Armatage, George. Cattle; Their Varieties and Management in Health and Disease. Rev. and enl. ed. London; Frederich Warne & Co., 1894. 240p.
First	Armsby, Henry P. Manual of Cattle-Feeding: A Treatise on the Laws of Animal Nutrition and the Chemistry of Feeding Stuffs in Their Application to the Feeding of Animals. New York; J. Wiley, 1880. 525p. (5th ed., 1896. 525p.)
First	Armsby, Henry P. The Nutrition of Farm Animals. New York; The Macmillan Co., 1917. 743p.

Ranking

First   Armsby, Henry P. The Principles of Animal Nutrition. 1st ed. New York; J. Wiley & Sons, 1903. 614p. (3d ed., rev., 1908.)

First   Arndt, Milton H. Battery Brooding: A Complete Exposition of the Important Facts Concerning the Successful Operation and Handling of the Various Types of Battery Brooders. New York; Orange Judd, 1931. 323p. (New and revised ed., 1932. 325p.)

First   Asdell, Sydney A. Patterns of Mammalian Reproduction. Ithaca, N.Y.; Comstock Publishing Co., 1946. 437p.

Second   Association of Breeders of Thorough-Bred Neat Stock. Herd Record; Short Horns. Hartford, Conn.; Williams, Wiley & Waterman, 1863. 86p.

Second   Atkinson, Morton E., and Grant M. Curtis. The Production of 300-Eggers and Better by Line Breeding. Dayton, Ohio; The Reliable Poultry Journal Pub. Co., 1923. 415p.

Third   Austin, Mary H. The Flock. Boston and New York; Houghton, Mifflin & Co., 1906. 266p.

Second   Axe, J. Wortley. The Horse, Its Treatment in Health and Disease. . . . London; The Gresham Pub. Co., 1905. 4 vols.

B

First   Babcock, Ernest B. Genetics in Relation to Agriculture. New York; McGraw-Hill, 1918. 675p. (2d ed., 1927. 673p.)

First   Bailey, Liberty H., ed. Cyclopedia of American Agriculture; A Popular Survey of Agricultural Conditions, Practices and Ideals in the United States and Canada. New York and London; The Macmillan Co., 1907–1909. 4 vols. (4th ed., 1912.)

Second   Bailey, Liberty H., ed. The Principles of Agriculture; A Text-Book for Schools and Rural Societies. New York and London; The Macmillan Co., 1898. 300p. (15th ed., rev., 1909. 336p.)

Second   Baker, Austin H. Live Stock: A Cyclopedia for the Farmer and Stock Owner. Special ed. Minneapolis; H. L. Baldwin Pub. Co., 1911. 1398p.

Second   Barger, Edgar H., and Leslie E. Card. Diseases and Parasites of Poultry. Philadelphia; Lea & Febiger, 1935. 354p. (5th ed., rev. by E. H. Barger, L. E. Card and B. S. Pomeroy, 1958. 408p.)

Second   Barker, Sydney G. Wool Quality: A Study of the Influence of Various Contributory Factors, Their Significance and the Technique of Their Measurements. London; H.M.S.O., 1931. 333p.

First   Barnes, Will C. Western Grazing Grounds and Forest Ranges; A History of the Livestock Industry as Conducted on the Open Ranges of the Arid West. . . . Chicago; The Breeder's Gazette, 1913. 390p.

Second   Barrows, Anna. Eggs: Facts and Fancies about Them. Boston; D. Lothrop, 1890. 159p.

Second   Bartlett, Edwin S. Sheep Shearing. Chicago; Breeder Publications, 1938. 127p.

Third   Bates, Cadwallader J. The History of Improved Short-Horn or Durham Cattle, and of the Kirklevington Herd. Newcastle-upon-Tyne, U.K.; R. Red-

Ranking

           path, 1871. 371p. (Rev. ed., 1897, as Thomas Bates and the Kirklevington Shorthorns. 513p.)

Second   Bateson, William. Materials for the Study of Variation, Treated with Special Regard to Discontinuity in the Origin of Species. London and New York; Macmillan, 1894. 598p.

Third   Bateson, William. Problems of Genetics. New Haven, Conn.; Yale University Press, 1913. 258p.

Third   Beeler, Maxwell N. Marketing Purebred Livestock. New York; The Macmillan Co., 1929. 393p.

First   †Bement, Caleb N. The American Poulterer's Companion. New York; Saxton & Miles, 1845. 379p. (New ed., enl. New York; Harper & Bros., 1871. 304p.)

First   †Bement, Caleb N. The American Poultry Book: Being a Practical Treatise of the Management of Domestic Poultry . . . by Micajah R. Cock. New York; Harper & Bros., 1843. 179p.

Second   Benesch, Franz, and John G. Wright. Veterinary Obstetrics: Including Certain Aspects of the Physiology and Pathology of Reproduction in Domestic Animals. Baltimore; William Wood & Co., 1938. (Later ed., Williams & Wilkins, 1951. 459p.) (Translation of Die Geburtshilfe bei Rind und Pferd.)

First   †Benjamin, Earl W. Marketing Poultry Products. New York; J. Wiley & Sons, 1923. 328p. (5th ed., 1960. 327p.)

Second   Bennett, Frank P. Wool and Sheep Facts. Boston and New York; The American Wool and Cotton Reporter, 1895.

First   †Bennett, John C. The Poultry Book: A Treatise on Breeding and General Management of Domestic Fowls. Boston; Phillips, Sampson & Co., 1850. 310p. (Reprinted, 1851.)

Third   Biddell, Herman. Heavy Horses; Breeds and Management. London; Vinton & Co., 1894. 219p. (Live Stock Handbooks no. 3) (4th ed., by Herman Biddell, C. I. Douglas, Thomas Dykes et al., 1905.)

First   †Biester, Harry E., and Louis Devries, eds. Diseases of Poultry. Ames; Iowa State College Press, 1943. 1005p. (6th ed., edited by M. S. Hofstad, 1972. 1176p.)

Third   Biggle, Jacob. Biggle Horse Book. Philadelphia; W. Atkinson Co., 1894. 121p. (10th ed., 1913. 136p.)

First   †Biggle, Jacob. Biggle Poultry Book. Philadelphia; W. Atkinson, 1895. 160p. (10th ed., 1917. 176p.)

Second   Black, William L. A New Industry, or Raising the Angora Goat, and Mohair, for Profit. Fort Worth, Tex.; Keystone Printing Co., 1900. 486p.

Third   Blew, William C. Light Horses; Breeds and Management. 2d ed. London; Vinton & Co., 1894. 226p. (Live Stock Handbooks no. 2)

Second   Blount, William P., ed. Diseases of Poultry. Baltimore; Williams & Wilkins, 1947. 562p.

Second   Bradley, O. Charnock. The Structure of the Fowl, rev. by Tom Grahame. 1st ed. London; A. & C. Black, 1915. 153p. (4th ed., Edinburgh; Oliver & Boyd, 1960. 143p.)

Ranking

Third   Bresslau, Ernst. The Mammary Apparatus of the Mammalia in the Light of
             Ontogenesis and Phylogenesis. London; Methuen, 1920. 145p.
First   Briggs, Hilton M. Modern Breeds of Livestock. New York; Macmillan,
             1949. 772p. (4th ed., 1980. 802p.)
Second   Brisbin, James S. The Beef Bonanza; Or, How to Get Rich on the Plains.
             Philadelphia; J. B. Lippincott & Co., 1881. 222p. (Later ed., Norman;
             University of Oklahoma Press, 1959. 208p.)
First   Brody, Samuel. Bioenergetics and Growth. New York; Reinhold, 1945.
             1023p.
Second   Brown, Edward M. Poultry Breeding and Production. London; Caxton,
             1929. 2 vols.
First   Brown, Edward M. Races of Domestic Poultry. London; E. Arnold, 1906.
             234p.
Second   Brown, George A. Sheep Breeding in Australia. . . . 2d ed. Melbourne;
             Walker, 1890. 496p. (3d ed., as Australian Merino Studs, 1904. 389p.)
Third   Brown, George A. Studies in Stock Breeding. An Inquiry into the Various
             Phonomena Connected with the Breeding of the Domestic Animals.
             Melbourne; Walker, May & Co., 1902. 426p.
Third   Brown, William Robinson. The Horse of the Desert. New York; The Der-
             rydale Press, 1929. 218p. (Later ed., New York; Macmillan, 1948. 218p.)
Second   Bull, Sleeter. The Principles of Feeding Farm Animals. New York; Mac-
             millan, 1916. 397p. (Rev. ed., written with W. E. Carroll, Danville, Ill.;
             Interstate, 1949. 400p.)
First   †Burnham, George P. Burnham's New Poultry Book: A Practical Treatise
             on Selecting, Housing and Breeding Domestic Fowls, and Raising Poultry
             and Eggs for Market. New York; American News Co. and Boston; N. E.
             News Co., 1871. 343p. (Reprinted in 1877.)
First   †Burnham, George P. The History of the Hen Fever: A Humorous Record.
             San Diego, Calif; Frank E. Marcy, 1935. 301p. (2d ed., Boston; J. French
             and Co. and New York; J. C. Derby, 1955. 326p.)
Second   Burnham, George P. Secrets in Fowl Breeding. Melrose, Mass.; 1876. 58p.
             (A companion treatise to Diseases of Domestic Poultry.)
Second   Burrows, Harold. Biological Actions of Sex Hormones. Cambridge, U.K.;
             University Press, 1945. 514p. (2d ed., rev. and reset, 1949. 615p.)
Second   Busbey, Hamilton. The Trotting and the Pacing Horse in America. New
             York and London; Macmillan, 1904. 369p.

                                        C
First   Caldwell, William H. The Guernsey, a Portrayal of the Advancement of
             Guernsey Cattle in America. Peterborough, N.H.; The American Guernsey
             Cattle Club, 1941. 393p.
Third   Carlson, George L. Studies in Horse Breeding. 2d ed. Norfolk, Nebr.; The
             author, 1910. 321p.
First   †Card, Leslie E., and Melvin Henderson. Farm Poultry Production. Dan-
             ville, Ill.; The Interstate Printing Co., 1933. 202p. (4th ed., 1948. 230p.)
Third   Carman, Harry J., ed. American Husbandry. New York; Columbia Univer-

Ranking

sity Press, 1939. 582p. (Columbia University Studies in the History of American Agriculture no. 6) (Author may have been John Mitchell or Arthur Young.)

First   Carrier, Lyman. The Beginnings of Agriculture in America. New York; McGraw-Hill Book Co., 1923. 323p. (C. V. Piper, consulting editor.)

Third   Carrington, W. T., et al. Live-Stock. 4th ed. London; n.d. 156p. (8th ed., Vinton & Co., 1919.) (Morton's Handbooks of the Farm no. 2)

Second   Carter, William H. The Horses of the World. Washington, D.C.; National Geographic Society, 1923. 118p.

Second   Castle, William E. The Genetics of Domestic Rabbits. Cambridge; Harvard University Press, 1930. 31p.

Second   Castle, William E. Heredity in Relation to Evolution and Animal Breeding. New York and London; D. Appleton & Co., 1911. 184p. (Based on a course of 8 lectures delivered, Nov. and Dec. 1910, before the Lowell Institute, Boston, as well as on a course of 5 lectures delivered before the Graduate School of Agriculture held under the auspices of the Association of Agricultural Colleges and Experiment Stations at Ames, Iowa, July 1910.)

Second   Castle, William E. Mammalian Genetics. Cambridge; Harvard University Press, 1940. 169p.

Third   Chandler, Asa C. Animal Parasites and Human Disease. New York; Wiley, 1918. 570p. (10th ed., by Asa C. Chandler and Clark P. Read, 1961. 822p.)

Second   Chauveau, Auguste. The Comparative Anatomy of the Domesticated Animals . . . trans. from 2d rev. and enl. ed. and edited by George Fleming. London; J. & A. Churchill, 1873. 957p. (1st American ed., New York; D. Appleton & Co., 1873. 957p. Later eds. in 1886 and 1905.)

Second   Clarke, William J. Fitting for Show Ring and Market. Chicago; Draper Pub. Co., 1900. 248p.

Third   Clarke, William J. Modern Sheep: Breeds and Management. Chicago; American Sheep Breeder Co., 1907. 333p.

First   Clemen, Rudolf A. The American Livestock and Meat Industry. New York; Ronald Press Co., 1923. 872p.

First   Clemen, Rudolf A. By-Products in the Packing Industry. Chicago; University of Chicago Press, 1927. 410p.

Third   Coburn, Foster D. Swine Husbandry. New York; O. Judd Co., 1877. 275p. (3d ed., rev. and enl., 1903. 311p.)

Third   Coburn, Foster D. Swine in America; A Text-Book for the Breeder, Feeder and Student. New York; O. Judd Co., 1909. 614p. (Rev. ed., 1922. 583p.) (Also available in Portuguese.)

Third   Cochrane, Effie R. The Milch Cow in England. London; Faber & Faber, 1946. 348p.

Third   Coffey, Joel S., and Lyman E. Jackson. Livestock Management. Philadelphia; J. B. Lippincott, 1940. 500p. (Rev., 1949.)

Second   Coffey, Walter C. Productive Sheep Husbandry. Philadelphia and London; J. B. Lippincott Co., 1918. 479p. (3d ed., rev. Chicago and Philadelphia; J. B. Lippincott Co., 1937. 479p.)

Ranking

Second   Coleman, John, ed. The Cattle of Great Britain. London; The Field Office, 1875. 162p.
First   Coleman, John, ed. The Cattle, Sheep and Pigs of Great Britain . . . with illustrations from the original drawings by Harrison Weir. 2d ed. London; H. Cox, 1887. 491p.
Second   Commonwealth Bureau of Animal Breeding and Genetics. The Technique of Artificial Insemination. Edinburgh and London; Oliver & Boyd, 1933. 56p.
Second   Copeland, Lynn. Development of the Jersey Breed. Ann Arbor, Mich.; Edwards Brothers, 1926. 207p.
Third   Cowie, Alfred T. Pregnancy Diagnosis Tests: A Review. Edinburgh; Commonwealth Bureaux of Animal Breeding and Genetics, Dairy Science, Animal Health, 1948. 283p. (Commonwealth Agricultural Bureaux. Joint Publication no. 13)
First   Craig, John A. Judging Live Stock. Des Moines, Iowa; The author, Kenyon Printing & Mfg. Co., 1901. 193p. (27th ed., 1920. 187p.)
Third   Craig, John A. Sheep-Farming in North America. New York; The Macmillan Co., 1913. 302p. (Reissued, 1918.)
Third   Craig, Robert A. Common Diseases of Farm Animals. Philadelphia and London; J. B. Lippincott Co., 1915. 334p. (4th ed., rev., 1927. 332p.)
Third   Craig, Robert A. Diseases of Swine, with Special Reference to the Preventive Measures of Disease. New York; O. Judd Co., 1906. 191p.
First   Crew, Francis A. Animal Genetics: An Introduction to the Science of Animal Breeding. Edinburgh; Oliver & Boyd, 1925. 420p.
Second   Crew, Francis A. The Genetics of Sexuality in Animals. Cambridge, U.K.; University Press, 1927. 188p.
Second   Cronwright Schreiner, Samuel. The Angora Goat . . . published under the auspices of the South African Angora Goat Breeders' Assoc. London and New York; Longmans, Green & Co., 1898. 296p.
Second   Curtis, George W. Horses, Cattle, Sheep and Swine. College Station, Tex.; The author, 1888. 269p.
Second   Curtis, Robert S. The Fundamentals of Live Stock Judging and Selection. Philadelphia and New York; Lea & Febiger, 1915. 455p. (3d ed., thoroughly rev., Philadelphia; 1925. 472p.)

D

Second   Dale, Edward E. The Range Cattle Industry. Norman; University of Oklahoma Press, 1930. 216p. (Later ed., 1960. 207p.)
Third   Dalziel, Hugh. The Diseases of Dogs, Their Pathology, Diagnosis, and Treatment. New and rev. ed. New York; Jesse Haney & Co., 187–? 136p. (4th ed., rev. and enl. by Alexander C. Piesse. London; 1915? 144p.)
First   Darwin, Charles. The Origin of Species by Means of Natural Selection. New York; D. Appleton, 1889. 2 vols. (Edited by J. W. Burrow. Harmondsworth, U.K.; Penguin Books, 1985. 477p.)
First   Darwin, Charles. The Variation of Animals and Plants Under Domestication. Authorized ed. New York; Orange Judd & Co., 1868. 2 vols. (Reissued, New York; Appleton, 1900.)

Ranking

Second	Daumas, Melchior J. The Horses of the Sahara, and the Manners of the Desert . . . trans. by James Hutton. London; W. H. Allen, 1863. 355p.
Third	Davenport, Arthur C. The American Live Stock Market; How It Functions. Chicago; Drovers Journal Print, 1922. 174p.
Second	Davenport, Charles B. Inheritance in Poultry. Washington, D.C.; Carnegie Institution of Washington, 1906. 136p. (Carnegie Institution of Washington, Publication no. 52; Papers of the Station for Experimental Evolution no. 7)
Third	Davenport, Eugene. Domesticated Animals and Plants. Boston; Ginn & Co., 1910. 321p.
Second	Davenport, Eugene. Principles of Breeding. Boston and New York; Ginn & Co., 1907. 727p.
Third	Davidson, Hamish R. The Production and Marketing of Pigs. London, New York and Toronto; Longmans, Green & Co., 1948. 535p. (3d ed., London; 1966. 516p.)
Second	Dawson, Henry C. The Hog Book; Embodying the Experience of Fifty Years in the Practical Handling of Swine in the American Cornbelt. Chicago; The Breeder's Gazette, 1911. 414p.
Second	Day, George E. Productive Swine Husbandry. Philadelphia and London; J. B. Lippincott, 1913. 330p. (Rev. ed., Philadelphia, Chicago and London; 1924. 384p.)
Third	Day, George E. Swine; A Book for Students and Farmers. Des Moines, Iowa; The Kenyon Press, 1906. 108p.
Second	Day, William. The Horse, How to Breed and Rear Him. London; R. Bentley, 1888. 453p.
Second	De Voe, Thomas F. The Market Book. New York; Printed for the author, 1862. 2 vols. (Reprinted by B. Franklin, 1969.)
Second	Denhardt, Robert M. The Horse of the Americas. 1st ed. Norman; University of Oklahoma Press, 1948. 286p. (New ed., rev. and enl., 1975. 343p.)
Third	Devon Cattle Breeders' Society. Devon Cattle. Wellington, U.K.; Bryant, 192–. 27p. (Later ed., Exeter, Engl; Pollard, 1957. 96p.)
Third	Dietrich, William. Swine: Breeding, Feeding, and Management. Chicago; Sanders Pub. Co., 1910. 312p.
Third	Dimon, John. American Horses and Horse Breeding. Hartford, Conn.; The author, 1895. 449p.
Second	Dinsmore, Wayne, and John Hervey. Our Equine Friends. Chicago; Horse and Mule Association, 1944. 32p.
Second	Dixon, Edmund S. Ornamental and Domestic Poultry: Their History and Management. London; Gardeners' Chronicle, 1848. 345p. (Reprinted from the Gardeners' Chronicle and Agricultural Gazette, with additions. 2d ed., rev. and enl., 1850. 404p.)
Second	Dobie, J. Frank. The Longhorns . . . illustrated by Tom Lea. Boston; Little, Brown & Co., 1941. 388p. (Reissued, Austin; University of Texas Press, 1980.)
Second	Dollar, John A. A Handbook of Horse-Shoeing. New York; W. R. Jenkins, 1898. 438p.
Third	Doncaster, Leonard. Heredity in the Light of Recent Research. Cambridge, U.K.; University Press, 1910. 140p. (3d ed., 1921. 163p.)

Ranking

Third   Dowell, Austin A., and Knute Bjorka. Livestock Marketing. 1st ed. New York and London; McGraw-Hill, 1941. 534p.

First   Dukes, Henry H. The Physiology of Domestic Animals. Ann Arbor, Mich.; Edwards Brothers, 1933. 391p. (10th ed., edited by Melvin J. Swenson, Ithaca, N.Y.; Comstock Pub. Associates, 1984. 922p.)

Second   Dutch-Friesian Herd Book Association of America. Some Information Concerning the North Holland or Friesian Breed of Black and White Piebald Cattle, edited by S. Hoxie. 2d ed., rev. Utica, N.Y.; Curtiss & Childs, 1884. 56p.

Second   Dykstra, Ralph R. Animal Sanitation and Disease Control. Danville, Ill.; Interstate, 1942. 558p. (6th ed., 1961. 858p.)

E

First   East, Edward M. Inbreeding and Outbreeding; Their Genetic and Sociological Significance. Philadelphia and London; J. B. Lippincott Co., 1919. 285p.

Second   Eckles, Clarence H. Dairy Cattle and Milk Production. New York; Macmillan, 1911. 342p. (5th ed., rev., by Ernest L. Anthony, 1956. 587p.)

Second   Eckles, Clarence H. Milk and Milk Products. 1st ed. New York; McGraw-Hill Book Co., 1929. 379p. (4th ed., 1951. 454p.)

Second   Edmonds, James L., William E. Carroll, William G. Kammlade, William B. Nevens, and Roscoe R. Snapp. Producing Farm Livestock. New York; J. Wiley & Sons; London; Chapman & Hall, 1932. 439p.

Third   Eliot, Jared. Essays upon Field Husbandry in New England, edited by Harry J. Carman and Rexford G. Tugwell. New York; Columbia University Press, 1934. 261p.

Second   Espe, Dwight L. Secretion of Milk. Ames, Iowa; Collegiate Press, 1938. 265p. (4th ed., written by D. L. Espe and Vearl R. Smith, 1952. 291p.)

Second   Ewing, Perry V., ed. The Golden Hoof; A Practical Sheep Book. Chicago; Sheep Breeder, 1936. 256p.

First   †Ewing, William R. Handbook of Poultry Nutrition. 1st ed. South Pasadena, Calif.; 1941. 1518p. (4th rev. ed., 1951.)

F

Third   Farley, Frank W. Raising Beef Cattle on Farm and Range, edited by John M. Hazelton. Kansas City, Mo.; Walker Pub., 1931. 179p.

Second   Farrington, Edward H., and Fritz W. Woll. Testing Milk and Its Products. 1st ed. Madison, Wis.; Mendota Book Co., 1897. 236p. (27th ed., 1928. 280p.)

Second   The Feathered World. Ducks, the Standard and Most Authoritative Work upon All Varieties of Waterfowl Yet Published. London; The Feathered World, 1926. 140p.

First   †Felch, Isaac K. Poultry Culture. Chicago; Donohue, Henneberry & Co., 1885. 438p. (Reprinted, 1903.)

Third   Feldman, William H. Avian Tuberculosis Infections. Baltimore; Williams & Wilkins Co., 1938. 483p.

Ranking

Third   Finlay, Gerald F. Recent Developments in Cattle Breeding. Edinburgh; Oliver & Boyd, 1924. 62p. (Prepared for the Scottish Cattle Breeding Conference.)

Second   Fisher, Ronald A. The Genetical Theory of Natural Selection. Oxford; The Clarendon Press, 1930. 272p. (2d ed., rev., New York; Dover Publications, 1958. 291p.)

Third   Fishwick, Victor C. Pigs; Their Breeding, Feeding and Management. 3d ed., rev. London; C. Lockwood & Son, 1949. 252p. (9th ed., rev., 1965. 267p.)

Second   Flint, Charles L. Milch Cows and Dairy Farming. New York; A. O. Moore; Boston; A. Williams & Co., 1858. 416p. (New ed., Boston; Crosby & Nichols, 1864. 426p.)

Second   Flower, William H. The Horse; A Study in Natural History. New York; D. Appleton, 1892. 196p.

Second   Foster, Michael. A Text Book of Physiology . . . from the 3d and rev. English ed. Philadelphia, H. C. Lea's & Son, 1880. 1030p. (7th ed., New York; Macmillan, 1896. 1351p.)

Third   Foster, Michael. Physiology. New York; D. Appleton & Co., 1874. 132p. (Editions also in 1879 and 1883.)

Third   Fraser, Allan. Farming for Beef. London; C. Lockwood, 1950. 144p.

Second   Fraser, Allan. Sheep Farming. London; C. Lockwood & Son, 1937. 178p. (7th ed., 1965. 154p.)

Third   Fraser, Allan, and John T. Stamp. Sheep Husbandry. London; Lockwood, 1949. 297p. (5th ed., as Sheep Husbandry and Diseases, 1968. 438p.)

Third   Fraser, Wilber J. Dairy Profit. Danville, Ill.; Interstate, 1940. 270p. (Rev. ed., 1949. 316p.)

First   Fraser, Wilber J. Dairy Farming: Most Milk and Profit per Acre. New York; J. Wiley & Sons; London; Chapman & Hall, 1930. 333p.

Third   Fraser, Wilber J. Profitable Farming and Life Management. Danville, Ill.; Interstate Printers, 1937. 416p. (2d ed., rev., 1948. 418p.)

G

Second   Galton, Francis. Natural Inheritance. London and New York; Macmillan, 1889. 259p.

Second   Garner, Frank H. The Cattle of Britain. London and New York; Longmans, Green & Co., 1944. 158p.

Second   Gay, Carl W., ed. The Breeds of Live-Stock by Live-Stock Breeders. New York; The Macmillan Co., 1916. 483p. (Original material was prepared for the Cyclopedia of American Agriculture, vol. III.)

Second   Gay, Carl W. The Principles and Practice of Judging Live-Stock. New York; The Macmillan Co., 1914. 413p.

Second   Gay, Carl W. Productive Horse Husbandry. 1st ed. Philadelphia and London; J. B. Lippincott Co., 1914. 331p. (4th ed., rev., 1932. 335p.)

Third   Gerrard, Frank. Meat Technology; A Practical Textbook for Student and Butcher. 1st ed. London; L. Hill, 1945. 304p. (3d ed., 1964. 352p.)

Second   Gibbs, Charles S. A Guide to Sexing Chicks. New York; Orange Judd Pub. Co., 1935. 63p.

Ranking

Second   Gilbert, Frank A. Mineral Nutrition of Plants and Animals. 1st ed. Norman; University of Oklahoma Press, 1949. 131p.
Second   Gilbey, Walter. Thoroughbred and Other Ponies with Remarks on the Height of Racehorses Since 1700 . . . being a rev. ed. of Ponies: Past and Present. London; Vinton & Co., 1903. 156p.
Second   Gilfillan, Archer B. Sheep. Boston; Little, Brown, 1929. 272p.
Second   Gill, Leonard U., ed. The Book of the Rabbit. London; Bazaar Office, 1881. 440p. (2d ed., rev. and enl., by Kempster W. Knight. London; L. U. Gill, 1889. 484p.)
First   Gilmore, Lester O. Dairy Cattle Breeding, edited by R. W. Gregory. Philadelphia; Lippincott, 1952. 604p.
Second   Goldschmidt, Richard B. The Material Basis of Evolution. New Haven, Conn.; Yale University Press; London; H. Milford, Oxford University Press, 1940. 436p.
Second   Goldschmidt, Richard B. The Mechanism and Physiology of Sex Determination. London; Methuen & Co.; New York; George H. Doran Co., 1923. 259p.
Second   Goldschmidt, Richard B. Physiological Genetics. 1st ed. New York and London; McGraw-Hill Book Co., 1938. 375p.
Third   Goodale, Stephen L. The Principles of Breeding: Or, Glimpses at the Physiological Laws Involved in the Reproduction and Improvement of Domestic Animals. Boston; Crosby, 1861. 164p.
Third   Goodwin, J. P., ed. Britain Can Breed It; Live Stock of the British Isles Reviewed. London; Farmer and Stock-Breeder, 1948. 128p. (2d ed., 1949. 164p.)
Second   Gorman, John A. The Western Horse; Its Types and Training. Danville, Ill.; The Interstate, 1939. 278p. (5th ed., edited by Gaydell M. Collier, 1967. 452p.)
First   Goubaux, Armand, and Gustave Barrier. The Exterior of the Horse . . . trans. from French 2d French ed. and edited by Simon J. Harger. 2d ed. Philadelphia; J. B. Lippincott Co., 1892. 916p.
Second   Gould, Sylvester E. Trichinosis. 1st ed. Springfield, Ill.; C. C. Thomas, 1945. 356p.
First   Gow, Robert M. The Jersey: An Outline of Her History During Two Centuries—1734–1935. New York; American Jersey Cattle Club, 1936. 539p.
Second   Gowen, John W. Manual of Dairy Cattle Breeding. Baltimore; Williams & Wilkins Co., 1925. 113p.
Second   Gowen, John W. Milk Secretion: The Study of the Physiology and Inheritance of Milk Yield and Butter-Fat Percentage in Dairy Cattle. Baltimore; Williams & Wilkins Co., 1924. 363p.
Second   Gray, Lewis C. History of Agriculture in the Southern United States to 1860. Washington, D.C.; Carnegie Institution of Washington, 1933. 1086p. 2 vols. (Reprinted, Gloucester, Mass.; Peter Smith, 1958.)
Second   Grotenfelt, Gosta. The Principles of Modern Dairy Practice from a Bacteriological Point of View . . . authorized American ed. by F. W. Woll. 1st ed. New York; J. Wiley & Sons, 1894. 285p. (3d ed., rev., 1902. 286p.)

Ranking

Second   Gruneberg, Hans. Animal Genetics and Medicine. New York; P. B. Hoeber, 1947. 296p.

Second   Gruneberg, Hans. The Genetics of the Mouse. Cambridge, U.K.; The University Press, 1943. 412p. (2d ed., rev. and enl., The Hague; Martinus Nijhoff, 1952. 650p.)

Third   Gullickson, Thor W. Feeding Dairy Cattle. Saint Paul, Minn.; Webb Book Pub. Co., 1943. 223p.

Second   Guthrie, Edward S. The Book of Butter: A Text on the Nature, Manufacture and Marketing of the Product. New York; Macmillan, 1918. 270p.

H

Third   Hadley, Frederick B. The Horse in Health and Disease; A Text-Book Pertaining to Veterinary Science for Agricultural Students. Philadelphia and London; W. B. Saunders, 1915. 261p.

Third   Hadley, Frederick B. Principles of Veterinary Science; A Text-Book for Use in Agricultural Schools. Philadelphia and London; W. B. Saunders Co., 1920. 420p. (5th ed., Philadelphia; 1954. 546p.)

Second   Hagan, William A. The Infectious Diseases of Domestic Animals; With Special Reference to Etiology, Diagnosis, and Biologic Therapy. 1st ed. Ithaca, N.Y.; Comstock Pub. Co., 1943. 665p. (7th ed., rev. by James H. Gillespie and John F. Timoney, 1981. 581p.)

First   Hagedoorn, Arend L. Animal Breeding. London; C. Lockwood & Son, 1939. 304p. (6th ed., edited and annotated by Allan Fraser, 1962. 371p.)

Third   Halnan, Edward T. The Scientific Principles of Poultry Feeding. London; H.M.S.O., 1944. 60p. (Ministry of Agriculture and Fisheries Bulletin no. 7)

Second   Halnan, Edward T., and Frank H. Garner. The Principles and Practice of Feeding Farm Animals. London; Longmans, Green & Co., 1940. 359p. (5th ed., rev. and partly rewritten by Alfred Eden. London; Estates Gazette, 1966. 382p.)

Third   Hamerton, Philip G. Chapters on Animals . . . with 20 illustrations by J. Veyrassat and Karl Bodmer. Boston; Roberts Brothers, 1874. 253p. (Rev. ed. as Chapters on Animals; Dogs, Cats and Horses. Boston; D. C. Heath & Co., 1900. 88p.) (Heath's Home and School Classics no. 4)

Third   Hamilton, Samuel W. Profitable Turkey Management. 1st ed. Cayuga, N.Y.; Beacon Milling Co., 1934. 95p. (9th ed., 1954. 160p.)

Second   Hammer, Bernard W. Dairy Bacteriology. New York; J. Wiley & Sons; London; Chapman & Hall, 1928. 473p. (4th ed., by B. W. Hammer and Frederick J. Babel, 1957. 614p.)

First   Hammond, John. The Artificial Insemination of Cattle. Cambridge, U.K.; W. Heffer, 1947. 61p.

First   Hammond, John. Farm Animals; Their Breeding, Growth, and Inheritance. New York; Longmans, Green & Co., 1940. 199p. (3d ed., London; E. Arnold, 1960. 199p.)

First   Hammond, John. Growth and the Development of Mutton Qualities in the

Ranking

	Sheep; A Survey of the Problems Involved in Meat Production. Edinburgh and London; Oliver & Boyd, 1932. 597p.
First	Hammond, John. The Physiology of Reproduction in the Cow. Cambridge, U.K.; University Press, 1927. 226p.
First	Hammond, John. Reproduction in the Rabbit. Edinburgh and London; Oliver & Boyd, 1925. 210p.
Third	Harper, Merritt W. Breeding of Farm Animals. New York; Orange Judd Co., 1914. 335p. (Reissued, 1923.)
Second	Harper, Merritt W. The Training and Breaking of Horses. New York; The Macmillan Co., 1912. 387p.
Second	Harris, Albert W. The Blood of the Arab, the World's Greatest War Horse. Chicago; Priv. print., The Arabian Horse Club of America, 1941. 176p.
Second	Harris, Joseph. Harris on the Pig; Breeding, Rearing, Management, and Improvement. New York; Orange Judd Co., 1870. 250p. (Rev. and enl., 1889. 318p.)
Second	Harrison, Edwin S. Judging Dairy Cattle . . . with photographs by Henry A. Strohmeyer, Jr., and John T. Carpenter, Jr. New York; J. Wiley & Sons; London; Chapman & Hall, 1940. 132p.
First	†Hartman, Roland C., and G. S. Vickers. Hatchery Management. New York; Orange Judd Pub. Co., 1932. 386p. (Revised and reset, 1946. 404p.)
First	†Hartman, Roland C. Keeping Chickens in Cages: A Description of the Outdoor Individual Cage System of Poultry Management as Developed Mainly in Southern California. Redlands, Calif, 1950. 181p. (4th ed., 1956. 304p.)
Second	Harvey, William C., and Harry Hill. Milk Production and Control. London; H. K. Lewis, 1936. 555p. (4th ed., 1967. 711p.)
Second	Hawk, Philip B. Practical Physiological Chemistry. Philadelphia; P. Blakiston's Sons & Co., 1907. 416p. (14th ed., as Physiological Chemistry, edited by Bernard L. Oser. New York; Blakiston Division, McGraw-Hill, 1965. 1472p.)
Second	Hawkesworth, Alfred. Australasian Sheep and Wool. 3d ed., rev. and enl. Sydney; Brooks & Co., 1911. 483p. (7th ed., 1948. 509p.)
Second	Hayes, John L. The Angora Goat; Its Origin, Culture and Products. Cambridge, U.K.; University Press, 1882. 178p.
Third	Hayes, M. Horace. Points of the Horse. 2d ed. London; W. Thacker & Co., 1897. 736p. (7th ed., rev. New York; Arco Pub. Co., 1969. 541p.)
Third	Hayes, M. Horace. Veterinary Notes for Horse Owners. 4th ed., rev. and enl. London; W. Thacker & Co., 1891. 828p. (17th ed., rev. by Peter D. Rossdale. New York; Prentice Hall Press, 1987. 740p. Subtitle varies.)
Second	Haynes, Sheppard K. Practical Pigeon Production; A Practical Manual and Reliable Handbook on Squab Production as a Profitable Enterprise. New York; Orange Judd Pub. Co., 1944. 263p.
Second	Hays, Frank A., and Gay T. Klein. Poultry Breeding Applied. Mount Morris, Ill.; Poultry-Dairy Pub. Co., 1943. 192p. (2d ed., Mount Morris, Ill.; Watt Pub. Co., 1952. 250p.)
First	Hazard, Willis P. The Jersey, Alderney, and Guernsey Cow: Their History, Nature and Management. Philadelphia; Porter & Coates, 1872. 142p.

Ranking

Third   Hazelton, John M. History and Handbook of Hereford Cattle and Hereford Bull Index. Kansas City; Hereford Journal Co., 1925. 391p. (3d ed., Walker Pub., 1935. 512p.)

Second   Hegner, Robert W. College Zoology. Rev. ed. New York; The Macmillan Co., 1926. 645p. (10th ed., by Richard A. Boolootian and Karl A. Stiles. New York; Macmillan; London; Collier Macmillan, 1981. 803p.)

Second   Hegner, Robert W. The Germ-Cell Cycle in Animals. New York; The Macmillan Co., 1914. 346p.

Second   Helm, Henry T. American Roadsters and Trotting Horses. Chicago; Rand, McNally & Co., 1878. 552p.

Second   Helser, Maurice D. Farm Meats. New York; Macmillan Co., 1923. 274p.

Third   Henley, Walter de. Walter of Henley's Husbandry: Together with an Anonymous Husbandry, Seneschaucie, and Robert Grossetestes's Rules . . . trans. by Elizabeth Lamond. London and New York; Longmans, Green, 1890. 171p.

First   Henry, William A. Feeds and Feeding, A Hand-Book for the Student and Stockman. 2d ed. Madison, Wis.; The author, 1898. 657p. (1st–9th eds., written by W. A. Henry; 10th–14th ed., by W. A. Henry assisted by Frank B. Morrison; 15th–20th ed., rev. and rewritten by F. B. Morrison. 22d ed., published in Ithaca, N.Y., and Clinton, Iowa; Morrison Pub. Co., 1956. 1165p.)

Second   Herbert, Henry W. Frank Forester's Horse and Horsemanship of the United States and British Provinces of North America. New York; Stringer & Townsend, 1857. 2 vols. (Rev., cor., enl., and continued to 1871, by S. D. Bruce and B. G. Bruce. New York; G. E. Woodward, 1871.)

Second   Herman, Harry A., and Fred W. Madden. The Artificial Insemination of Dairy Cattle. Columbia, Mo.; Lucas Bros., 1947. 95p.

Third   Hesse, Richard. Ecological Animal Geography; An Authorized, Rewritten Edition Based on Tiergeographie auf Oekologischer Grundlage. New York; J. Wiley & Sons, Inc.; London; Chapman & Hall, 1937. 597p.

First   Heuser, Gustave F. Feeding Poultry. New York; J. Wiley & Sons; London; Chapman & Hall, 1946. 543p.

Second   Hill, Charles L. The Guernsey Breed. Waterloo, Iowa; F. L. Kimball Co., 1917. 417p.

Second   Hill, John W. The Management and Diseases of the Dog. New York; W. R. Jenkins, 1881. 383p. (5th ed., London; S. Sonnenschein & Co.; New York; The Macmillan Co., 1900. 531p.)

First   Hinman, Robert B., and Robert B. Harris. The Story of Meat. Chicago; Swift & Co., 1939. 291p. (2d printing, 1942.)

Second   Hoerle, Gustav A. The Angora Goat, Its Habits and Culture. New York; T. A. Wright, 1886. 32p.

First   †Hoffmann, Edmund, and Hugh A. Johnson. Successful Broiler Growing. Mt. Morris, Ill.; Watt Pub. Co., 1946. 186p. (3d ed, 1954. 256p.)

Second   Hogan, Walter. The Call of the Hen; Or the Science of the Selection and Breeding of Poultry. Petaluma, Calif.; The Petaluma Daily Courier, 1913. 126p. (Rev. by W. Hogan and Thomas E. Quisenberry. Kansas City, Mo.; American Poultry School, 1928. 135p.)

Ranking

Second   Holmes-Pegler, Henry. The Book of the Goat. 3d ed., rewritten and enl. London; L. U. Gill, 1886. 222p. (9th ed., rev. and enl. London; The Bazaar, Exchange and Mart; Columbia, Mo.; American Supply House, 1965. 255p.)

Second   Hook, Bryan. Milch Goats and Their Management. London; Vinton, 1896. 115p.

Second   Hopkins, John A., Jr. Economic History of the Production of Beef Cattle in Iowa. Iowa City; The State Historical Society of Iowa, 1928. 248p.

First   Horlacher, Levi J. Sheep Production. 1st ed. New York; McGraw-Hill Book Co., 1927. 418p.

Second   Horlacher, Levi J., and Carsie Hammonds. Sheep. Danville, Ill.; The Interstate, 1942. 348p.

Second   Horne, Thomas H. The Complete Grazier, originally written by William Youatt. London; Printed for B. Crosby & Co., 1805. 510p. (14th ed., rewritten and enl. by William Fream. London; C. Lockwood, 1900. 1086p.)

Second   Horse and Mule Association of America. Judging Horses and Mules. Chicago; Horse and Mule Association of America, 1935. 30p.

Second   Houck, Ulysses G. The Bureau of Animal Industry of the United States Department of Agriculture: Its Establishment, Achievements and Current Activities. Washington, D.C.; The author, Hayworth Printing Co., 1924. 390p.

First   Houghton, Frederick L. Holstein-Friesian Cattle. Brattleboro, Vt.; Press of the Holstein-Friesian Register, 1897. 371p.

Second   Housman, William. Cattle, Breeds and Management. London; 1897. 270p. (8th ed., Vinton, 1919.) (Live Stock Handbooks no. 4)

Second   Housman, William. The Improved Shorthorn. London; W. Ridgway, 1876. 60p.

Second   Howden, Peter. The Horse: How to Buy and Sell . . . Giving the Points Which Distinguish a Sound from an Unsound Horse. New York; Orange Judd, 1882. 131p.

Second   Howell, William H. A Text-Book of Physiology, for Medical Students and Physicians. Philadelphia; Saunders, 1905. 905p. (13th ed., rev. Philadelphia and London; Saunders, 1936. 1150p. 14th ed. published as A Textbook of Physiology.)

Second   Huidekoper, Rush S. Age of the Domestic Animals. Chicago; Eger, 1904. 217p.

Second   Hull, Thomas G. Diseases Transmitted from Animals to Man. Springfield, Ill., and Baltimore; C. C. Thomas, 1930. 350p. (6th ed., compiled and edited by William T. Hubbert, William F. McCulloch and Paul R. Schnurrenberger. Springfield, Ill.; C. C. Thomas, 1975. 1206p.)

Second   Hultz, Fred S. Corriedale Sheep, the Dual-Purpose Breed. Laramie, Wy.; American Corriedale Association, 1940. 123p.

Second   Hultz, Fred S. Range Beef Production in the Seventeen Western States. New York; J. Wiley & Sons; London; Chapman & Hall, 1930. 208p.

Second   Hultz, Fred S. Range Sheep and Wool in the Seventeen Western States. New York; J. Wiley & Sons; London; Chapman & Hall, 1931. 374p.

Ranking

Second	Hunter, John M., and John C. Scholes. Profitable Duck Management. 8th ed. Cayuga, N.Y.; Beacon Milling Co., 1950. 76p. (9th ed., 1954. 94p.)
Second	Hunting, William. The Art of Horse-Shoeing; A Manual for Farriers. American ed., rev. & enl. by the author. New York; W. R. Jenkins, 1898. 129p.
Second	Hunziker, Otto F. The Butter Industry. La Grange, Ill.; The author, 1920. 710p. (3d ed., rewritten and enl., 1940. 780p.)
Second	Hunziker, Otto F. Condensed Milk and Milk Powder. LaFayette, Ind.; The author, 1914. 262p. (7th ed., completely rev., 1949. 583p.)
First	†Hurd, Louis M. Practical Poultry Farming. New York; Macmillan Co., 1928. 405p. (4th ed., 1956. 575p. Also translated into German.)
First	†Hutt, Frederick B. Genetics of the Fowl. New York; McGraw-Hill, 1949. 590p.
Second	Huxley, Julian. The Individual in the Animal Kingdom. Cambridge, U.K.; University Press; New York; G. P. Putnam's Sons, 1912. 167p.
Second	Huxley, Julian, ed. The New Systematics. Oxford, U.K.; University Press, 1940. 583p. (Reprinted, Hampton, U.K.; Classey for the Systematics Association, 1971.)
Second	Huxley, Julian. Problems of Relative Growth. New York; MacVeagh, The Dial Press, 1932. 276p.

I

Third	Ingham, Ray W. Grass Silage and Dairying. New Brunswick, N.J.; Rutgers University Press, 1949. 88p.
Third	International Association of Milk Dealers. Laboratory Manual; Methods of Analysis of Milk and Its Products. Chicago; 1933. 461p. (2d ed., Washington, D.C.; Milk Industry Foundation, 1949. 629p.)
Second	International Congress of Animal Production, 5th, Paris, 1949; Communications and Reports. Paris; 1949. 3 vols. (Text in English, French, German or Italian; with summaries in the various languages. Published by the Congress under its earlier name: International Congress of Animal Husbandry.)
Second	Ives, Paul P. Domestic Geese and Ducks; A Complete and Authentic Handbook and Guide for Breeders, Growers and Admirers of Domestic Geese and Ducks. New York; Orange Judd Pub. Co., 1947. 372p.

J

Second	Jackson, Homer W. Profitable Culling and Selective Flock Breeding. Quincy, Ill.; Reliable Poultry Journal Pub. Co., 1920. 118p. (3d ed., Dayton, Ohio; 1923. 320p.)
Second	Jenkinson, John W. Vertebrate Embryology; Comprising the Early History of the Embryo and Its Foetal Membranes. Oxford, U.K.; Clarendon Press, 1913. 267p.
Second	Jennings, Robert. Cattle and Their Diseases Embracing Their History and Breeds, Crossing and Breeding, and Feeding and Management. . . . Philadelphia; J. E. Potter, 1864. 340p.

Ranking

Second   Jennings, Robert. Sheep, Swine, and Poultry. Philadelphia; J. E. Potter, 1864. 170p.

Third   Jobson, E. H. Angora Goat Raising. St. Louis, Mo.; 1900. 29p.

Third   Johnstone, James H. The Horse Book; A Practical Treatise on the American Horse Breeding Industry as Allied to the Farm. Chicago; Sanders Pub. Co., 1908. 299p. (Reissued, Chicago; The Breeder's Gazette, 1914. 289p.)

Third   Jones, C. Bryner, ed. Live Stock of the Farm. London; Gresham Pub. Co., 1915–1916. 6 vols.

Third   Jones, Donald F. Genetics in Plant and Animal Improvement. New York; Wiley, 1925. 568p.

Second   Jordan, Whitman H. The Feeding of Animals. New York; Macmillan, 1901. 450p. (Rev. ed., 1917. 473p.)

Second   Judkins, Henry F. The Principles of Dairying, Testing and Manufactures. New York; J. Wiley & Sons, 1924. 279p. (3d ed., rev. by Merrill J. Mack. New York; J. Wiley & Sons; London; Chapman & Hall, 1941. 315p.)

First   Jull, Morley A. Poultry Breeding. New York; J. Wiley & Sons; London; Chapman & Hall, 1932. 376p. (3d ed., New York; Wiley, 1952. 398p.)

First   †Jull, Morley A. Poultry Husbandry. 1st ed. New York; McGraw-Hill Book Co., 1930. 639p. (3d ed., 1951. 526p.)

First   Jull, Morley A. Raising Turkeys, Ducks, Geese, Game Birds. New York and London; McGraw-Hill Book Co., 1947. 467p.

K

First   Kammlade, William G. Sheep Science, edited by R. W. Gregory. Chicago and Philadelphia; J. B. Lippincott Co., 1947. 534p.

Second   Kaupp, Benjamin F. The Anatomy of the Domestic Fowl. Philadelphia and London; W. G. Saunders Co., 1918. 373p.

Third   Kaupp, Benjamin F., and Raymond C. Surface. Poultry Sanitation and Disease Control; The Complete Guide to Sanitation and Treatment of Disease. Chicago; Kaupp & Surface, 1939. 420p. (4th ed., rev. and enl., Minneapolis; 1950. 493p.)

Second   Kelley, Ralph B. Principles and Methods of Animal Breeding. New York; Wiley, 1946. 296p. (3d ed., rev., Sydney; Angus & Robertson, 1960. 358p.)

Second   Kellner, Oscar J. The Scientific Feeding of Animals . . . authorised translation by William Goodwin. Toronto; Macmillan, 1914. 404p.

Third   Kelly, Ernest, and Clarence E. Clement. Market Milk. New York; J. Wiley & Sons, 1923. 445p. (2d ed., 1931. 489p.)

Third   Kenan, William R. History of Randleigh Farm. Lockport, N.Y.; W. R. Kenan, Jr., 1935. 116p. (9th ed., 1959. 230p.)

Second   Kiddy, Charles A., and Harold D. Hafs, eds. Sex Ratio at Birth—Prospects for Control; A Symposium, July-August 1970, Pennsylvania State University. . . . Champaign, Ill.; American Society of Animal Science, 1971. 104p. (Organized under the auspices of the American Society of Animal Science.)

Second   King, Helen D. Studies on Inbreeding. Philadelphia; The Wistar Institute of

Ranking

Anatomy and Biology, 1919. 175p. (Reprinted from the May, July, October, 1918, and August, 1919, issues of the Journal of Experimental Zoology.)

Third   Kinsley, Albert T. Swine Practice. Chicago; American Veterinary Pub. Co., 1921. 374p. (Veterinary Practitioners' Series no. 2)

Third   Klein, Gay T. Starting Right with Turkeys . . . edited by Ed Robinson. New York; The Macmillan Co., 1946. 120p. (The Havemore Plan Reference Library no. 1)

Second   Kleinheinz, Frank. Sheep Management; A Handbook for the Shepherd and Student. Madison, Wis.; The author, 1911. 225p. (6th ed., 1927. 306p.)

Second   Krogh, August. The Comparative Physiology of Respiratory Mechanisms. Philadelphia; University of Pennsylvania Press, 1941. 172p.

Second   Kupper, Winifred. The Golden Hoof: The Story of the Sheep of the Southwest. 1st ed. New York; A. A. Knopf, 1945. 203p.

L

Third   Lamon, Harry M. Poultry Breeding and Selection. Washington, D.C.; The author, 1932. 100p. (Written as a part of the Poultry Course of the National Poultry Institute, Washington, D.C.)

Second   Lamon, Harry M., and Alfred R. Lee. Poultry Feeds and Feeding. New York; Orange Judd Pub. Co., 1922. 247p.

Third   Lamon, Harry M., and Joseph W. Kinghorne. Practical Poultry Production. St. Paul, Minn.; Webb Pub. Co., 1920. 365p. (Rev. ed., 1930. 438p.)

Third   Lamon, Harry M., and Rob R. Slocum. Ducks and Geese. New York; Orange Judd Pub. Co., 1922. 231p.

Second   Lamon, Harry M., and Rob R. Slocum. The Mating and Breeding of Poultry. New York; Orange Judd Co., 1923. 341p. (Reissued, 1927.)

First   Larson, Carl W., and Fred S. Putney. Dairy Cattle Feeding and Management. New York; Wiley, 1917. 471p. (3d ed., written by Harry O. Henderson, 1938. 557p.)

Second   Lattig, Herbert E. Dairy Cattle. Danville, Ill.; Interstate, 1935. 96p. (7th ed., by Julius E. Nordby, 1961. 135p.)

Second   Leese, A. S. A Treatise on the One-Humped Camel. Lincoln, Nebr.; Haynes, 1927. 382p.

Second   Leggett, William F. The Story of Wool. Brooklyn, N.Y.; Chemical Pub. Co., 1947. 304p.

Third   Lerner, I. Michael. Genetic Homeostasis. Edinburgh and London; Oliver & Boyd, 1954. 134p.

Second   Levi, Wendell M. Making Pigeons Pay. New York; Orange Judd Pub. Co., 1946. 263p. (Rev. ed., Sumter, S.C.; Levi Pub. Co., 1968.)

First   †Levi, Wendel M. The Pigeon. Columbia, S.C.; R. L. Bryan Co., 1941. 512p. (2d ed., rev. Sumter, S.C.; Levi Pub. Co., 1957. 667p.)

First   †Lewis, Harry R. Productive Poultry Husbandry. Philadelphia and London; J. B. Lippincott Co., 1913. 536p. (8th ed., rev., Chicago and Philadelphia; 1933. 588p.)

Second   Lewis, William M. The People's Practical Poultry Book. New York; Excel-

Ranking

sior Pub. House, 1871. 223p. (Later ed., 1895, as How to Raise Poultry for Pleasure and Profit.)

First   Lillie, Frank R. The Development of the Chick; An Introduction to Embryology. New York; H. Holt, 1908. 472p. (2d ed., rev., 1919.)

Second   Linsley, Daniel C. Morgan Horses. New York; C. M. Saxton, Barker, 1860. 340p.

Second   Linsley, John S. Jersey Cattle in America. New York; Burr Printing House, 1885. 741p.

Second   Linton, Robert G. Animal Nutrition and Veterinary Dietetics. Edinburgh; W. Green & Son, 1927. 399p. (3d-4th eds. by John T. Abrams. 4th ed., 1961. 826p.)

First   †Lippincott, William A. Poultry Production. Philadelphia; Lea & Febiger, 1914. 476p. (12th ed. by Malden C. Nesheim, Richard E. Austic, and Leslie E. Card, 1979. 399p.)

Third   Little, Ralph B., and Wayne N. Plastridge, eds. Bovine Mastitis. 1st ed. New York and London; McGraw-Hill Book Co., 1946. 546p.

Second   Long, Harold C. Plants Poisonous to Live Stock. Cambridge, U.K.; University Press, 1917. 119p.

Second   Long, James. The Book of the Pig; Its Selection, Breeding, Feeding, and Management. London; L. U. Gill, 1886. 360p. (3d ed., rev., London; The Bazaar, Exchange & Mart, 1916. 392p.)

First   Loomis, Frederic B. The Evolution of the Horse. Boston; Marshall Jones Co., 1926. 233p.

Third   Lovelock's American Standard of Excellence for Pure-Bred Cattle, Sheep and Swine, Being. . . . Salem, Va.; Printed and published for Frank A. Lovelock, 1893. 143p.

First   Low, David. The Breeds of the Domestic Animals of the British Islands Described by David Low. London; Longman, Orme, Brown, Green & Longmans, 1842. 2 vols. in 1. (Rewritten as On the Domestic Animals of the British Islands, with additions, 1853. 767p.)

Third   Lowe, Bruce. Breeding Racehorses by the Figure System . . . edited by William Allison. New York; W. R. Jenkins, 1898. 262p.

First   Lush, Jay L. Animal Breeding Plans. Ames; Iowa State College Press, 1937. 350p. (3d ed., 1945. 443p.)

Second   Lusk, Graham. The Elements of the Science of Nutrition. Philadelphia and London; W. B. Saunders, 1906. 326p. (4th ed., 1928. 844p.)

Second   Lydekker, Richard. The Horse and Its Relatives. New York; Macmillan Co., 1912. 286p.

First   Lydekker, Richard. The Ox and Its Kindred. London; Methuen, 1912. 271p.

First   Lydekker, Richard. The Sheep and Its Cousins. London; Allen, 1912. 315p.

Second   Lydekker, Richard. Wild Oxen, Sheep and Goats of All Lands, Living and Extinct. London; R. Ward, 1898. 318p. (Game Mammals of the World no. 2)

Third   Lydekker, Richard, et al. Natural History. New York; Appleton & Co., 1897. 771p.

Ranking

Third   Lyon, William E. First Aid Hints for the Horse Owner; A Veterinary Note Book. London; Constable, 1933. 127p. (6th ed., London; Collins, 1959. 151p.)

M

First   M'Combie, William. Cattle and Cattle-Breeders. 2d ed., rev. Edinburgh and London; Wm. Blackwood, 1869. 135p. (4th ed., enl., edited by James MacDonald, Edinburgh; 1896. 157p.)

Second   MacDonald, Duncan G. Cattle, Sheep and Deer. 5th ed. London; Steel & Jones, 1872. 745p.

Second   Macdonald, James, and James Sinclair. History of Aberdeen-Angus Cattle. Rev. ed. by James Sinclair. London; Vinton & Co., 1910. 682p.

Second   Macdonald, James. History of Hereford Cattle. London; Vinton, 1886. 380p. (Rev. ed. by James Sinclair, 1909. 501p.)

Second   MacEwan, Grant, and A. H. Ewen. The Science and Practice of Canadian Animal Husbandry. Toronto; T. Nelson & Sons, 1936. 462p.

Second   MacEwan, John W. G. The Breeds of Farm Live-Stock in Canada. Toronto and New York; T. Nelson & Sons, 1941. 526p.

Second   Mackenzie, Kenneth J. Cattle and the Future of Beef-Production in England. Cambridge, U.K.; University Press, 1919. 168p.

Second   Mahadevan, P. Dairy Cattle Breeding in the Tropics. Farnham Royal, U.K.; Commonwealth Agricultural Bureaux, 1958. 88p. (Commonwealth Bureau of Animal Breeding and Genetics, Technical Communication no. 11)

Second   Malden, Walter J. British Sheep and Shepherding. London; MacDonald & Martin, 1915. 239p.

Second   Malden, Walter J. Pig Keeping for Profit. London; Kegan Paul, Tranch, Trubner & Co., 1896. 120p.

First   Malin, Donald F. The Evolution of Breeds. Des Moines, Iowa; Wallace Pub. Co., 1923. 278p.

First   †Marsden, Stanley J., and J. Holmes Martin. Turkey Management. 1st ed. Danville, Ill.; The Interstate, 1939. 708p. (6th ed., 1955. 999p.)

Second   Marshall, Francis H., and E. T. Halnan. Physiology of Farm Animals. Cambridge, U.K.; The University Press, 1920. 339p. (3d ed., 1945.)

Second   Marshall, Frederick R. Breeding Farm Animals. Chicago; The Breeder's Gazette, 1912. 287p.

Third   Martin, George A. The Family Horse: Its Stabling, Care, and Feeding. New York; Orange Judd, 1911. 153p.

Second   Masui, Kiyoshi, and Juro Hashimoto. Sexing Baby Chicks . . . trans. by Hachiro Okumura. Vancouver, B.C.; Journal Print. Co., 1933. 91p. (Copyrighted by the Chick Sexing Association of America, Vancouver, Canada.)

Second   Mathews, Albert P. Physiological Chemistry; A Text-Book and Manual for Students. New York; Wood, 1915. 1040p. (5th ed., 1931. 1233p.)

Second   Matthews, Joseph M. The Textile Fibers, Their Physical, Microscopical and Chemical Properties. 3d ed., rewritten. New York; J. Wiley & Sons, 1907. 480p. (6th ed., 1954. 1283p.)

Ranking

First   Maynard, Leonard A. Animal Nutrition. 1st ed. New York and London;
            McGraw-Hill Book Co., 1937. 483p. (7th ed., by L. A. Maynard, John K.
            Loosli, Harold F. Hintz and Richard G. Warner, 1979. 602p.)
Second   Mayo, Nelson S. The Care of Animals; A Book of Brief and Popular Ad-
            vice on the Diseases and Ailments of Farm Animals. New York and Lon-
            don; The Macmillan Co., 1903. 459p. (2d ed., New York; Macmillan,
            1905. Later eds. as The Diseases of Animals.)
Second   Mayr, Ernst. Systematics and the Origin of Species from the Viewpoint of a
            Zoologist. Based on the Jesup Lectures delivered at Columbia University,
            March 1941, edited by L. C. Dunn. New York; Columbia University Press,
            1942. 334p.
Second   McAtee, Waldo L., ed. The Ring-Necked Pheasant and Its Management in
            North America. Washington, D.C.; The American Wildlife Institute, 1945.
            320p.
Second   McCandlish, Andrew C. The Feeding of Dairy Cattle. New York; J. Wiley
            & Sons, 1922. 281p.
First   McCay, Clive M. Nutrition of the Dog. Ithaca, N.Y.; Comstock Pub. Co.,
            1944. 140p.
Second   McCollum, Elmer V. The Newer Knowledge of Nutrition. New York; Mac-
            millan Co., 1918. 199p. (5th ed., entirely rewritten by E. V. McCollum,
            Elsa Orent-Keiles, and Harry G. Day, 1939. 701p.)
Second   McDowell, John C., and Albert M. Field. Dairy Enterprises. London and
            Philadelphia; J. B. Lippincott Co., 1930. 471p. (1946 ed., by A. M. Field
            and J. C. McDowell, edited by R. W. Gregory.)
Second   McFall, Robert J. The World's Meat. New York and London; D. Appleton
            & Co., 1927. 624p.
Third   McIntosh, Donald. Diseases of Swine: Written as a Text Book for the Vet-
            erinary Surgeon, Student and Swine Grower. Chicago; Donohue & Henne-
            berry, Printers, 1897. 230p.
First   †McGrew, Thomas F. The Bantam Fowl: A Description of all Standard
            Breeds and Varieties of Bantams. Quincy, Ill.; Reliable Poultry Journal
            Pub. Co., 1899. 44p. (2d ed., 1903. 67p.)
Second   McKay, George L., and Christian Larsen. Principles and Practice of Butter-
            Making. 1st ed. New York; J. Wiley & Sons; London; Chapman & Hall,
            1906. 329p. (4th ed., as Butter, by Claire C. Totman, G. L. McKay, and
            C. Larsen, 1939. 472p.)
Second   McKay, William J. The Evolution of the Endurance, Speed and Staying
            Power of the Racehorse. London; Hutchinson & Co., 1933. 318p. (2d ed.,
            1937. 319p.)
Third   McMeekan, Campbell P., et al. Principles of Animal Production. Auckland
            and London; Whitcombe & Tombs, 1943. 243p. (3d ed. rev., Christchurch;
            Whitcombe & Tombs, 1959. 318p.)
Third   Michigan State University. Reproduction and Infertility: Physiology, Anat-
            omy, Pathology, Biochemistry. Michigan State University Centennial Sym-
            posium, 1855–1955, June 1955. East Lansing; Michigan State University,
            1955. 112p.

Ranking

Second   Milburn, Matthew M. The Cow, Dairy Husbandry and Cattle Breeding. New York; C. M. Saxton, 1852. 109p.

Second   Milburn, Matthew M. The Sheep and Shepherding: Embracing the History, Varieties, Rearing, Feeding, and General Management of Sheep. London; Wm. S. Orr & Co.; Dublin; J. McGlashan, 1853. 124p.

Third   Miles, Manly. Stock-Breeding: A Practical Treatise on the Applications of the Laws of Development and Heredity to the Improvement and Breeding of Domestic Animals. New York; Appleton, 1879. 424p.

Second   Miller, Dudley. A Compilation of Articles on Holstein Cattle. Oswego, N.Y.; R. J. Oliphant, 1885. 135p.

Second   Miller, Timothy L. History of Hereford Cattle, Proven Conclusively the Oldest of Improved Breeds . . . with which is incorporated A History of the Herefords in America, by Wm. H. Sotham. Chillicothe, Mo.; T. F. B. Sotham, 1902. 592p.

First   †Miner, T. B. Miner's Domestic Poultry Book: A Treatise on the History, Breeding, and General Management of Foreign and Domestic Fowls. Rochester, N.Y.; Geo. W. Fisher and New York; A. S. Barnes and Co., 1853. 256p.

Third   Mojonnier, Timothy. The Technical Control of Dairy Products; A Treatise on the Testing, Analyzing, Standardizing and the Manufacture of Dairy Products. 1st ed. Chicago; Mojonnier Bros. Co., 1922. 909p. (2d ed., 1925. 936p.)

Second   Monier-Williams, Gordon W. Trace Elements in Food. New York; J. Wiley, 1949. 511p.

Second   Moore, Merton, and Elton M. Gildow. Developing a Profitable Dairy Herd. Seattle; Wood & Reber, 1945. 192p. (Later ed., Chicago; Windsor Press, 1953. 224p.)

Third   More Game Birds in America, Inc. More Game Birds by Controlling Their Natural Enemies. Rev. ed. New York; More Game Birds in America, 1936. 63p.

Second   More Game Birds in America, Inc. More Upland Game Birds; Why Game Birds Have Decreased, How They Can Be Restored. New York; More Game Birds in America, 1938. 47p.

Second   More Game Birds in America, Inc. Pheasant Breeding Manual. Rev. ed. New York; More Game Birds in America, 1936. 63p. (Rev. ed., 1939.)

Second   More Game Birds in America, Inc. Quail Breeding Manual . . . prepared under the direction of Arthur M. Bartley. New York; More Game Birds in America, 1936. 46p. (Rev. ed., 1939. 55p.)

Second   Morgan, Thomas H. Embryology and Genetics. New York; Columbia University Press, 1934. 258p.

Second   Morgan, Thomas H. The Physical Basis of Heredity. Philadelphia; Lippincott, 1919. 305p.

Second   Morgan, Thomas H. The Scientific Basis of Evolution. New York; W. W. Norton & Co., 1932. 286p.

Third   Morrison, Robert. The Individuality of the Pig. Its Breeding, Feeding, and Management. London; John Murray, 1926. 377p.

Ranking

Second   Mumford, Frederick B. The Breeding of Animals. New York; Macmillan, 1917. 310p.

Second   Mumford, Herbert W. Beef Production. Urbana, Ill.; Published by the author, 1907. 209p. (7th ed., 1908.)

Third   Murray, Alexander J. Cattle and Their Diseases, with an Introduction on the Breeding and Management of Cattle. Chicago; J. H. Sanders, 1887. 270p.

N

First   National Cattle Breeders' Association. British Pedigree Cattle. London; 1947. 110p.

Third   National Sheep Breeders' Association. British Pure-Bred Sheep. Brentford, U.K.; W. Pearce & Co., St. Georges Press, 1946. 142p.

Second   Needham, Joseph. Chemical Embryology. Cambridge, U.K.; The University Press, 1931. 3 vols.

Second   Nelson, Edward W. Wild Animals of North America, Intimate Studies of Big and Little Creatures of the Mammal Kingdom . . . with natural-color portraits from paintings by Louis Agassiz Fuertes, track sketches by Ernest T. Seton. Washington, D.C.; The National Geographical Society, 1918. 612p. (Rev., new ed., 1930. 254p.)

Second   Nelson, John A., and G. Malcolm Trout. Judging Dairy Products. Milwaukee, Wis.; Olsen Pub. Co., 1934. 145p. (3d ed., rev., 1951. 480p.)

Third   Newbigin, Marion I. Plant and Animal Geography. London; Methuen & Co., 1936. 298p.

First   Newburgh, Louis H., ed. Physiology of Heat Regulation and the Science of Clothing . . . prepared at the Request of the Division of Medical Sciences, National Research Council. Philadelphia; Saunders, 1949. 457p.

Second   Newman, Horatio H. The Biology of Twins (Mammals). Chicago; University of Chicago Press, 1917. 186p. (Later ed., 1924.)

Second   Newman, Horatio H. Evolution, Genetics, and Eugenics. Chicago; University of Chicago Press, 1925. 639p. (First published, 1921, as Readings in Evolution, Genetics, and Eugenics. 3d ed., also published under original title, New York; Greenwood Press, 1969. 620p.)

First   Nichols, James E. Livestock Improvement in Relation to Heredity and Environment. 1st ed. Edinburgh and London; Oliver & Boyd, 1944. 208p. (2d ed., rev., 1945.)

Second   Nolan, James J. Ornamental, Aquatic, and Domestic Fowl, and Game Birds; Their Importation, Breeding, Rearing, and General Management. Dublin; The author, 1850. 191p.

First   Nordby, Julius E. Livestock Judging Handbook. Danville, Ill.; The Interstate, 1937. 288p. (Later ed., 1960. 411p.)

Second   Nordby, Julius E. Selecting, Fitting and Showing Swine. Danville, Ill.; Interstate, 1939. 104p. (6th ed., 1961. 95p.)

Second   Nordby, Julius E., and Herbert E. Lattig. Horse: Selecting, Fitting and Showing. Danville, Ill.; Interstate, 1937. (4th ed., as Selecting, Fitting and Showing Horses, 1948. 120p.)

Second   Nordby, Julius E., and Herbert E. Lattig. Selecting, Fitting and Showing Beef Cattle. Danville, Ill.; Interstate, 1936. 132p.

Ranking

Third   Norton, Laurence J., and Laurell L. Scranton. The Marketing of Farm Prod-
            ucts; Principles and Problems for Students of Vocational Agriculture. Dan-
            ville, Ill.; Interstate Printing Co., 1932. 384p. (Rev. ed., 1949. 458p.)
Third   Nourse, Edwin G., and Joseph G. Knapp. The Cooperative Marketing of
            Livestock. Washington, D.C.; The Brookings Institution, 1931. 486p. (The
            Institute of Ecomonics of the Brookings Institution no. 40)

O

First   Olson, Thomas M. Elements of Dairying. New York; The Macmillan Co.,
            1939. 570p.
Third   Orla-Jensen, Sigurd. Dairy Bacteriology. Trans. from the 2d Danish ed.,
            with additions and revisions by P. S. Arup. Philadelphia; P. Blakiston's Son
            & Co., 1921. 180p. (2d English ed., 1931. 198p.)
Third   Orr, William. The Physiological and Genetical Aspects of Sterility in Do-
            mesticated Animals. Edinburgh; Oliver & Boyd, 1932. 80p.
Second   Osborn, Henry F. The Age of Mammals in Europe, Asia and North Amer-
            ica. New York; The Macmillan Co., 1910. 635p.
Second   Osgood, Ernest S. The Day of the Cattleman. Minneapolis; University of
            Minnesota Press, 1929. 283p. (Reprinted, Chicago; University of Chicago
            Press, 1957.)

P

Third   Parker, T. Jeffery, and William A. Haswell. A Textbook of Zoology. Lon-
            don and New York; Macmillan & Co., 1897. 2 vols. (6th ed., London;
            1940. Vol. 1 rev. by Otto Lowenstein, vol. 2 by C. Forster-Cooper.)
Second   Paterson, David D. Statistical Technique in Agricultural Research. 1st ed.
            New York and London; McGraw-Hill Book Co., 1939. 263p.
First   †Patten, Bradley M. The Early Embryology of the Chick. Philadelphia;
            Blakiston's Son & Co., 1920. 167p. (5th ed., New York; McGraw-Hill,
            1971. 284p.)
First   Patten, Bradley M. The Embryology of the Pig. 2d ed. Philadelphia;
            Blakiston Co., 1931. 327p. (3d ed., 1948. 352p.)
Second   Pavlov, Ivan P. The Work of the Digestive Glands, Lectures by J. P.
            Pavlow . . . trans. into English by W. H. Thompson. London; Charles
            Griffin, 1902. 196p. (2d English ed., London; Griffin; Philadelphia; J. B.
            Lippincott, 1910.)
Second   Peake, Ora B. The Colorado Range Cattle Industry. Glendale, Calif.; The
            Arthur H. Clark Co., 1937. 357p.
Third   Pearl, Raymond. Modes of Research in Genetics. New York; Macmillan,
            1915. 182p.
Second   Pearl, Raymond. The Nation's Food; A Statistical Study of a Physiological
            and Social Problem. Philadelphia and London; W. B. Saunders Co., 1920.
            274p.
Third   Pearse, Arthur S. Animal Ecology. 2d ed. New York; McGraw-Hill, 1939.
            642p.
Second   Pearse, Evan H. Sheep, Farm and Station Management. Sydney, Melbourne

Ranking

	and London; The Pastoral Review, 1920. 405p. (7th ed. as Sheep and Property Management.)
Third	Pearson, James H. Livestock; Educational Procedures in Marketing. Chicago; National Live Stock Producer, 1937. 101p.
Third	Peck, Charles L. Profitable Dairying; A Practical Guide to Successful Dairy Management. New York; O. Judd Co., 1906. 174p.
Second	Perry, Enos J. Among the Danish Farmers. Danville, Ill.; Interstate, 1939. 191p.
Second	Perry, Enos J., ed. The Artificial Insemination of Farm Animals. New Brunswick, N.J.; Rutgers University Press, 1945. 265p. (4th ed., rev., 1968. 473p.)
Third	Peters, Walter H. Swine Questions Answered. St. Paul, Minn.; Webb Book Pub. Co., 1927. 141p.
Second	Peters, Walter H., and George P. Deyoe. Raising Livestock. 1st ed. New York; McGraw-Hill, 1946. 450p. (2d ed., by W. H. Peters, G. P. Deyoe and William A. Ross, 1954. 540p.)
Second	Peters, Walter H., and Robert H. Grummer. Livestock Production. 1st ed. New York; McGraw-Hill, 1942. 450p. (2d ed., 1954. 540p.)
First	Petersen, William E. Dairy Science; Its Principles and Practice in Production, Management and Processing . . . edited by R. W. Gregory. Chicago and Philadelphia; J. B. Lippincott Co., 1939. 679p. (2d ed., 1950. 695p.)
First	Phillips, Ralph W. Breeding Livestock Adapted to Unfavorable Environments. Washington, D.C.; Food and Agriculture Organization, 1948. 182p. (FAO Agricultural Studies no. 1)
Second	Phillips, Ralph W., ed. Improving Livestock under Tropical and Subtropical Conditions; Report of an FAO Meeting . . . Lucknow, U.P., India, February 1950. Washington, D.C.; Food and Agricultural Organization, 1950. 55p. (FAO Development Paper, Agriculture no. 6)
First	Phillips, Ralph W., Ray G. Johnson, and Raymond T. Moyer. The Livestock of China. Washington, D.C.; U.S. Govt. Print. Off., 1945. 174p.
Second	Pickard, James N., and Francis A. Crew. The Scientific Aspects of Rabbit Breeding. Idle, Bradford and London; Watmoughs, 1931. 122p.
Second	Pincus, Gregory, and Kenneth V. Thimann, eds. The Hormones: Physiology, Chemistry, and Applications. New York; Academic Press, 1948. 5 vols. (Vols. 4–5, edited by Gregory Pincus, Kenneth V. Thimann and E. B. Astwood.)
Second	Pirtle, Thomas R. History of the Dairy Industry. Chicago; Mojonnier Bros. Co., 1926. 645p.
Second	Plumb, Charles S. Beginnings in Animal Husbandry. St. Paul, Minn.; Webb Pub. Co., 1912. 393p. (Also, 1921.)
First	Plumb, Charles S. Judging Farm Animals. New York; Orange Judd Co., 1916. 590p.
Second	Plumb, Charles S. Little Sketches of Famous Beef Cattle. Columbus, Ohio; The author, 1904. 99p.
Third	Plumb, Charles S. Registry Books on Farm Animals; A Comparative Study. Columbus; Ohio State University Press, 1930. 306p.

Ranking

First   Plumb, Charles S. Types and Breeds of Farm Animals. 1st ed. Boston and New York; Ginn, 1906. 563p. (Rev. ed., 1920. 820p.)

Second   Potter, Ermine L., ed. Western Live-Stock Management. New York; Macmillan Co., 1917. 462p. (Reissued, 1930.)

Second   Powell-Owen, William. Poultry Breeding and Production. 3d ed. London; Poultry World, 1944. 152p. (5th ed., 1955. 136p.)

Second   Powers, Stephen. The American Merino: For Wool and for Mutton. A Practical Treatise on the Selection, Care, Breeding, and Disease of the Merino Sheep in All Sections of the United States. New York; O. Judd Co., 1887. 368p. (Reissued, 1911.)

Second   Practical Angora Goat Raising. San Jose, Calif.; C. P. Bailey & Sons Co., 1905. 97p.

First   Prentice, E. Parmalee. American Dairy Cattle, Their Past and Future. New York and London; Harper & Bros., 1942. 453p.

First   Prentice, E. Parmalee. Breeding Profitable Dairy Cattle; A New Source of National Wealth. Boston; Houghton Mifflin Co., 1935. 261p.

Second   Prentice, E. Parmalee. The History of Channel Island Cattle: Guernseys and Jerseys. Williamstown, Mass.; Mount Hope Farm, 1940. 100p.

First   Prescott, Maurice S. Holstein-Friesian History. Lacona, N.Y.; The Corse Press, 1930. 254p. (Diamond jubilee ed., Lacona, N.Y.; Holstein-Friesian World, 1960. 557p.)

Third   Pringle, Robert O. The Live-Stock of the Farm. 2d ed. Edinburgh and London; W. Blackwood and Sons, 1875. 430p. (3d ed., rev., 1886. 385p.)

Second   Profitable Game Bird Managment. 1st–9th eds. Cayuga, N.Y.; Beacon Milling Co., 1934–58. (Title varies: 1934, Practical Game Bird Production. 1st–7th eds. prepared by Thomas Rae; 8th–9th by Philip T. Grant.)

Second   Prothero, Rowland E. (Baron Ernle). The Pioneer and Progress of English Farming. London and New York; Longmans, Green & Co., 1888. 290p. (Later published as English Farming, Past and Present. 6th ed., London; Heinemann, F. Cass, 1961. 559p.)

First   Punnett, Reginald C. Heredity in Poultry. London; Macmillan, 1923. 204p.

Second   Punnett, Reginald C. Mendelism. Cambridge, U.K.; Macmillan & Bowes, 1905. 63p. (7th ed., London; Macmillan & Co., 1927. 236p.)

Third   Pycraft, William P. A History of Birds. London; Methuen & Co., 1910. 458p.

R

Third   Raine, William M., and Will C. Barnes. Cattle. Garden City, N.Y.; Doubleday, Doran & Co., 1930. 340p.

Second   Randall, Henry S. Fine Wool Sheep Husbandry. New York; O. Judd Co., 1863. 189p.

Second   Randall, Henry S. The Practical Shepherd: A Complete Treatise on the Breeding, Management and Diseases of Sheep. 2d ed. Rochester, N.Y.; D. D. T. Moore; Philadelphia; J. B. Lippincott & Co., 1843. 454p. (31st ed., New York; American News, 1863. 452p.)

Second   Randall, Henry S. Sheep Husbandry; With an Account of the Different

Ranking

Breeds. . . . New York; Bangs Brothers, 1852. 320p. (New ed., New York; O. Judd. 538p.)

Second Reaman, George E. History of the Holstein-Friesian Breed in Canada. Toronto; Collins, 1946. 568p.

Second Reliable Poultry Journal Publishing Company. The Leghorns, Brown, White, Black Buff and Duckwing. Quincy, Ill.; Reliable Poultry Journal Pub. Co., 1904. 73p.

Second Rice, Elmer C. The National Standard Squab Book. 2d ed. Boston; 1902. 80p. (58th ed., Melrose, Mass.; Squab Pub. Co., 1944. 720p.)

First   †Rice, James E., and Harold E. Botsford. Practical Poultry Management. New York; J. Wiley & Sons, Inc., 1925. 506p. (5th ed., 1949. 614p.)

First   Rice, Victor A. Breeding and Improvement of Farm Animals. 1st ed. New York; McGraw-Hill Book Co., 1926. 362p. (6th ed., 1967. 477p.)

Third   Richards, Irmagarde. Modern Milk Goats; Status of the Milk Goat Industry. Philadelphia and London; J. B. Lippincott, 1921. 271p.

Second Richardson, H. D. Domestic Pigs: Their Origin and Varieties, Management with a View to Profit . . . New ed., enl. London; W. S. Orr, 1852. 148p. (Later rev. and extended ed., with illustrations on wood by W. Oldham and Harrison Weir, London; F. Warne & Co., 1872. 152p.)

Second Richardson, William N. The Rabbit; How to Select, Breed and Manage the Rabbit for Pleasure or Profit. Syracuse, N.Y.; C. C. De Puy, 1896. 34p. (7th ed., 1916. 64p.)

Second Richmond, Henry D. Dairy Chemistry: A Practical Handbook for Dairy Chemists and Others Having Control of Dairies. London; C. Griffin & Co., 1899. 384p. (5th ed., rev. by J. G. Davis and F. J. Macdonald, 1953. 603p.)

First   Ridgeway, William. The Origin and Influence of the Thoroughbred Horse. Cambridge, U.K.; University Press, 1905. 538p.

Third   Rikard-Bell, Hal M. The Handbook of Modern Pig Farming. London; H. F. & G. Witherby, 1937. 128p.

Second Ritzman, Ernest G., and Francis G. Benedict. Nutritional Physiology of the Adult Ruminant. Washington, D.C.; Carnegie Institution of Washington, 1938. 200p. (Carnegie Institution of Washington Publication no. 494)

Third   Roadhouse, Chester L., and James L. Henderson. The Market-Milk Industry. 1st ed. New York and London; McGraw-Hill Book Co., 1941. 624p. (2d ed., 1950. 716p.)

Second Robbins, William J., et al. Growth. New Haven, Conn.; Yale University Press; London; H. Milford, Oxford University Press, 1928. 189p.

First   Roberts, Isaac P. The Horse. New York and London; Macmillan Co., 1905. 401p.

Second Robertson, T. Brailsford. The Chemical Basis of Growth and Senescence. Philadelphia and London; J. B. Lippincott Co., 1923. 389p.

First   †Robinson, John H. The Growing of Ducks and Geese for Profit and Pleasure. Dayton, Ohio; Reliable Poultry Journal Pub. Co., 1924. 447p.

Second Robinson, John H. Our Domestic Birds; Elementary Lessons in Aviculture. Boston and New York; Ginn, 1913. 317p. (Reprinted as Our Domestic

Ranking

	Birds; A Popular Primer of Aviculture. Dayton, Ohio; Reliable Poultry Journal Pub. Co., 1924.)
Second	Robinson, John H. Principles and Practice of Poultry Culture. Boston and New York; Ginn & Co., 1912. 611p. (Reissued, Dayton, Ohio; Reliable Poultry Journal Pub. Co., 1925. 584p.)
Second	Robinson, Louis. Wild Traits in Tame Animals: Being Some Familiar Studies in Evolution. Edinburgh; W. Blackwood & Sons, 1897. 329p.
Second	Rogers, Lore A. Fundamentals of Dairy Science, by Associates of Lore A. Rogers in the Research Laboratories of the Bureau of Dairy Industry, U.S. Department of Agriculture. New York; Chemical Catalog Co., 1928. 543p. (2d ed., Reinhold Pub. Corp., 1935. 616p.)
First	†Romanoff, Alexis L., and Anastasia J. Romanoff. The Avian Egg. New York; J. Wiley, 1949. 918p.
Second	Ross, Harold E. The Care and Handling of Milk. New York; Orange Judd Pub. Co; London; Paul, Trench, Troubner & Co., 1927. 362p. (2d ed., rev. and enl. New York; Orange Judd, 1939. 417p.)
Second	Rushworth, William A. The Sheep . . . a Historical and Statistical Description of Sheep and Their Products. Buffalo, N.Y.; Buffalo Review Co., 1899. 496p.
Second	Russell, James E. Heredity in Dairy Cattle: Lessons in Breeding and Herd Development for 4H and FFA Dairy Clubs and Other Beginners. Peterborough, N.H.; American Guernsey Cattle Club, 1945. 135p.

S

First	Saddle and Sirloin Club, Chicago. A Biographical Catalog of the Portrait Gallery of the Saddle and Sirloin Club, by Edward N. Wentworth. Chicago; Union Stock Yards, 1920. 343p.
Third	Salmon, Daniel E. The Diseases of Poultry. Washington, D.C.; G. E. Howard & Co., 1899. 248p.
Third	Salmon, Daniel E., Dr. Murray, et al. Special Report on Diseases of Cattle and on Cattle Feeding, by Daniel E. Salmon, Dr. Murray et al. Washington, D.C.; U.S. Bureau of Animal Industry, 1892. 496p. (Rev. ed., 1942. 507p.)
Second	Sammis, John L. Cheese Making; A Book for Practical Cheesemakers, Factory Patrons, Agricultural Colleges and Dairy Schools. 6th ed. of Cheesemaking, by John W. Decker, entirely rewritten. Madison, Wis.; Mendota Book Co., 1918. 225p. (12th ed., rev. Cheese Maker Book Co., 1948. 333p.)
Second	Sampson, Arthur W. Livestock Husbandry on Range and Pasture. New York; J. Wiley; London; Chapman & Hall, 1928. 411p.
Second	Sanders, Alvin H. At the Sign of the Stock Yard Inn. Chicago; Breeder's Gazette Print, 1915. 322p.
First	Sanders, Alvin H. The Cattle of the World. Washington, D.C.; National Geographic Society, 1926. 142p.
First	Sanders, Alvin H. A History of Aberdeen-Angus Cattle. Chicago; New Breeder's Gazette, 1928. 1042p.

Ranking

Second   Sanders, Alvin H. A History of the Percheron Horse. Chicago; Breeder's Gazette Print, 1917. 602p.

First   Sanders, Alvin H. Short-Horn Cattle; A Series of Historical Sketches, Memoirs and Records of the Breed and Its Development in the United States and Canada. Chicago; Sanders Pub. Co., 1900. 902p. (3d ed., 1916. 840p.)

First   Sanders, Alvin H. The Story of the Herefords. Chicago; Breeder's Gazette, 1914. 1087p.

Second   Sanders, James H. The Breeds of Live Stock, and the Principles of Heredity. Chicago; J. H. Sanders Pub. Co., 1887. 480p.

Second   Sanders, James H. Horse-Breeding; Being the General Principles of Heredity Applied to the Business of Breeding Horses. . . . Rev. ed. Chicago; J. H. Sanders Pub. Co., 1885. 249p. (Later ed., 1905. 428p.)

Second   Sanford, Albert H. The Story of Agriculture in the United States. Boston and New York; D. C. Heath & Co., 1916. 394p.

Second   Schneider, Burch H. Feeds of the World, Their Digestibility and Composition. Morgantown; Agricultural Experiment Station, West Virginia University, 1947. 299p.

Second   Schoenheimer, Rudolf. The Dynamic State of Body Constituents. Cambridge; Harvard University Press, 1942. 78p. (2d ed., 1946. 78p.)

Second   Scott, William B. A History of Land Mammals in the Western Hemisphere . . . illustrated with 32 plates and more than 100 drawings by Bruce Horsfall. New York; Macmillan, 1913. 693p. (Rev. ed., illustrated by B. Horsfall and Charles R. Knight, 1937. 786p.)

Third   Scottish Cattle Breeding Conference, Edinburgh 1924. Cattle Breeding; Proceedings . . . edited by G. F. Finlay. Edinburgh and London; Oliver & Boyd, 1925. 495p.

Third   Self, Margaret C. The Horseman's Encyclopedia. New York; Barnes, 1946. 519p. (New and rev. ed., 1963. 428p.)

Third   Self, Margaret C. Horses; Their Selection, Care and Handling. New York; A. S. Barnes & Co., 1945. 170p.

Second   Seton, Ernest T. Life-Histories of Northern Animals; An Account of the Mammals of Manitoba . . . with drawings by the author. New York; C. Scribner's Sons, 1909. 2 vols.

Second   Shaler, Nathaniel S. Domesticated Animals: Their Relation to Man and to His Advancement in Civilization. New York; C. Scribner's Sons, 1895. 267p.

Second   Shaw, Thomas. Animal Breeding. New York and Chicago; O. Judd Co., 1906. 406p.

Second   Shaw, Thomas. The Feeding and Management of Live Stock . . . a series of lectures. 2d ed. St. Anthony Park, Minn.; Webb Pub. Co., 1902. 99p.

Second   Shaw, Thomas. Feeding Farm Animals. New York; O. Judd Co., 1908. 536p. (Reprinted, 1912.)

Second   Shaw, Thomas. Management and Feeding of Cattle. New York; Orange Judd, 1909. 461p.

Second   Shaw, Thomas. Sheep Husbandry in Minnesota. St. Paul, Minn.; Webb, 1900. 205p.

Ranking

First   Shaw, Thomas. The Study of Breeds in America; Cattle, Sheep and Swine. New York and Chicago; Orange Judd Co., 1901. 371p.

Second   Sheldon, John P. Dairy Farming: Being the Theory, Practice, and Methods of Dairying. London, Paris and New York; Cassell, Petter, Galpin & Co., 1879. 570p. (Issued in parts.)

Second   Shepard, Silas M. The Hog in America, Past and Present. Indianapolis, Ind.; Swine Breeders' Journal, 1886. 262p. (Reprinted, Wilmington, Del.; Scholarly Resources, 1974.)

Third   Shepherd, William. Prairie Experiences in Handling Cattle and Sheep. London; Chapman & Hall, 1884. 215p. (U.S. imprint: New York; O. Judd, 1885. Reprinted, Freeport, N.Y.; Books for Libraries Press, 1971.)

Third   Shields, Joan, and Harry Shields. The Modern Dairy Goat. London; C. Arthur Pearson, 1949. 172p. (Reissued, 1972.)

Second   Shull, A. Franklin. Heredity. 1st ed. New York; McGraw-Hill Book Co., 1926. 287p. (4th ed, 1948. 311p.)

Second   Sidky, A. R. The Buffalo of Egypt. 2d ed. Cairo; Govt. Press, 1955. 2 vols.

Second   Sidney, Samuel. The Book of the Horse. London and New York; Cassell, Petter & Galpin, 1875. 604p. (Classic ed., reissued, New York; Bonanza Books, distributed by Crown Pub., 1985. 680p.)

Second   Sidney, Samuel. The Pig. New ed. London; G. Routledge, 1871. 135p.

First   Sinclair, James, ed. History of Shorthorn Cattle. London; Vinton & Co., 1907. 895p.

Second   Sinclair, James. History of the Devon Breed of Cattle. London; Published for the Devon Breeders' Society by Vinton, 1893. 392p.

Second   Sinclair, James. Sheep: Domestic Breeds and Their Treatment. New ed. London; Vinton & Co., 1896. 144p.

Second   Sinclair, John G. Anatomy of the Fetal Pig. Ames, Iowa; Collegiate Press, 1936. 80p.

First   Sinnott, Edmund W., and L. C. Dunn. Principles of Genetics. New York, etc.; McGraw-Hill, 1925. 431p. (5th ed., 1958. 459p.)

Second   Sisson, Septimus. A Text-Book of Veterinary Anatomy. Philadelphia and London; W. B. Saunders Co., 1910. 826p. (Superseded by The Anatomy of the Domestic Animals. 4th ed., rev. by James D. Grossman, 1953. 972p.)

Second   Skeavington, George, and John Sherer. The Horse and Modern Veterinary Practice; Dogs, Cattle, Sheep, Pigs, Poultry, etc. London; London Printing & Pub. Co., 1871. 1016p.

Second   Smith, Frederick. A Manual of Veterinary Physiology. London; Bailliere, Tindall & Cox; New York; W. R. Jenkins, 1892. 414p. (5th ed., Chicago; A. Eger, 1921. 892p.)

Second   Smith, Howard R. Profitable Stock Feeding; A Book for the Farmer. Lincoln, Nebr.; The author, 1905. 413p. (16th ed., St. Paul, Minn.; 1919. 420p.)

Second   Smith, Robert M. The Physiology of the Domestic Animals; A Text-Book for Veterinary and Medical Students and Practitioners. Philadelphia and London; F. A. Davis, 1890. 938p.

Ranking

First   Smith, William W. The Elements of Live Stock Judging. Philadelphia and Chicago; J. B. Lippincott Co., 1927. 147p.

First   Smith, William W. Pork Production. New York; Macmillan, 1922. 492p. (3d ed., 1952. 616p.)

First   Snapp, Roscoe R., and Alvin L. Neumann. Beef Cattle. 3d ed. New York; J. Wiley & Sons, 1939. 684p. (5th ed., 1960.)

First   Snedecor, George W. Statistical Methods Applied to Experiments in Agriculture and Biology. Ames, Iowa; Collegiate Press, 1937. 341p. (4th ed., 1946. 485p.)

Second   Snyder, Laurence H. The Principles of Heredity. Boston and New York; D. C. Heath & Co., 1935. 385p. (5th ed., written by L. H. Snyder and Paul R. David, Boston; 1957. 507p.)

Third   Sommer, Hugo H. Market Milk and Related Products. Madison, Wis.; The author, 1938. 699p. (3d ed., 1952. 750p.)

Second   Sommer, Hugo H. The Theory and Practice of Ice Cream Making. Madison, Wis.; The author, 1932. 628p. (6th ed., 1951. 723p.)

Second   Southwell, Byron L., John T. Wheeler, and A. O. Duncan. Swine Production in the South. Danville, Ill.; Interstate, 1940. 307p.

Second   Spearing, Jack. Fitting and Showing Dairy Cattle. Ames; Iowa State College Press, 1952. 97p.

Third   Speed, John G. The Horse in America. New York; McClure, Phillips & Co., 1905. 287p.

Third   Spencer, Sanders. The Pig: Breeding, Rearing, and Marketing. London; C. A. Pearson, 1919. 184p.

Second   Spencer, Sanders. Pigs; Breeds and Management. London; Vinton, 1897. 180p. (4th ed., 1905.) (Live Stock Handbooks no. 5)

Second   Spooner, William C. The History, Structure, Economy, and Diseases of the Sheep. . . . London; Cradock & Co., 1844. 463p.

Second   Stewart, Elliott W. Feeding Animals. Lake View, N.Y.; The author, 1883. 521p. (5th ed., 1890. 558p.)

Second   Stewart, Henry. The Domestic Sheep: Its Culture and General Management. 2d ed. Chicago; American Sheep Breeder Press, 1898. 371p. (2d ed., 1900. 383p.)

Second   Stewart, Henry. The Shepherd's Manual. A Practical Treatise on the Sheep. New ed., rev. and enl. New York; O. Judd Co., 1882. 264p.

Third   Stong, Philip D. Horses and Americans. New York; Frederick A. Stokes Co., 1939. 333p.

Second   Storer, John. The Wild White Cattle of Great Britain. New ed. London and New York; Cassell, Petter, Galpin & Co., 1879. 384p.

First   †Sturkie, Paul D. Avian Physiology. Ithaca, N.Y.; Comstock Pub. Associates, 1954. 423p. (4th ed. edited by P.D. Sturkie. New York; Springer-Verlag, 1986. 516p.)

Second   Sturtevant, Alfred H. An Introduction to Genetics. Philadelphia and London; W. B. Saunders Co., 1939. 391p.

Third   Sturtevant, E. Lewis. The Dairy Cow; A Monograph on the Ayrshire Breed of Cattle. Boston; A. Williams & Co., 1875. 252p.

Ranking

Third   Summerhays, Reginald S. The Observer's Book of Horses and Ponies. London and New York; F. Warne, 1949. 239p. (Rev. ed., 1961. 255p.)

Second   Swift, Raymond W., and Cyrus E. French. Energy Metabolism and Nutrition. Washington, D.C.; Scarecrow Press, 1954. 264p.

T

First   †Taylor, Lewis W., ed. Fertility and Hatchability of Chicken and Turkey Eggs. New York; J. Wiley, 1949. 423p.

Second   Taylor, Louis. The Horse America Made, the Story and Analysis of the World's Greatest Saddle Horse. . . . Louisville, Ky.; The American Saddle Horse Breeders Assoc., 1944. 243p.

Second   Taylor, William G. The Saddle Horse, His Care, Training, and Riding. New York; Holt & Co., 1925. 270p.

Second   Tegetmeier, William B. Pheasants for Coverts and Aviaries. London; H. Cox, 1873. 124p. (Reissued, edited by Eric Parker, London; The Field, 1931. 268p.)

First   Tegetmeier, William B. The Poultry Book: Comprising the Breeding and Management of Profitable and Ornamental Poultry, Their Qualities and Characteristics . . . with coloured illustrations by Harrison Weir. London; George Routledge & Sons; New York; A. D. Betts, 1867. 356p. (New ed., greatly enl., London and New York; G. Routledge, 1873. 390p.)

Second   Tegetmeier, William B., and C. L. Sutherland. Horses, Asses, Zebras, Mules, and Mule Breeding. London; H. Cox, 1895. 166p.

Second   Thom, Charles, and Walter W. Fisk. The Book of Cheese. New York; Macmillan Co., 1918. 392p.

Second   Thomas, James F. H. Sheep. London; Faber & Faber, 1945. 196p.

Third   Thompson, George F. A Manual of Angora Goat Raising. Chicago; American Sheep Breeder Co. Press, 1903. 236p.

Second   Thomson, J. Arthur. The Biology of Birds. New York; Macmillan, 1923. 436p.

Second   Thomson, J. Arthur. Heredity. London; J. Murray, 1908. 602p.

Second   Thurston, Robert H. The Animal as a Machine and a Prime Motor, and the Laws of Energetics. 1st ed. New York; J. Wiley & Sons, 1894. 97p.

First   Titus, Harry W. The Scientific Feeding of Chickens. Danville, Ill.; Interstate, 1941. 110p. (5th ed., by H. W. Titus and James C. Fritz, 1971. 336p.)

First   Tomhave, William H. Meats and Meat Products. Philadelphia and Chicago; J. B. Lippincott, 1925. 418p.

Third   Tothill, John D. Agriculture in the Sudan. London; Oxford University Press, 1948. 974p.

Second   Towne, Charles W., and Edward N. Wentworth. Pigs from Cave to Corn Belt. 1st ed. Norman; University of Oklahoma Press, 1950. 305p.

Second   Towne, Charles W., and Edward N. Wentworth. Shepherd's Empire . . . with drawings by Harold D. Bugbee. 1st ed. Norman; University of Oklahoma Press, 1945. 364p.

Ranking

Second   Trevathan, Charles E. The American Thoroughbred. New York and London; Macmillan, 1905. 495p.
Third   Trippensee, Reuben E. Wildlife Management. 1st ed. New York; McGraw-Hill Book Co., 1948. 2 vols.
Second   Trow-Smith, Robert. A History of British Livestock Husbandry, 1700–1900. London; Routledge & Kegan Paul, 1959. 351p.
Third   Turnbow, Grover D., and Lloyd A. Raffetto. Ice Cream; A Textbook for Student and Manufacturer. New York; J. Wiley & Sons; London; Chapman & Hall, 1928. 407p. (2d ed., by G. D. Turnbow, Paul H. Tracy and L. A. Raffetto, as The Ice Cream Industry, 1947. 654p.)
First   Turner, Charles W. The Comparative Anatomy of the Mammary Glands, with Special Reference to the Udder of Cattle. Columbia, Mo.; University Cooperative Store, 1939. 373p.

U

Second   Udall, Denney H. The Practice of Veterinary Medicine. Ithaca, N.Y.; Udall, 1933. 267p. (5th rev. ed., 1947. 751p.)
Second   United States Bureau of Animal Industry. Special Report on Diseases of the Horse, by Drs. Pearson et al. Rev. ed. Washington, D.C.; U.S. Govt. Print. Off., 1907. 608p. (Rev. ed., 1942. 584p.)

V

Third   Van Es, Leunis. The Principles of Animal Hygiene and Preventive Veterinary Medicine. New York; J. Wiley & Sons; London; Chapman & Hall, 1932. 768p.
Second   Van Slyke, Lucius L. Modern Methods of Testing Milk and Milk Products. New York; Orange Judd Co., 1906. 214p. (3d ed., rev., 1927. 344p.)
Second   Van Slyke, Lucius L., and Walter V. Price. Cheese; A Treatise on the Manufacture of American Cheddar Cheese and Some Other Varieties. New York; Orange Judd Pub. Co.; London; K. Paul, Trench, Trubner & Co., 1927. 364p. (Rev. and enl., 1952. 522p.)
Second   Vasey, George. Delineations of the Ox-Tribe; Or, the Natural History of Bulls, Bisons, and Buffaloes. London; G. Biggs, 1851. 192p.
First   Vaughan, Henry W. Breeds of Live Stock in America. Columbus, Ohio; R. B. Adams & Co., 1931. 780p.
First   Vaughan, Henry W. Types and Market Classes of Live Stock. Columbus, Ohio; R. B. Adams, 1915. 448p. (4th rev., 21st ed. Columbus, Ohio; College Book Co., 1941. 607p.)
Third   Vesey-FitzGerald, Brian S., ed. The Book of the Horse. Los Angeles; Borden Pub. Co., 1947. 879p. (London; Nicholson & Watson, 1949. 879p.)
Second   Von Bergen, Werner, ed. American Wool Handbook. 1st ed. New York; American Wool Handbook Co., 1938. 864p. (3d ed., enl., New York; Interscience, 1963.)
First   †Von Culin, E. C. The Art of Incubation and Brooding: A Guide to Profitable Poultry Raising. Delaware City, Del.; E. & C. Von Culin, 1894. 166p.

Ranking

W

Second   Waddington, Conrad H. An Introduction to Modern Genetics. London; B. Allen & Unwin, 1939. 441p.

Second   Wallace, John H. Horse of America in His Derivation, History, and Development. New York; The author, 1897. 575p.

First   Wallace, Robert. Farm Live Stock of Great Britain. 2d ed. Edinburgh; Oliver & Boyd, 1889. 333p. (5th ed., rev. and enl. 1923. 868p.)

Third   Walsh, John H., and James I. Lupton. The Horse, in the Stable and the Field. London and New York; Routledge, Warne & Routledge, 1861. 622p. (15th ed., rev. by Harold Leeney, London; George Routledge & Sons, 1899. 687p.)

Second   Warfield, William. The Theory and Practice of Cattle-Breeding. Chicago; J. H. Sanders Pub. Co., 1889. 390p.

First   Warren, George F. Farm Management. New York; Macmillan, 1913. 590p. (Also trans. into Russian, 1929.)

Third   Washburn, Robert M. Productive Dairying. Philadelphia and London; J. B. Lippincott Co., 1917. 432p. (3d ed., rev., Capetown; G. Winderley; Philadelphia; Printed by J. B. Lippincott, 1925.)

Second   Watson, George C. Farm Poultry; A Popular Sketch of Domestic Fowls for the Farmer and Amateur. New York and London; The Macmillan Co., 1901. 341p. (13th ed., rev., 1920. 369p.)

Third   Watson, James. The Dog Book. New York; Doubleday, Page & Co., 1906. 2 vols.

Second   Watson, James A., and James A. More. Agriculture, the Science and Practice of British Farming. Edinburgh; Oliver & Boyd, 1924. 656p. (11th ed., rev. and enl. by James A. McMillan, 1962. 818p.)

Third   Watson, James A., and May E. Hobbs. Great Farmers . . . illustrated. London; Selwyn & Blount, 1937. 287p.

Second   Watson, James A., James Cameron, and G. H. Garrad. The Cattle-Breeder's Handbook. London; Ernest Benn, 1926. 144p.

Second   Watson, John, et al., eds. The Best Breeds of British Stock; A Practical Guide for Farmers and Owners of Live Stock in England and the Colonies. London; W. Thacker, 1898. 130p.

Second   Watson, Stephen J. Feeding of Livestock. London and New York; T. Nelson & Sons, 1949. 325p.

Second   Weir, Harrison. The Poultry Book. . . . American ed., edited by Willis G. Johnson et al. New York; Doubleday, Page & Co., 1903. 2 vols. (1915 ed. published in Garden City, N.Y. 1311p.)

Second   Weisman, Abner I. Spermatozoa and Sterility; A Clinical Manual. New York; Hoeber, 1941. 314p.

Second   Weisman, August. The Germ-Plasm; A Theory of Heredity . . . trans. by W. Newton Parker and Harriet Ronnfeldt. New York; C. Scribner's Sons, 1898. 477p. (Reissued, 1902.)

Second   Weld, Mason C. The Percheron Horse in America. New York; O. Judd, 1886. 142p.

First   Wentworth, Edward N. America's Sheep Trails; History, Personalities. Ames; Iowa State College Press, 1948. 667p.

Ranking

Third   Wentworth, Lady. British Horses and Ponies. London; W. Collins, 1944. 46p.

Second   Whitney, Leon F. The Basis of Breeding. New Haven, Conn.; Earle C. Fowler Pub., 1928. 260p. (Rev. ed., 1933. 249p.)

Second   Widmer, Jack. Practical Animal Husbandry. New York; Scribner's Sons, 1949. 159p.

Second   Widmer, Jack. Practical Beef Production. New York; C. Scribner's Sons, 1946. 93p.

Second   Widmer, Jack. Practical Horse Breeding and Training. New York; C. Scribner's Sons, 1942. 114p.

First   †Wier, Harrison. The Poultry Book. Am. ed., edited by W. G. Johnson and G. O. Brown. New York; Doubleday, Page & Co., 1903. 2 vols. (Reprint, 1904, 1915. 1311p.)

Second   Wilcox, Earley V. Farm Animals: Horses, Cows, Sheep, Swine, Goats, Poultry, etc. New York; Doubleday, Page & Co., 1906. 357p.

Third   Wilder, Fred. The Modern Packing House. Chicago; Nickerson & Collins, 1905. 581p.

Third   Williams, J. Whitridge. Obstetrics; A Text-book for the Use of Students and Practitioners. 4th ed., rev. and enl. New York and London; D. Appleton, 1917. 1029p. (18th ed., 1989. 984p.)

Second   Williams, Walter L. The Diseases of the Genital Organs of Domestic Animals. Ithaca, N.Y.; The author, 1921. 856p. (3d ed., 1943. 641p.)

Third   Willoughby, Edward F. Milk, Its Production and Uses. London; C. Griffin & Co., 1903. 259p.

First   Wilson, James. The Evolution of British Cattle and the Fashioning of Breeds. London; Vinton & Co., 1909. 147p.

Third   Wilson, John M., ed. The Rural Cyclopedia. Edinburgh; A. Fullarton & Co., 1854–1857. 4 vols.

First   Wing, Henry H. Milk and Its Products. New York; Macmillan Co., 1897. 280p. (11th ed., 1907. 311p.)

Second   Wing, Joseph E. Sheep Farming in America. New and rev. ed. Chicago; Sanders Pub. Co., 1905. 332p. (3d ed., 1912. 367p.)

First   †Winter, A. R., and E. M. Funk. Poultry Science and Practice . . . edited by R. W. Gregory. Chicago and Philadelphia; J. B. Lippincott, 1941. 739p. (4th ed., 1956. 662p.)

First   Winters, Laurence M. Animal Breeding. New York; Wiley, 1925. 309p. (5th ed., 1954. 420p.)

Third   Woll, Fritz W. Productive Feeding of Farm Animals. Philadelphia and London; J. B. Lippincott Co., 1915. 362p. (4th ed. rev., 1925. 385p.)

Second   Wood, Thomas B. Composition and Nutritive Value of Feedingstuffs. 1st ed. Cambridge, U.K.; Cambridge University (Pitt Press), 1917.

Second   Wood, Thomas B. Animal Nutrition. London; Clive, 1924. 226p. (2d ed., 1927.)

Third   Wood, Thomas B., and L. F. Newman. Beef Production in Great Britain. Liverpool; R. Silcock & Sons, 1928. 67p.

Third   Woodruff, Hiram W. The Trotting Horse of America; How to Train and

Ranking

Drive Him. New York; J. B. Ford, 1868. 412p. (19th ed., rev. and enl., Philadelphia; Porter & Coates, 1874. 477p.)

First   Wriedt, Christian. Heredity in Live Stock. London; Macmillan & Co., 1930. 179p.

Second   Wright, Lewis. The Book of Poultry. Popular ed. London and New York; Cassell, 1885. 591p. (Later popular ed., rev., 1891.)

Second   Wright, Lewis. The Practical Poultry Keeper. New York; Orange Judd Co., 1869. 252p. (Later ed., 1905. London and New York; Cassell, 1920. 315p.)

Second   Wrightson, John. Sheep; Breeds and Management. 2d ed. London; Vinton, 1895. 235p. (8th ed., 1919.) (Live Stock Handbooks no. 1)

Y

Second   Yapp, William W. Dairy Cattle Judging and Selection. New York; J. Wiley, 1959. 324p.

First   Yapp, William W., and William B. Nevens. Dairy Cattle: Selection, Feeding and Management. New York; J. Wiley, 1926. 378p. (4th ed., 1955. 420p.)

Second   Youatt, William. The Horse. London; Baldwin & Cradock, 1938. 472p. (Later ed., rev. and enl. by Walker Watson, New York; Longmans, Green & Co., 1915. 589p.)

Second   Youatt, William. The Pig: A Treatise on the Breeds, Management, Feeding, and Medical Treatment, of Swine. London; Cradock & Co., 1847. 164p. (Later rev. ed., New York; C. M. Saxton, 1852. 175p.)

First   Youatt, William. Sheep: Their Breeds, Management, and Diseases. New York; C. M. Saxton, 1848. 159p. (Later new ed., New York; O. Judd Co., 1885. 159p.)

Second   Youatt, William, and W. C. L. Martin. Cattle . . . edited by A. Stevens. New York; C. M. Saxton, 1851. 469p. (Later new ed., written by W. Youatt, London; Simpkin, Marshal, 1889. 600p.)

Second   Youatt, William, and W. C. L. Martin. The Hog. . . . New York; Orange Judd, 1865. 231p.

Z

First   Ziegler, Percival T. The Meat We Eat. Danville, Ill.; Interstate, 1944. 377p. (10th ed., written by John R. Romans and P. T. Ziegler, 1974. 776p.)

This evaluation provides 108 monographs which should be considered of paramount importance for preservation. The second ranked 362 should be considered of importance but should not be processed ahead of the first-ranked items. Similarly, the third ranked titles may be delayed the longest time from the point of view of scholarly, historical value.

The publishers of these historical monographs break out in this fashion:

Commercial publishers	80.7%
University departments and presses	9.9
Societies and organizations	7.1
National or international governments	2.3
	100.0%

The low governmental numbers must be viewed as exclusive of the mass of pamphlets, bulletins, and reports issued by these bodies. The influence of this type of material on all of the publishing of the period is great, consitituting about 50% of all documents. However, we are dealing here only with monographs and mostly those of major size.

The different commercial publishers number 170, of which 142 are represented by only one or two titles. The most heavily represented commercial publishers in descending importance are Macmillan, Wiley, Orange Judd, Lippincott, Interstate and Vinton. All others have ten or fewer titles. Cambridge University Press has the earliest university press title, 1882, and the greatest number, fourteen. Iowa State College Press is next with seven.

This was a period of active publication by animal associations and clubs, of which twenty-seven are represented, 7.1% of all the monographs. The names of the groups are interesting: American Sheep Breeder Co., More Game Birds in America, American Guernsey Cattle Club, Horse and Mule Association, American Corriedal Association, Chick Indexing Association of America, National Cattle Breeders Association (U.K.), and State Historical Society of Iowa.

The range of years represented in the list is 1805 through 1958. The median year is 1922.

Beekeeping

As a supplement to the animal science literature, the beekeeping literature has been citation analyzed and coordinated with the expert advice of Roger A. Morse, Professor of Apiculture at Cornell University, to whom we are greatly indebted. The following list of monographs has been developed as those titles within the specified time span which should be conserved. With the publication of Langstroth's *Hive and the Honey-Bee* and Moses Quinby's *Mysteries of Bee-Keeping Explained*, both in 1853, a century of prolific publishing in beekeeping was underway on both sides of the Atlantic. This list of ninety-eight titles includes a few published in England but is predominantly American in coverage, and is intended as a selective list of the most prominent of the many publications which appeared from the middle of the nineteenth century to the middle of the twentieth century.

The weighting, tally and rankings are the same as used for the animal science and health monographs.

Readers are referred to the works of Eva Crane and to that of Fusonie and Fusonie for additional bibliographic details in beekeeping. The literature in this area is of great historical interest to entomologists as well as agriculturalists.

Historically Important Monographs in Beekeeping, 1860–1949

Ranking

Second   Abbott, Charles P. Queen Breeding for Amateurs. Petts Wood, Eng; 1947. 48 p. (New and rev. ed., Petts Wood; Bee Craft, 1951. 60p.)

Second   Alexander, E. W. Alexander's Writings on Practical Bee Culture . . . edited and compiled by H. H. Root. 3d ed. Medina, Ohio; A. I. Root Co., 1910. 98p.

Second   Allen, M. Yate. European Bee Plants and Their Pollen. Alexandria, Egypt; The Bee Kingdom League, 1936. 148p.

First   Alley, Henry. The Beekeeper's Handy Book; Or, Twenty-Two Years' Experience in Queenrearing. . . . Wenham, Mass.; The author, 1883. 184p. (3d ed., rev. and enl., 1885. 269p.)

Second   Alley, Henry. The National Beekeeper's Directory. Salem, Mass.; Salem Press Publ. and Printing, 1889. 139p.

Second   Alley, Henry. Thirty Years Among the Bees. Salem, Mass.; Salem Press, 1891. 72p. (Rev. ed., 1893. 88p.)

Third   Atkins, E. W. How to Succeed with Bees. 2d ed. Madison, Wis.; Democrat Printing Co., 1924. 96p. (13th ed., 1942.)

First   Beck, Bodog F. Bee Venom Therapy. New York and London; D. Appleton-Century Co., 1935. 238p.

Third   Beck, Bodog F. Honey and Health. 1st ed. New York; R. M. McBride & Co., 1938. 272p.

Third   Bent, Eric R. Swarm Control Survey. Aldershot; Gale & Polden, The Wellington Press, 1946. 87p.

Second   Betts, Annie D. The Diseases of Bees: Their Signs, Causes and Treatment. Camberley, Eng.; The Apis Club, 1940. (2d ed., 1951. 69 p.)

Second   Betts, Annie D. Practical Bee Anatomy. Benson, Eng.; The Apis Club, 1923. 88p.

Third   Brown, J. P. H. Bee-Keeping for Beginners. Augusta, Ga.; Richards & Shaver, 1898. 110p.

First   Cheshire, Frank R. Bees and Bee-Keeping; Scientific and Practical. London; L. U. Gill, 1886–1888. 2 vols.

First   Comstock, Anna. How to Keep Bees, A Handbook for the Use of Beginners. New York; Doubleday, Page, 1905. 228p. (Rev. ed., Garden City, N.Y.; Doubleday, Page, 1920. 230p.)

Ranking

First	Cook, Albert J. Manual of the Apiary. Lansing, Mich.; 1876. 59p. (5th ed., rev. and enl., Chicago; T. G. Newman, 1880. 302p.)
Second	Cowan, Thomas W. British Bee-Keeper's Guide Book to the Management of Bees in Moveable Comb Hives, and the Use of the Extractor. 1st ed. London; Houlston, 1881. 135p. (25th ed., London; British Bee Journal Office, 1924. 226p.)
Second	Cowan, Thomas W. The Honey Bee: Its Natural History, Anatomy, and Physiology. London; Houlston, 1890. 220p. (2d ed., 1904.)
Second	Dadant, Camille P. Dadant System of Beekeeping. Hamilton, Ill.; American Bee Journal, 1920. 115p. (2d ed., 1932. 117p. Also trans. into Spanish, Italian, French and Russian.)
Second	Dadant, Camille P. First Lessons in Beekeeping. Hamilton, Ill.; American Bee Journal, 1918. 167p. (10th ed., 1935. Also trans. into Spanish.)
Second	Dadant, Maurice G. Outapiaries and Their Management. Hamilton, Ill.; American Bee Journal, 1919. 124p. (2d ed., rev., 1932. 126p.)
Second	Digges, Joseph R. The Irish Bee Guide. Leitrim, Ireland; Irish Bee Journal Office, 1904. 220p. (11th ed., published as The Practical Bee Guide. Dublin; Talbot Press, 1943. 313p.)
First	Doolittle, Gilbert M. Scientific Queen-Rearing as Practically Applied. Chicago; T. G. Newman, 1889. 163p. (6th ed., Hamilton, Ill.; American Bee Journal, 1915. 126p.)
First	Doolittle, Gilbert M. A Year's Work in an Out-Apiary. 2d ed. Medina, Ohio; A. I. Root Co., 1908. 61p. (5th ed., published as Management of Out-Apiaries, 1922. 65p.)
Third	Douglass, Benjamin W. Every Step in Beekeeping. Indianapolis; Bobbs-Merrill Co., 1921. 177p.
Second	Flower, Ada B. Beekeeping up to Date. London and New York; Cassell & Co., 1925. 109p. (8th ed., London; 1942.)
First	Grout, Roy A., ed. The Hive and the Honeybee; A new book on beekeeping to succeed Langstroth on the Hive and the Honeybee. Hamilton, Ill.; Dadant & Sons, 1946. 633p. (Extensively rev. ed., 1975. 740p.)
Third	Hamilton, William. The Art of Bee-Keeping. York; Herald Printing Works, 1945. 182p.
Second	Harbison, John S. The Bee-Keeper's Directory. San Francisco; H. H. Bancroft & Co., 1861. 440p.
Second	Harbison, W. C. Bees and Bee-Keeping: A Plain, Practical Work. . . . New York; Saxton, 1860. 288p.
Second	Hawkins, Kennith. Beekeeping in the South. Hamilton, Ill.; American Bee Journal, 1920. 120p.
Second	Heddon, James. Success in Bee-Culture as Practiced and Advised. Dowagiac, Mich.; Times Print, 1885. 128p.
Third	Herrod-Hempsall, William. The Anatomy, Physiology and Natural History of the Honey Bee. 2d ed. London; The British Bee Journal, 1943. 172p.
Third	Herrod-Hempsall, William. The Bee-Keeper's Guide to the Management of Bees in Movable Comb Hives, Illustrated. 1st ed. London; The British Bee Journal, 1938. 169p. (8th ed., rev., 1947.)

Ranking

First   Herrod-Hempsall, William. Bee-Keeping New and Old. London; The British Bee Journal, 1930. 2 vols.

Third   Hooper, M. M. Common Sense Beekeeping. London; Link House Publications, 1939. 96p. (3d ed., 194–? 78 p.)

Third   Hopkins, Isaac. The Illustrated Australasian Bee Manual and Complete Guide to Modern Bee Culture in the Southern Hemisphere. 3d ed. Auckland, N.Z.; 1886. 335p. (5th ed., Wellington; Gordon & Gotch, 1911. 173p.)

Second   Howes, Frank N. Plants and Beekeeping. London; Faber & Faber, 1945. 224p. (New and rev. ed., London and Boston; Faber, 1979.)

Second   Huber, Francois. New Observations upon Bees . . . trans. from the French by Camille P. Dadant. Hamilton, Ill.; American Bee Journal, 1926. 230p.

First   Hutchinson, William Z. Advanced Bee-Culture, Its Methods and Management. Flint, Mich.; The Review Print, 1891. 87p. (4th ed., Medina, Ohio; A. I. Root Co., 1911. 205p.)

First   Kelley, Walter T. How to Grow Queens for 15 Cents Each. Paducah, Ky.; 19––. 20p.

Third   Kelsey, Wilfred E. The Spell of the Honey Bee. London; Chapman & Hall, 1945. 263p. (2d ed., rev., 1947. 274p.)

Third   Kidder, K. P. Kidder's Guide to Apiarian Science. . . . Burlington, Vt.; S. B. Nichols; Chicago; R. Blanchard, 1858. 175p.

First   King, N. H., and Homer A. King. The Bee-Keeper's Text-Book with Alphabetical Index. Cleveland, Ohio; Viets & Savage, 1864. 128p. (23d ed., New York; King & Slocum, 1876. 139p.)

Third   Kretchmer, E. The American Bee-Keepers' Guide. Chicago; Wabash Steam Printing House, 1872. 244p.

First   Langstroth, Lorenzo L. Langstroth on the Hive and the Honey-Bee; A Bee Keeper's Manual. Northampton; Hopkins, Bridgman, 1853. 384p. (Photoreprint of the 1853 ed., Medina, Ohio; A. I. Root Co., 1977. 378p.)

Second   Lawson, John A. Honeycraft in Theory and Practice. London; Chapman & Hall, 1931. 228p. (Later ed., 1945. 164p.)

Second   Lockard, John R. Bee Hunting. Columbus, Ohio; A. R. Harding Publ. Co., 1908. 72p. (Reissued, 1956.)

Second   Lovell, John H. The Flower and the Bee; Plant Life and Pollination. New York; C. Scribner's Sons, 1918. 286p.

Second   Lovell, John H. Honey Plants of North America. Medina, Ohio; A. I. Root Co., 1926. 408p.

Third   Lyon, D. Everett. Biggle Bee Book. Philadelphia; W. Atkinson Co., 1909. 136p. (Reprinted, 1913.)

Third   Lyon, D. Everett. How to Keep Bees for Profit. New York; Macmillan Co., 1910. 329p.

Third   Mace, Herbert. Modern Bee-Keeping. London; Wyman & Sons, 1927. 225p. (Rev. ed., Harlow, Eng.; Bee-Keeping Annual Office, 1933.)

Third   Maeterlinck, Maurice. The Life of the Bee . . . trans. by Alfred Sutro. New York; Dodd, Mead and Co., 1901. 427p. (Rev. ed., 1946. 278p.)

Second   Manley, Robert O. Honey Farming. London; Faber & Faber, 1946. 293p.

Ranking

Second   Manley, Robert O. Honey Production in the British Isles. Reading and London; Bradley & Son, 1936. 343p.

First   Miller, Charles C. Fifty Years Among the Bees. Medina Ohio; A. I. Root Co., 1911. 340p. (Enlarged from the author's Forty Years Among the Bees. Memorial ed., 1920. 328p.)

First   Miller, Charles C. Forty Years Among the Bees. Chicago; B. W. York & Co., 1903. 327p. (2d ed., 1906. 336p.)

First   Miller, Charles C. A Thousand Answers to Beekeeping Questions . . . as Answered by Him in the Columns of the American Bee Journal, compiled by Maurice G. Dadant. Hamilton, Ill.; American Bee Journal, 1917. 276p.

Second   Miner, T. B. The American Bee Keeper's Manual. 4th ed. New York; Saxton, 1857. 349p.

Third   Mitchell, N. C. First Lessons in Bee Culture. Indianapolis; Indianapolis Printing & Publ. House, 1871. 96p.

Third   Morley, Margaret W. The Honey-Makers. Chicago; A. C. McClurg, 1899. 424p.

Third   Morse, Josephine. Following the Bee Line. Chicago; Thomas S. Rockwell Co., 1931. 127p.

Third   Neighbor, Alfred. The Apiary. 3d ed., enl. and rev. London; Kent & Co., 1878. 359p.

Second   Nelson, James A. The Embryology of the Honey Bee. Princeton, N.J.; Princeton University Press, 1915. 282p.

Second   Newman, Thomas G. Bees and Honey; Or, the Management of an Apiary for Pleasure and Profit. 3d ed. Chicago; The American Bee Journal, 1882. 158p. (Rev., 1892. 192p.)

First   Pellett, Frank C. American Honey Plants. Hamilton, Ill.; American Bee Journal, 1920. 297p. (5th ed., edited by Dadant & Sons, Hamilton, Ill.; Dadant, 1976. 467p.)

Second   Pellett, Frank C. Beginner's Bee Book. Philadelphia and London; J. B. Lippincott, 1919. 179p.

First   Pellett, Frank C. History of American Beekeeping. Ames, Iowa; Collegiate Press, 1938. 213p.

Second   Pellett, Frank C. Practical Queen Rearing. 3d ed. Hamilton, Ill.; American Bee Journal, 1918. 103p. (6th ed., Quincy, Ill.; pub. by Jost & Kiefer Printing Co. for Dadant & Sons, 1945. 102p.)

Second   Pellett, Frank C. Productive Bee-Keeping. Philadelphia and London; J. B. Lippincott Co., 1916. 302p. (4th ed., rev., 1928.)

Second   Pellett, Frank C. The Romance of the Hive. New York and Cincinnati; Abingdon Press, 1931. 203p.

First   Phillips, Everett F. Beekeeping: A Discussion of the Life of the Honeybee and the Production of Honey. New York; Macmillan, 1928. 490p. (Continued by John E. Eckert and Frank R. Shaw, 1960. 536p.)

First   Quinby, Moses. Mysteries of Bee-Keeping Explained: Being a Complete Analysis of the Whole Subject. New York; M. Saxton & Co., 1853. 376p. (New and rev. ed., New York; Orange Judd Co., 1919. 271p.)

First   Root, Amos I. The ABC of Bee Culture. 1st ed. Medina, Ohio; A. I. Root Co., 1879. 163p. (Eds. of 1899–1905, 1945–, rev. by E. R. Root; eds. of

Ranking

	1908–1940, by A. I. Root and E. R. Root; later eds. as The ABC and XYZ of Bee Culture. Also trans. into French, German, Spanish and Russian.)
Third	Rowe, Henry G. Starting Right with Bees. . . . 1st ed. Medina, Ohio; A. I. Root Co., 1922. 128p. (Largely rewritten by E. R. Root. 11th ed., rev. and edited by Walter Barth, 1956. 100p.)
Third	Sechrist, Edward L. Honey Getting. Hamilton, Ill.; American Bee Journal, 1944. 128p. (2d ed., Roscoe, Calif.; Earthmaster Publications, 1947. 82p.)
Third	Sharp, Dallas L. The Spirit of the Hive. New York and London; Harper & Bros., 1925. 240p.
Third	Simmins, Samuel. A Modern Bee-Farm and Its Economic Management. London; T. Pettitt & Co., 1887. 195p. (Rev. ed., Heathfield, Eng.; The author, 1928. 506p.)
Second	Sladen, Frederick W. Queen-Rearing in England. 2d ed. London; Madgwick, Houlston & Co., 1913. 86p.
First	Smith, Jay. Queen Rearing Simplified. Medina, Ohio; A. I. Root Co., 1923. 119p.
Second	Snelgrove, Louis E. The Introduction of Queen Bees. 1st ed. Paulton and London; Printed by Purnell & Sons, 1940. 205p. (3d ed., 1948.)
Second	Snelgrove, Louis E. Queen Rearing. 1st ed. Bleadon; I. Snelgrove, 1946. 344p.
Second	Snelgrove, Louis E. Swarming; Its Control and Prevention. London; Privately printed, 1934. 95p. (9th ed., 1946. 100p.)
First	Snodgrass, Robert E. Anatomy and Physiology of the Honeybee. 1st ed. New York; McGraw-Hill, 1925. 327p.
Third	Stuart, Frank S. Bee-Keeping Practice. London; C. Arthur Pearson, 1945. 206p.
Third	Sturges, Arthur M. Practical Beekeeping. London and New York; Cassell & Co., 1924. 307p.
Third	Tinker, G. L. Bee-Keeping for Profit, How to Get the Largest Yields of Comb and Extracted Honey. Flushing, Mich.; Rulison's Printing House, 1890. 47p. (Rev. and enl. ed., Chicago; G. W. York & Co., 1893. 130p.)
Third	Townsend, E. D. The Townsend Bee Book, or How to Make a Start in Bees. Medina, Ohio; A. I. Root Co., 1910. 87p. (Rev., 1914. 82p.)
Third	Wadey, H. J. The Bee Craftsman; A Short Guide to the Life Story and Management of the Honey-Bee. Chatham; 1943. 115p. (5th ed., Petts Wood, Eng; Bee Craft, 1949. 117p.)
First	Watson, Lloyd R. Controlled Mating of Queen Bees. 1st ed. Hamilton, Ill.; American Bee Journal, 1927. 50p.
Third	Webster, W. B. The Book of Bee-Keeping. London; L. U. Gill, 1888. 103p. (6th ed., London; Bazaar, Exchange & Mart, 192–? 104p.)
Third	Wedmore, Edmund B. A Manual of Beekeeping for English-Speaking Beekeepers. London; E. Arnold, 1932. 413p. (2d ed. rev., 1945. 389p.)
Third	Wedmore, Edmund B. The Ventilation of Bee-Hives. Kent, Eng.; Bee Craft, 1947. 115p.
Third	Whitehead, Stanley B. Honey Bees and Their Management. London; Faber & Faber, 1946. 153p.

Ranking

First   Wilder, J. J. Southern Bee Culture. Cordele, Ga.; 1908. 143p.
First   Wilder, J. J. Wilder's System of Beekeeping. Waycross, Ga.; 1927. 96p.

B. The Popular Periodicals of the United States

An important medium for the dissemination of agricultural information to the farmer was the early agricultural periodicals. John S. Skinner's *American Farmer*, which began publication in Baltimore in 1819, was one of the earliest and most significant of these. Early farm periodicals were clearinghouses of general agricultural information and borrowed liberally from each other. Before 1834, farm periodicals presented information without regard for system or organization. After that date, periodicals began to gather and organize information under particular headings. For example, the *Cultivator* (Albany, N.Y., 1834–1865) developed columns of particular interest to farmers such as "Cattle Husbandry," "Horticulture," "Poultry Yard," and "Veterinary." These specialized columns reveal the developing specialized interests among farmers during the mid-1800s. To some extent, farmers in various parts of the country were already specialized by 1810. In the South, for example, tobacco and cotton were primary crops. In the West, grain crops, corn, cattle, hogs and sheep were dominant.

Specialized agricultural literature, or literature which focused on a specific type of farm activity, began to appear with some regularity in the United States around 1870 and became significant by 1880. James F. Evans and Rodolfo N. Salcedo, in their *Communications in Agriculture: The American Farm Press* (1974), indicate that one-third of all farm periodicals published in 1880 were specialized in subject matter; by 1920 the specialized accounted for 42%. This specialization occurred as agriculture progressed in the nineteenth century from subsistence to commercial in nature. The farmer was no longer merely raising crops and animals for the survival of a family but was now able to offer a significant portion of his produce for sale in the available markets. In order for specialized agricultural publications to exist, there had to be a large and prosperous industry in the particular specialization to support that literature. Other necessary criteria included a reliable readership that would provide a substantial market for the publications, advertisers to provide financial support to publishers, and interesting, accurate, and pertinent information to relay to the reader.

Although horticulture was the first specialized agricultural subject field to have its own periodicals, dairy periodicals were an early class of specialized animal agricultural publications. *The Western Reserve Farmer and Dairyman* (Jefferson, Ohio) was the first periodical devoted specifically to dairying. It began publication in 1852 and lasted for less than one year. Another early dairy publication was *The Dairyman's Record*. It began at Little Falls, N.Y., in 1859, appeared as the *Dairy Farmer* in 1860, and ceased publication in 1862. It too, like *The Western Reserve Farmer,* suffered from a lack of material for publication, as well as lack of advertisers and a resistance on the part of farmers to "book learning." These first "dairy" periodicals were actually not very different from the general agricultural periodicals of the time except that they tended to emphasize dairying to a greater degree. Overall, few successful dairy periodicals were created before 1883. One notable exception was *Hoard's Dairyman* (Ft. Atkinson, Wis.), which began publication in 1870 and is still being published today with a vigorous circulation of 190,000. Other early dairy periodicals which continued well into the twentieth century include *The Jersey Bulletin* (Indianapolis, Ind., 1883–1953) and the *Milk Reporter* (Sussex, N.J., 1881–1928).

Of the specialized farm periodicals that appeared during the 1870–1880s, most were devoted to general livestock, poultry, and beekeeping. Breeders' associations became active after 1870, and by the late 1870s several livestock breeds had enough advocates to support separate periodicals. *The National Livestock Journal* (Chicago, 1870–1889), the *Monthly Bulletin of the American Jersey Cattle Club* (Newport, R.I., and New York, 1877–1881), *The Guernsey Breeder's Journal* (Westchester, Pa., 1885–1887), and the *Holstein-Friesian Register* (Brattleboro, Vt., 1886–1928) were four early, important livestock publications. Early popular periodicals devoted to the swine industry include *Swine Breeder's Journal* (Indianapolis, Ind., 1882–1928), *American Swineherd* (Chicago, 1885+, meaning to date), and *Western Swine Breeder* (Lincoln, Nebr., 1894–1907). Early specialized sheep publications include the *American Sheep Breeder and Wool Grower* (Chicago, 1883+) and the *Shepherd's Criterion* (Chicago, 1891–1909).

The number of United States agricultural periodicals increased rapidly in the late 1800s; from 176 in 1881, to 316 in 1890, to 415 in 1900. Farmers were making use of the practical and useful information obtained from reading and from other sources. Current issues kept them in touch with the latest prices and changes in market conditions.

From 1900 to 1928, the output per person in agriculture increased by 47%, making the American farmer the world's greatest agricultural producer per worker. At no other time in history has the farmer contributed as much to prosperity and national advancement. *Batten's Agricultural Direc-*

tory of 1908 states: "The phenominal (*sic*) crops of recent years, and which have played so great a part in advancing the farmer, have sometimes been credited to unusual weather conditions or luck. The man who knows the facts will tell you it was neither of these but that the independent and imperial position of the farmer today is a direct result of his awakening to newer methods and machinery; greater attention to the adaptation of crops to soils; improved facilities for marketing; and intelligent cooperation. The authoritative farm paper has also played its important part, and it has never occupied so influential a position with its host of readers."

Batten's further reported that in 1908 there were a total of 458 agricultural periodicals published in the United States directed to the nation's farm dwellers, "an army of nearly thirty-one millions of people who are actually at the fountain-head of this country." Clearly the farmer's role in the development of the country was being recognized by publishers and the improving eduction of the rural population increased the farmer's search for information on market conditions as well as improved methods of raising and caring for his crops and livestock. In 1908 the average U.S. farm received nearly three periodicals, and each periodical had an average circulation of over 33,000. The farmers' "information age" was in its nascent period.

Popular, general distribution periodicals offer one of the best historical records in American agriculture. Their value is rated highly by animal scientists who need to find historical records, as well as by agricultural historians.

The citation analysis of source documents as outlined in Section A does not offer help in identifying and determining the historical value of popular literature. Citation analysis deals with scholarly and scientific publications and the references to the popular periodical literature are few. It does, of course, identify the scholarly journals which are discussed in Section C. Other methods had to be used to identify popular journals in animal science and to establish their relative historical merits. Journal lists, library catalogs, and historical writings concerned with agricultural periodicals and agricultural history were used. This literature served as the source for a compilation of U.S. popular animal science and related industry periodicals.

Lists were prepared from these sources, divided into distinct subjects such as beef cattle and swine, and then sent to animal scientists for comments and title-by-title evaluations. The titles are presented here in two lists, one for all of animal science, and a second for bees and beekeeping. Scientists with extensive knowledge provided the rankings in the list of historically important animal science periodicals following.

Popular Periodical Reviewers

Donald E. Becker
  Animal Nutrition
  University of Illinois
Tony J. Cunha, Prof. Emeritus
  Animal Science
  University of Florida
John K. Loosli, Prof. Emeritus
  Animal Nutrition
  Cornell University
Lon D. McGillard
  Animal Science
  Michigan State University
T. Wayne Perry
  Animal Science
  Purdue University

Wilson G. Pond
  USDA Children's Nutrition
  Research Center, Baylor
  College of Medicine, Houston
John L. Skinner
  American Poultry Historical
  Society, University of
  Wisconsin, Madison
Clair E. Terrill
  USDA Agricultural Research
  Service, Beltsville, Maryland
George W. Trimberger
  Prof. Emeritus, Dairy
  Husbandry, Cornell University

We express our thanks to these consultants for their contribution in helping evaluate and produce this list.

It should be noted again that this list is primarily publications of United States origin and of the popular rather than the scientific journals in the field of animal husbandry and animal science. These more popular titles may contribute to a broader understanding of the culture and the times in which they were published.

The scale in the right-hand column indicates:

1 = Top-ranked periodicals with primary preservation priority.

2 = Periodicals of lesser importance, but worthy of preservation.

An asterisk (*) indicates that end date information is incomplete.

Historically Important Popular and Trade Periodicals in Animal Science and Health, 1850–1950

American Association of Instructors and Investigators in Poultry Husbandry, Journal. New Brunswick, N.J.; v.1–7, 1914–1921//.   1

American Berkshire Association, Bulletin. Springfield, Ill.; v.1–3, 1907–1909//. (NAL has v.1–2, 1879–1880.)   2

American Berkshire Record. Springfield, Ill.; American Berkshire Assoc., v.1–60, 1876–1923//.   1

American Cattle Producer. Denver; American National Livestock Assoc., v.1– 1919–. Began as Producer, v.1–15, 1919–1934.   2

American Cheesemaker. Grand Rapids, Mich.; v.1–32, 1886–1917//.   2

American Chester-White Record. Dayton, Ohio; American Chester-White Record Assoc., v.1–17, 1885–1912//.   1

American Creamery and Poultry Produce Review. New York; v.1–89, 1895–1939//.   1

American Dairy Products Review. New York; v.1–15, 1939–1953//. Also known as American Dairy Products Manufacturing Review. 1939–1948 as American Butter Review. 1948–1950 as American Butter and Cheese Review.   1

American Dairyman. New York; v.1–61, 1877–1907//.   1

American Duroc-Jersey Record. Springfield, Ill.; American Duroc-Jersey Swine Breeders' Assoc., v.1–58, 1885–1923//.   1

American Egg and Poultry Review. New York; v.1– 1940–. Supersedes in part American Produce Review.   2

American Fancier. Johnstown and New York; Blunck & Drevenstedt, v.1–38, 1893–1909//.   2

American Fancier and Stock-Keeper. Boston; v.1–81, 1889–1928//? Began as American Stock Keeper.   1+

American Farmer, Live Stock and Poultry Raiser. Philadelphia and Indianapolis; Solon L. Goode, v.1–26, 1884–1911//. Also known as American Poultry Raiser and Livestock Journal.   2

American Farming. Chicago; v.1–27, 1906–1932//.   2

American Gamekeeper. Woodglen, N.J., and East Bangor, Pa.; v.1–8, 1894–1902.   2

American Hampshire Herdsman. Peoria, Ill.; Hampshire Swine Registry, v.1– 1926–.   1

American Hatchery News. Kansas City, Mo.; v.1– 1925–.   1

American Horsebreeder. Boston; v.1–53, 1882–1935//.   1

American Jersey Cattle Club, Monthly Bulletin. Newport, R.I.; v.1–4, 1877–1881//.   1

American Poland-China Record. Cedar Rapids, Iowa; American Poland-China Record Co., v.1–90, 1879–1923//.   1

American Poultry Advocate. Syracuse, N.Y.; v.1–36, 1892–1927//.   2

American Poultry Association, News. Fort Wayne, Ind.; v.1– 1925–.   2

American Poultry Association, Quarterly. Fort Wayne, Ind., and Davenport, Iowa; v.1–8, 1925–1944//.   2

American Poultry Association, Proceeding. Buffalo, N.Y., etc.; v.1–41, 1974–1916//?   1

American Poultry Journal. Chicago; v.1–90, 1874–1959//.   1

American Poultry World. Buffalo, N.Y.; American Poultry Pub. Co., v.1–8, 1909–1917//.   2

American Poultry Yard. Hartford, Conn.; v.1–11, 1878–1888//.   2

American Poultryman. East Palestine and Springfield, Ohio; 1883–. Merged with Ohio Poultry Journal, and Record and Ladies Poultry Journal.   2

American Poultryman. Lincoln, Nebr.; v.1–20, 1894–1915//. Began as Poultry Gazette.   2

American Sheep-Breeder and Wool Grower. Chicago; v.1–48, 1883–1928.   1

American Shropshire Sheep Record. Lafayette, Ind., etc.; v.1–32, 1885– 1922//.   1

American Standard of Perfection. Buffalo, N.Y.; 1878–. Continues American Standard of Excellence.   2

American Stock Farm and Advance Farmer. Winona, Minn.; J. H. Johnston, v.1–46, 1880–1907//.   2

American Stock Journal, and Farmers' and Stock Breeders' Advertiser. Parkesburg, Pa.; v.1–18, 1866–1881//?   1

American Stockman. Kansas City, Mo.; G. M. Bishop, v.1–12, 1901– 1912//?   2

American Stockman and Farmer. Chicago; v.1–3, 1878–1881//.   2

American Swine and Poultry Journal. Cedar Rapids, Iowa; v.1– 1874–.   1

American Swineherd. Chicago; v.1–46, 1884–1929//.   2

American Yorkshire Record. St. Paul, Minn.; American Yorkshire Club, v.1–5, 1901–1915//.   1

Anglo-American Stockman. Toronto and Buffalo, N.Y.; v.1– 1905?-1907.   2

Animal Husbandry. Freeport and Chicago; v.1–8, 1910–1914//.   2

Arizona Cattleman and Farmer. Tucson, Ariz.; v.1–14, 1917–1931//.   2

Aviculture. Los Angeles, etc.; Avicultural Society of America, v.1– 1933–.   1

Avicultural Magazine. London; Avicultural Society . . . , v.1– 1894–.   1

Avicultural Magazine. New York; Avicultural Society of America, v.1– 1929–.   1

Ayrshire Digest. Brandon, Vt.; Ayrshire Breeders' Assoc., v.1– 1915–.   1

Berkshire Bulletin. Springfield, Ill.; American Berkshire Assoc., v.1–3, 1919–1921//.   2

Berkshire News. Lebanon, Ind., etc.; American Berkshire Assoc., v.1– 1935–.   2

Berkshire World. Springfield, Ill.; American Berkshire Assoc., v.1–18, 1909–1926//.   2

Big Four Poultry Journal. Chicago; v.1–26, 1898–1917//.   2

Blooded Stock Farmer. Oxford, Pa.; C. E. Morrison, v.1–19, 1896– 1913//.   2

Breeder and Dairyman. Harrisburg, Pa.; v.1–15, 1922–1937//.   1

Breeder and Sportsman. San Francisco; D. L. Hackett and J. DeWitt, v.1– 72, 1882–1919//.   2

Breeder's Gazette. Chicago; Sanders Pub. Co., v.1– 1881–.   1

Breeders World. New Albany, Ind.; v.1–16, 1925–1941//?   2

Breeders' Journal. Cleveland, Ohio; American Assoc. of Trotting Horse Breeders, v.1–22, 1912–1933.   2

British Berkshire Herd Book. Salisbury, Eng.; British Berkshire Society, v.1–42, 1885–1926//.   1

Brown Swiss Bulletin. Beloit, Wis.; v.1– 1922–.   1

Brown Swiss Record. Oswego, N.Y., and Beloit, Wis.; 1908–1940//.   2

Brownell's Dairy Farmer. Detroit, Mich.; v.1–9, 1909–1917//.   2

The Business Hen and Busy Bee. St. Paul, Minn.; v.1– Apr. 1899–.   2

Butcher Worker. New York; v.1– 1937–.   2
Butcher Workman. Syracuse, N.Y.; Amalgamated Meat Cutters and   2
    Butcher Workmen of North America, v.1–4, 1911–1914; nsv1, 1915–.
Butchers Advocate. New York; 1886–1932//. Also known as Butchers Ad-   1
    vocate and National Butcher, and National Butcher.
Butter, Cheese and Egg Journal. Milwaukee, Wis.; v.1–19, Jan. 1910–   2
    Mar. 1928.
Butterfat. Modesto, Calif.; v.1– 1920–.   2
Butter-Fat. Vancouver, B.C.; Fraser Valley Producers Assoc., v.1– 1922– 2

Cackle and Crow. Guilford, Conn.; v.1–35, 1926–1956//.   1
California Agriculturist and Live Stock Journal. San Jose, Calif.; v.1–8, 2
    1870–1877//.
California Cultivator. Los Angeles; v.1–95, 1877–1948//.   1
California Dairyman. Los Angeles; California Milk-Producers Assoc.,   1
    v.1– 1922–.
California Wool Grower. San Francisco, Calif.; v.1–27, 1925–1952?   2
Canada Poultry Journal. Brooklin, Brantford and Toronto, Ont.; v.1–5,   2
    1875–1879//?
Canadian Dairy and Ice Cream Journal. Toronto; v.1– 1923–.   1
Canadian National Poultry Record. Ottawa; v.1– 1925–.   2
Canadian Poultry Journal. Toronto, Ont.; v.1–19, 1915–1934//.   2
Canadian Poultry News. Owen Sound, Ont.; v.1–19, 1898–1919//?   2
Canadian Poultry Review. Toronto, Ont.; Donovan Ltd., v.1–99, 1887–   1
    1975.
Carolina Poultry and Livestock Review. North Carolina; v.1–4, 1932–   2
    1935.
Cattleman. Fort Worth, Texas; v.1– 1914–.   1
Central Poland China Record. Indianapolis, Ind.; Central Swine Record   2
    Assoc. of Indiana, v.1–26, 1880– 1911//.
Certified Milk. Brooklyn, N.Y.; American Assoc. of Medical Milk Com-   2
    missions; Certified Milk Producers' Assoc. of America, v.1– 1926–.
Chanticleer; The Modern Poultryman. Guildford, Eng.; Southern Counties   2
    Poultry Society, v.1–13, 1927–1939//.
Cheese Reporter. Sheboygan, Wis.; v.1– 1876–.   1
Chester White Journal. Peoria, Ill., etc.; Chester White Swine Record As- 1
    soc., v.1– 1910–.
Chester White Swine Record. Rochester, Ind.; Chester White Swine Rec-   2
    ord Assoc., v.18–28, 1913–1923//.
Chicago Poultry Letter. Chicago; J. S. L. Hall, v.1– 1886–.   1
Commercial Poultry. Chicago; v.1–19, 1890–1910//.   2
Co-op Chicken News. Bellingham, Wash.; Cooperative Chick Assoc.,   2
    1935–Jan. 1956.
The Co-operative Poultry Post. Hartford, Conn.; H. H. Stoddard, v.1–   2
    1884–.
Cooperative Poultryman. Los Angeles; Poultry Producers of Southern Cali- 2
    fornia, v.1–28, 1925–1963. Continues Calawhite Egg Bulletin.

Cow Bell. Edmonton, Alberta, Can.; v.1–16, 1927–1942//.   2

The Creamery Gazette. Ames and Des Moines, Iowa; v.?–25, 1895–   2
1900//.

Creamery Journal. Waterloo, Iowa; v.1–61, 1890–1950//.   1

Dairy Farmer. Little Falls, N.Y.; v.1–2, 1860–1862//.   1

Dairy Farmer. Waterloo and Des Moines, Iowa; v.1–27, 1903–1929//.   1

Dairy Foods Review. San Francisco; v.1– 1901–.   1

Dairy Gazette. Lincoln, Nebr. and Beatrice, Nebr.; v.1–12, 1897–1910//.   2

Dairy Goat Journal. Fairbury, Nebr.; v.1– 1923–.   2

Dairy Plant Production. Chicago; v.1–34, 1922–1955//.   2

Dairy Produce. Chicago; v.1–49, 1894–1942//.   1

Dairy Record. St. Paul, Minn.; v.1–86, 1900–1985. Changed title to   1
Dairy Foods, v.87, 1986.

Dairy World. Chicago; v.1–25, 1884–1905//.   2

Dairy World. Chicago; v.1–33, 1922–1954//.   1

Dairyman. Montreal and Toronto; v.1–2?– 1884–1887.   2

Dairyman's Journal. Chicago; v.1–16, 1915–1929.   1

Dairyman's Monthly Review. Cincinnati, Ohio; v.1–15, 1923–1937//.   2

Dairymen's League News. New York, etc.; Dairymen's League Coopera-   2
tive Assoc., 1917–1922.

Dairymen's Price Reporter. Pittsburgh, Pa.; v.1– 1916–.   1

De Laval Monthly. New York; 1907–1955.   2

Dixie Poultry Breeder. Columbia, Tenn.; v.1–13, 1894–1907, v.1–13,   2
no.1 as Dixie Game Fowl. Also known as Dixie Poultry Breeder
Monthly.

Duroc Digest. Minneapolis; v.1–8, 1919–1923//.   2

Duroc Journal-Bulletin. Shenandoah, Iowa, etc.; v.1–29, 1904–1931//.   2

Duroc News. Morton and Peoria, Ill.; United Duroc Record Assoc., v.1–   1
1927–.

Duroc Swine Breeders' Journal. Indianapolis, Ind.; Morris Printing Co.,   1
v.1–48, 1882–1928//.

Eastern Poultryman. Freeport, Me.; v.1–6, 1899–1905//.   2

Elgin Dairy Report. Elgin, Ill.; v.1–31, 1890–1922//.   1

Everybody's Poultry Magazine. Hannover, Pa.; v.1–73, 1897–1968.   1+

Familiar Science and Fancier's Journal. Springfield, Mass.; v.1–6, 1874–   2
1879//, v.1–4 as Fanciers' Journal and Land and Water.

Fancier's Review. Chatham, N.Y.; v.1–14, 1888–1900//.   2

Fanciers' Gazette. Indianapolis, Ind.; v.1–24, 1883–1906//.   1

Fanciers' Journal. Philadelphia; v.1–10, 1888–1893//. Continued as Fan-   2
ciers' Journal and Sportsmen's Chronicle.

Fancy Fowls. Hopkinsville, Ky.; v.1–11, 1897–1907//.   2

Farm and Dairy. Toronto and Peterboro, Ont.; v.1–53, 1881–1934//.   1

Farm and Poultry Review. St. Louis; Farmer Off., 1900–.   1

Farm-Poultry. Boston; v.1–27, 1889–1916//.   1

Farm Stock and Home. Minneapolis; S. M. Owen, v.1–45, 1884–   1
1929//.

Farm Stock and Home Success. v.23– 1906. American Poultryman   2 merged with American Stock Farm to form this journal. v.1–23 as Ohio Poultry Journal.

Farmer and Stockman. Des Moines, Iowa, and Kansas City, Mo.; v.1–45, 1878–1922//.   1

Farmer and Stockman. Kansas City, Mo.; v.1–8, 1924–1931//.   2

The Feather. Washington, D.C.; v.1–17, 1895–1913//.   2

Feather Fancier. Georgetown, Ont.; v.1– 1945–   1

Feed Bag. Milwaukee, Wis.; Central Retail Feed Assoc.; v.1– 1925–.   2

Feeding and Marketing. Kansas City, Kans.; v.1–12, 1912–1919//.   2

A Few Hens. Boston; I. S. Johnson & Co., v.1–5, 1897–1902//.   2

Florida Poultry and Dairy Journal. Zephyrhills, Fla.; Florida State Poultry Producers Assoc., 1916–1951. Began as Florida Poultry and Stockman.   2

Florida Poultry Journal. Lakeland, Fla.; v.1– 1923–. Began as Poultry in Florida.   2

Game Breeder and Sportsman. New York; v.1–52, 1912–1947//?   2

Game Fanciers' Journal. Battle Creek, Mich.; v.1–32, 1879–1910//.   1

Geflugel-Zuchter. Hamburg, Wis.; v.1–44, 1890–1935//.   2

Georgia Poultry Herald. Blakely, Ga.; Herald Pub. Co., v.1–3, 1899–1902. Continued as Southern Poultry Courier.   2

Goat World. Baldwin Park, Calif., Vincennes, Ind., etc.; v.1–32, 1916–1947//.   1

The Golden Buffs and Breeders World. New Albany, Ind.; v.1–7, 1925–1932.   2

Goodall's Farmer. Chicago; v.1–38, 1873–1910//.   1

Grit and Steel. Gaffney, S.C.; 1899–.   1

Guernsey Breeders' Journal. Peterboro, N.H.; v.1– 1910–.   1

Hampshire Advocate, Live Stock and Poultry Record. Peoria, Ill.; v.1–15, 1909–1926//.   2

Harper-Adams Utility Poultry Journal. Newport, Eng.; National Poultry Institute, v.1–34, 1915–1949//.   1

Hatchery Tribune. Mount Morris, Ill.; v.1–19, 1927–1945.   1

Hoard's Dairyman. Fort Atkinson, Wis.; v.1– 1870–.   1

Hog Breeder. Chicago; v.1–29, 1933–1954//.   1

Holstein-Friesian Register. Brattleboro, Vt.; v.1–46, 1886–1928//.   1

Holstein-Friesian World. Syracuse, N.Y., etc.; v.1– 1904–.   2

Home Farm and Fancier. Nashville, Tenn.; new series, no.1– 1895–. Also known as Home, Farm and Factory.   2

Horse Review. Chicago; v.1–83, 1889–1932//.   1

Horse World. Buffalo, N.Y.; v.1–62, 1889–1920//.   2

Horseman and Fair World. Indianapolis, Ind.; v.1– 1877–.   1

Horseman and the Spirit of the Times. Chicago; v.1–35, 1881–1915//.   2

Ice Cream Trade Journal. New York; v.1– 1905–.   2

Illustrated Poultry Record. London; v.1–10, 1908–1917//.   2

Incubator and Brooder Journal. Palestine, Ill.; E. R. Alexander, v.1– 1897–.   2

Industrious Hen. Knoxville, Tenn.; v.1–14, 1904–1918//.   2

Inland Poultry Journal. Indianapolis and Spencer, Ind.; v.1–42, 1896–1937//.   1

Intermountain Poultry Advocate. Colorado Springs; v.1– 1911–.   2

International Plymouth Rock Journal. Union City, Mich.; v.1– 1909–, v.1–5 as National Barred Rock Journal.   1

International Review of Poultry Science. Rotterdam; v.1–13, 1928–1940//.   1

Interstate Milk Producers Review. Philadelphia; v.1– 1920–.   1

Inter-State Poultryman. Tiffin, Ohio; v.1–7, 1888–1900//.   2

Jersey Bulletin. Indianapolis; v.1–72, 1883–1953//.   1

Kentucky Farmer and Breeder. Lexington, Ky.; v.1–9, 1904–1912//.   2

Ladies Poultry Journal. Moberly, Mo.; v.1–5, 1903–1908//.   1

Leghorn World. Waverly, Iowa; v.1–25, 1916–1941//.   1

Live Stock and Dairy Journal. San Francisco and Sacramento, Calif.; v.1–16, 1903–1916//.   2

Live Stock Inspector. Woodward, Okla.; W. E. Bolton, v.1–8, 1895–1903//.   2

Live Stock Journal. Buffalo and New York; v.1–7, 1870–1876//.   2

Live Stock Journal. Cleveland, Ohio; v.1– 1898–1903.   2

Live Stock Journal. Indianapolis; v.1– 1889–1910*.   2

Live Stock Journal. Morganville, Kans.; v.1–3?, 1891–1894//.   2

Live Stock Journal. St. Louis; v.1–6?, 1879–1884//.   2

Live Stock Record. Sioux City, Iowa; v.1– 1901–1910*.   2

Live Stock Review. Cincinnati, Ohio; v.1– 1875–1908//.   2

Livestock Journal. Chicago; T. Butterworth, v.1–58, 1868–1915//.   1

Live Stock Tribune. Los Angeles; v.1–14, 1895–1909//.   2

Massachusetts Poultry Society, Journal. Amherst; v.1–2, 1916–1918//.   2

Massachusetts Poultryman. Gardner, Mass.; v.1–4, 1937–1940.   2

Meat; The Idea Magazine for Meat Packers and Related Manufacturers. Chicago; v.1– 1934–.   2

Meat and Live Stock Digest. Chicago; American Meat Institute, v.1–23, 1920–1943//.   2

Michigan Farmer and Livestock Journal. Detroit, Mich.; Lawrence Pub. Co., v.1– 1843–.   1

Michigan Milk Messenger. Detroit, Mich.; v.1–32, 1919–1951.   1

Michigan Poultry Breeder. Battle Creek, Mich.; v.1–25?, 1885–1910*.   2

Mid-West Fancier. Kansas City, Mo.; v.1–4, 1902–1907//?   2

Mid-Western Poultryman. Chicago; v.1– 1936–.   2

Milk Dealer. Milwaukee, Wis.; v.1–58, 1911–1968//.   1

Milk Magazine. Waterloo, Iowa; v.1–12, 1913–1924//.   2

Milk News. Chicago; v.1–33, 1892–1927//.   1

Milk Plant Monthly. Chicago; v.1–47, 1912–1958//.   1

The Milk Producer. Chicago; v.1– 1910–1910*.   2

Milk Products Journal. Milwaukee, Wis.; v.1– 1910–.   1

Milk Reporter. Sussex, N.J.; v.1–41, 1881–1928//.   1

Milking Shorthorn Journal. Independence, Iowa; v.1– 1919–.   1

Minnesota Dairyman. Northfield, Minn.; v.1–5, 1906–1910*.   2
Missouri Stock Journal. v.1–4, 1899–1902//.   2
Modern Poultry Breeder. Battle Creek, Mich.; v.1–48, 1885–1932//.   1
Modern Poultry Keeping. London; Poultry Assoc. of Great Britain, v.1–   1
  87, 1919–1963//.
National Butter, Cheese, and Egg Association Proceedings. Davenport,   2
  Iowa; v.1–14, 1874–1887//? Title varies.
National Egg Products Association Bulletin. Chicago; 1940–1950. Contin-   2
  ued as Eggtracts.
National Fanciers' Journal. Chicago; v.1–4, 1899–1902//.   2
National Farm Poultry Journal. Minneapolis; v.1–9, 1922–1930//. Began   2
  as Northwestern Poultry Journal.
National Farmer and Stock Grower. Louisville, Ky.; Philip H. Hale, v.1–   1
  53, 1899–1926//.
National Farmer; Diversified Farming, Dairying Sugar Beet Culture. Bay   2
  City, Mich.; v.1–18, 1899–1918//.
National Live Stock Bulletin. Boston and Washington, D.C.; Frank P.   2
  Bennett & Co., v.1–13, 1896–1908//?
National Live Stock Journal. Chicago; v.1–20, 1870–1889//.   2
National Pig Breeders' Association Herd Book. London; v.1– 1885–.   1
National Poland-China Journal. Winchester and Shelbyville, Ind.; v.1–12,   1
  1916–1926//.
National Poland-China Record. Dayton, Ohio; United Brethren Pub.   2
  House, v.28–45, 1906–1923//.
National Poultry and Small Stock Journal. St. Louis, Mo.; v.1–3, 1920–   2
  1922.
National Poultry, Butter and Egg Bulletin. Chicago; v.1–16, 1916–   1
  1932//.
National Poultry Journal. Fyfield, Eng.; v.1–6, 1930–1936//.   2
National Poultry Journal. London; National Utility Poultry Society, v.1–8,   2
  1920–1927//?
National Poultry Journal. Washington, D.C.; v.1–15, 1923–1937//.   2
National Poultry Journal. Harrisonburg, Va.; v.1–3, 1909–1911//.   2
National Poultry Magazine. Syracuse and Buffalo, N.Y.; 1903–1912//.   2
National Poultry Monitor. Ashland, Ohio; v.1–8, 1880–1887//.   2
National Poultry Organization Society, Journal. London; v.1–7, 1907–   2
  1913.
National Poultryman and Fanciers' Gazette. Indianapolis; v.1–24, 1883–   2
  1909//.
National Squab Magazine. Boston; v.1–10, 1909–1918.   2
National Stockman and Farmer. Pittsburgh, Pa.; Axtell-Rush Pub. Co.,   1
  v.1–44, 1877–1921//.
National Wool Grower. Salt Lake City, etc.; National Wool Growers' As-   1
  soc., v.1– 1911–.
Naturalist and Fanciers' Review. Blencoe, Iowa, and Albion, N.Y.; v.1–   2
  1899–.
Nevada Stockgrower. Reno, Nev.; v.1–14, 1919–1933//.   2

New England Dairyman. Boston; New England Milk Producers' Assoc., v.1– 1917–.   1

New England Poultry Journal. Hartford, Conn.; v.1–9, 1902–1911//?   2

New England Poultryman and Northeastern Breeder. Boston; v.1–33, 1925–1941//.   1

Northwest Dairyman. Northfield, Minn.; Minnesota Co-operative Dairies Assoc., v.1–13, 1906–1918//.   2

Northwest Dairyman and Farmer. Seattle, Wash.; v.1–47, 1887–1932//.   1

Northwest Poultry Journal. Salem, Oreg.; v.1–43, 1895–1938//. Began as Oregon Poultry Journal.   1

Northwestern Horseman and Stockman. Lake Crystal, Mankato and Minneapolis, Minn.; v.1–17, 1890–1904//?   2

Northwestern Stockman and Farmer. Helena, Mont.; Chas. H. Reifernath and Assoc.v.1–33, 1890–1923//.   2

Nulaid News. San Francisco; Poultry Producers of Central Calif., v.1–40, 1923–1962.   1

Ohio Poland-China Record. Cincinnati, Ohio; Ohio Poland-China Record Assoc., v.1–27, 1877–1905//.   2

Ohio Swine Journal. Kinsey and Dayton, Ohio; v.1–5?, 1886–1891//.   2

OK Poultry Culture. Mounds and Tulsa, Okla.; v.1–20, 1911–1931//. Began as OK Poultry Journal.   2

Orff's Farm and Poultry Review. Saint Louis; v.1–9, 1900–1909//.   2

Orpington Poultry Journal. Scotch Plains, N.J.; v.1–7, 1902–1908//?   2

Orpingtons. Zion, Ill.; v.1– 1925–.   2

Pacific Poultrycraft. Los Angeles; No.1–337, 1895–1939//. Also known as Pacific Polycraft, and Western Poultry Journal.   1

Pacific Poultryman. Seattle, Wash.; v.1–35, 1896–1931//.   1

Pet-Stock, Pigeon and Poultry Bulletin. New York; New York State Poultry Society, v.1–23, 1869–1893//? Also known as Poultry Bulletin.   1

Pittsburg Live Stock Journal. Pittsburgh, Pa.; v.1–11, 1899–1910*.   2

Plymouth Rock Monthly. Cedar Rapids and Waverly, Iowa; v.1–43, 1888–1931; 1932–1941//, v.1–35 as Western Poultry Journal.   1

Poland China Advocate. Shelbyville, Ind.; v.1–8, 1926–1934//.   2

Poland China Journal. Kansas City, Mo.; v.1–29, 1914–1943//.   1

Poland China World. Springfield, Ill.; v.1– 1913–.   1

Poultry, A Monthly Magazine. Freeport, Ill.; v.1–9, 1904–1913//. Continued as Poultry and Suburban Farmer.   2

Poultry and Egg National Board Reporter. Chicago; v.1–14, 1940–1954.   1

Poultry and Eggs Weekly; National Weekly of the Poultry, Turkey, Egg and Butter Industries. Kansas City, Mo.; v.1– 1920–; 1920–1954 as Produce Packer. Supersedes in part New York Packer.   2

The Poultry and Farm Journal. Minneapolis; v.1–12?, 1877–1888//.   2

Poultry and Farm Journal. Pueblo, Colo.; v.1– 1897–.   2

Poultry and Farm Supply World. Chicago; v.1–38, 1924–1961//.   1

Poultry and Horse Review. Burlington, Vt.; v.1– 1892–.   2

Poultry and Stock Review. Syracuse, N.Y.; v.1–2, 1890–1891//? Began as Farm Poultry and Stock Review.   2

Poultry and Suburban Farmer. Kalamazoo, Mich.; Freeport, Ill.; v.1–12, 1904–1916//.   2

Poultry and Turkey Journal of the Western States. Denver, Colo.   2

Poultry Argus. Polo, Ill.; Miller & Clinton, v.1– 1874–.   2

Poultry Craftsman. San Jose, Calif.; v.1–52, 1885–1938//. Also known as Pacific Poultry Breeder, and Poultry Craftsman and Breeder.   1

Poultry Culture. Kansas City, Mo.; v.1–23, 1897–1920//.   2

Poultry Culture. Tulsa, Okla.; v.1–21, 1911–1932//.   2

Poultry Digest. Hanover, Pa.; v.1– 1939–.   1

Poultry Digest. New York; v.1–6, 1906–1911//.   2

Poultry Facts. Springfield, Mo.; v.1–7, 1928–1935//?   2

Poultry Fancier. Hopkinsville, Ky., and Hanover, Pa.; v.1–20, 1897–1915//.   2

Poultry Farmer and Rabbit Breeder. Indianapolis; v.1–6, 1923–1928.   2

Poultry Farmer. London; v.1–157, 1889–1968//.   1+

Poultry Garden and Fruits. Manilla, N.Y.; Blackman & Dennison, v.1– 1892–.   2

Poultry, Garden and Home. Quincy, Ill.; v.1–40, 1894–1933//. 1894–1931 as Reliable Poultry Journal.   1+

Poultry, Garden and Home Advocate. Toronto; v.1–19, 1898–1917//. Began as Poultry Advocate.   2

Poultry Gazette. Topeka, Kans.; v.1–15, 1898–1910//.   2

Poultry Guide and Friend. Hammonton, N.J., etc.; v.1– 1881–1892//.   2

Poultry Herald. St. Paul, Minn.; v.1–71, 1888–1960//.   1+

Poultry Husbandry. Waterville, N.Y.; v.1–9, 1906–1914//.   2

Poultry Index. Stoughton, Mass.; v.1–3, 1911–1914//?   2

Poultry Industry. Boston; v.1–62, 1925–1954//. Began as Northeastern Poultryman.   1

Poultry Industry. Gouverneur, N.Y.; v.1–2, 1899–1901//.   2

Poultry Item. Sellersville, Pa.; v.1–44, 1893–1941//.   1+

Poultry Keeper. Quincy, Ill.; v.1–57, 1884–1941//.   1

Poultry Life. Portland, Oreg.; Oregon Poultry Producers Assoc., v.1–15, 1911–1925//.   2

Poultry Life of American. Belton, Tex. and Indianapolis; v.1–26, 1891–1917//. Began as National Fancier.   2

Poultry Monthly. Albany, N.Y.; Ferris Pub. Co., v.1–24, 1879–1902//.   2

Poultry Nation. Elyria, Ohio; v.1–8, 1875–1882//.   2

Poultry Outlook Letter. Mt. Morris, Ill.; Watt Pub. Co., v.1– 1936–, v. 1–11 as Poultry Industry Trade News.   2

Poultry Pointers. Grand Rapids, Mich.; v.1–8, 1908–1915//.   2

Poultry Post. Goshen, Ind.; Post Pub. Co., v.1–11, 1908–1918//.   2

Poultry Press. Connersville, Ind.; v.1– 1914–.   1+

Poultry Press. York, Pa.; v.1– 1870–.   2

Poultry Quarterly. Marietta, Ga.; Georgia State Poultry Breeders' Assoc., v.1–4, 1927–1930//.   2

Poultry Raiser. Chicago; v.1–3, 1884–1887//.   2

Poultry Record. Carey, Ohio; v.1–11, 1908–1918//.   2
Poultry Record. Farmington, Ill.; v.1–12, 1873–1878//.   2
Poultry Review. Elmira, N.Y.; v.1–10, 1904–1915//?   2
Poultry Review and Stock Journal. Washington, D.C.; G. Parish, v.1–5,   2
  1881–1883.
Poultry Science Association, Journal. New Brunswick, N.J.; v.1–7, 1914–   1
  1921//.
Poultry Standard. Stamford, Conn.; Poultry Standard Co., v.1–8, 1899–   2
  1906. Began as Eastern Farmer.
Poultry Success. Springfield, Ohio, etc.; v.1–45, 1889–1934//.   1
Poultry Supply Dealer. Chicago; v.1–6, 1926–1932//.   1
Poultry Topics and Western Poultry News. Lincoln, Nebr., and Warsaw,   2
  Mo.; v.1–27, 1891–1916//.
Poultry Tribune. Mount Morris, Ill.; v.1–75, 1895–1969. In several re-   1+
  gional eds. after 1918. Continued as Egg Industry.
Poultry World. Hartford, Conn.; H. H. Stoddard, v.1–26, 1872–1896//.   1
Poultry World, consolidated with The Farm and Poultry Digest. Heron   2
  Lake, Minn., etc.; v.1– 1904–1910//.
Poultry World. London; Poultry World, Ltd., v.1– 1907–.   1
Poultry Yard. Charlotte, N.C.; v.1– 1906–1910*   2
Poultryman. Petaluma, Calif.; v.1–35, 1895–1929//?   2
Poultryman. Vineland, N.J.; v.1–39, 1931–1969//.   1
Practical Dairyman and Agriculturist. Chatham, N.Y.; v.1–7?, 1872–   2
  1898//.
Practical Poultryman and Poultry Star. Whitney's Point and Fayetteville,   2
  N.Y.; v.1–19, 1887–1905//.
Profitable Poultry and Horticulture. Boston; v.1–5, 1910–1915//.   2
Progressive Poultry Journal and American Poultryman. Mitchell, S.Dak.;   2
  v.1–25, 1903–1920//.
Pure Milk News. Chicago; Pure Milk Assoc., v.1– 1926–. 1926–1954 as   2
  Pure Milk; News of Chicagoland Dairy Farmers.
Quality Milk Producer. Moline, Ill.; Quality Milk Assoc., v.1– 1950;   2
  nsv1–8, 1952–1959//. Superseded by Mississippi Valley Dairyman.
Record of Improved Essex Swine. New Augusta, Ind., etc.; American Es-   2
  sex Assoc., v.1–3, 1890–1896//.
Reliable Poultry Journal. Quincy, Ill.; v.1–38, 1894–1931//. Also known   1+
  as New Reliable Poultry Journal.
Rhode Island Red Journal. Waverly, Iowa; v.1–30, 1912–1941//.   1
Rider and Driver. New York; v.1– 1890–.   1
San Diego Poultry Journal. San Diego, Calif.; no.1– 1924–.   2
Shepherd's Criterion. Chicago; v.1–19, 1891–1909//.   2
Shorthorn World and Farm Magazine. Aurora, Ill.; v.1– 1915–.   1
Small-Yorkshire Swine Register. New York; American Small-Yorkshire   2
  Club, v.1–2, 1885–1890//.
South-Western Poland China Record. Gadsden, Tenn.; Southwestern Po-   2
  land-China Record Assoc., v.1–2, 1901–1905//.

Southern Dairy Products Journal. Atlanta, Ga.; v.1– 1927–.   1
Southern Poultry Journal. Dallas, Tex.; v.1–20, 1894–1914//.   2
Southern Poultry Journal. Pleasant Hill, Mo.; v.1–7, 1925–1931//.   2
Southern Poultryman. Dallas, Tex.; v.1–18, 1899–1906//?   2
Southwestern Stockman Farmer. Los Angeles; Frank H. Owen, v.1–49,   1
    1884–1932//.
Spotted Poland China Digest. Kansas City, Mo.; v.1–9, 1924–1933//.   2
Spotted Poland China Journal. Indianapolis, Ind.; v.1–10, 1915–1924//.   1
Standard and Poultry World. Quincy, Ill.; v.1–7, 1908–1913//.   2
Standard Chester White Record. Indianapolis, Ind.; Standard Chester   1
    White Record Assoc., v.1–16, 1890–1912//.
Standard Poultry Journal. Pleasant Hill, Mo.; v.1–7, 1925–1931//.   2
Stock Farm. Lexington, Ky.; National Trotting Horse Journal, v.1–58,   2
    1883–1912//.
Swine Grower. Geneva, Ill.; Official Journal of the O. I. C. and Chester   2
    White Record Assoc., v.1–9, 1917–1926//.
Swine Record. Peoria, Ill.; American Hampshire Swine Record Assoc.,   1
    v.1–16, 1906–1920//.
Texas Stock and Farm. Fort Worth, Texas; A. W. Grant, v.1–30, 1880–   2
    1911//.
Texas Stockman and Farmer. San Antonio, Texas; Vories P. Brown, v.1–   1
    34, 1881–1916//.
Thoroughbred Record. Lexington, Ky.; v.1– 1875–.   1
Trotter and Pacer. New York; v.1–84, 1894–1926//?   2
Turkey World. Chicago, Ill.; v.1– 1926–.   1+
U.S. Egg and Poultry Magazine. Chicago; 1926–1932, 1933–1952.   1
Wallace's Monthly. N.Y.; v.1–19, 1875–1894//.   2
Washcoegg. Seattle; Washington Co-operative Egg & Poultry Assoc.,   2
    v.1–37, 1923–1960//.
Western Breeders' Journal. Portland, Oreg.; v.1–66, 1879–1934//?   1
Western Breeders' Journal. Clay Center, Kans.; v.1–10, 1898–1908//.   2
Western Farm Life. Denver, Colo.; v.1– 1899–.   1
Western Garden and Poultry Journal. Des Moines, Iowa; v.1–10, 1890–   2
    1899//?
Western Milk Dealer and Dairy Counselor. Seattle, Wash.; v.1–15, 1918–   2
    1933//.
Western Poultry Journal. Los Angeles; v.1–13, 1915–1926//.   1
Western Poultry World. Denver, Colo.; v.1–12, 1902–1914//?   2
Western Poultryman. Salt Lake City, Utah; v.1–7, 1914–1920//?   2
Western Swine Breeder. Lincoln, Nebr.; v.1–15, 1894–1907//.   2
Western Swineherd. Geneseo, Ill.; v.1–7, 1884–1894//.   2
Wool Grower and Stock Register. Buffalo and Rochester, N.Y.; v.1–10,   2
    1849–1856//.
Wyandotte Herald. Waverly, Iowa; v.1–12, 1919–1931//. Merged into   1
    Poultry Culture.

These periodicals were chiefly published in the Northeast of the United States until about 1880, when primary publishing in this field shifted to the Midwest. Many of the periodicals in this list had an influence far beyond their place of publication. Some for strictly local or within-state use are not included in this compilation, nor are those of very short duration.

The second list, the list of beekeeping periodicals published prior to 1950, was derived from the citation and review process. Again we are indebted to Roger A. Morse, Professor of Apiculture, Cornell University, for his valuable advice in evaluating these titles.

The scale provided in the right-hand column indicates ranking as follows:
1 = Top-ranked periodicals with primary preservation priority.
2 = Periodicals of lesser importance, but worthy of preservation.

Historically Important Beekeeping Periodicals, 1850–1950

American Apiculturist. Wenham, Mass.; S. M. Locke & Co., v.1–13,   1
1883–1895//.

American Bee Gazette. New York; v.1, nos.1–3, 1866//?   2

American Bee Journal. Philadelphia; Dadant & Sons, v.1– 1861–.   1+

American Beekeeper. Falconer, N.Y.; W. T. Falconer Manfg. Co., v.1–   1
18, 1891–1908//.

American Beekeeper. Lebanon, Mo.; v.1–5, 1879–1883//.   2

American Honey Producer. Laramie, Wy.; American Honey Producers'   2
League, v.1–5, 1927–1931//.

American Honey Producers' League, League Bulletin. Ft. Collins, Colo.;   2
v.1–7, 1920–1927//.

Annals of Bee Culture. Louisville, Ky.; J. Morton & Co., 1869–1872//.   2

Australasian Bee Journal. Auckland, N.Z.; v.1–3, 1887–1889//?   2

Australasian Beekeeper. West Maitland, N.S.W.; Pender Bros., v.1–   1
1899–.

Australian Bee Bulletin. West Maitland, N.S.W.; E. Tipper, v.1–20,   2
1892–1911//.

Australian Bee Journal. Melbourne; Victorian Apiarists' Assoc., v.1–   1
1918–.

Bee Bulletin. Anderson, S.C.; Anderson County Beekeepers' Assoc., v.1,   2
nos.1–9, 1925//.

Bee Craft. Welwyn, Rochester, Eng.; British Beekeepers' Assoc., v.1–   1
1919–.

The Bee Hive. Andover, Conn.; v.1–5, 1886–1890//.   2

Bee Hive. Medina, Ohio; v.1–17, 1921–1940//.   1

Bee World. Gerrards Cross, Bucks, Eng.; International Bee Research As-   1+
soc., v.1– 1919–.

Bee-Keeper's Exchange. Canajoharie, N.Y.; Houck & Peet, v.1–5, 1879–   2
    1883//.
Bee-Keeper's Magazine. New York; H. A. King & Co., v.1–17, 1872–   2
    1889//.
Bee-Keepers' Review. Lansing, Mich.; National Beekeepers' Assoc., v.1–   1
    46, 1888–1933//.
Beecause. Watertown, Wis.; G. B. Lewis Co., v.1–21, 1922–1945//?   1
Beekeepers' Advance and Poultrymens' Journal. Mechanic Falls, Me.;   2
    v.1–18, 1887–1890//?
Beekeepers' Guide. Kendallville, Ind.; v.1–17, 1877–1893//.   1
Beekeepers' Instructor. Adelphi, Ohio; v.1–4, 1879–1882//.   2
Beekeepers' Journal and Agricultural Repository. Nevada, Ohio; v.1,   2
    nos.1–8, 1869.
Beekeepers' Journal and National Agriculturist, for the Apiary, Farm and   2
    Fireside. New York; v.1–17, 1872–1889//.
Beekeepers' Magazine. Barrytown, N.Y.; King & Aspinwall, v.1–17,   2
    1872–1889//.
Beekeepers' Magazine. Lansing, Mich.; Michigan Beekeepers' Assoc.,   1+
    v.1– 1938–.
Beekeepers' Record. London; v.1–72, 1882–1952.   1
Beekeepers' Review. Flint, Mich.; National Beekeepers Assoc., v.1–46,   1
    1888–1933//.
Beekeeping. Exeter, Eng.; Devon Beekeepers' Assoc., v.1– 1935–.   1
Bees. Hapeville, Ga.; American Bee Breeders Assoc., v.1–6, 1947–   2
    1953//.
British Bee Journal & Bee-Keepers Adviser. London; v.1– 1873–.   1+
California Apiculturist. Oakland and Los Angeles; v.1, nos.1–12, 1882//.   2
Canadian Bee Journal. Peterborough, Ont.; v.1–85, 1885–1974//.   1
Connecticut Honey Bee. Norwich, Conn.; Connecticut Beekeepers' As-   2
    soc., v.1– 1929–.
Dixie Beekeeper. Waycross, Ga.; v.1–11, 1919–1930//.   2
Frontier Bees and Honey. Spokane, Wash.; v.1–22, 1920–1941//.   2
Gleanings in Bee Culture. Medina, Ohio; A. I. Root Co., v.1– 1873–.   1+
Honey Producers' Cooperator. Los Angeles; California Honey Producers'   2
    Cooperative League, v.1–2, 1919–1921//.
Illinois State Beekeepers' Association Bulletin. Hamilton, Ill.; v.1– 1913–.   2
Irish Bee Journal. Lough Rynn; v.1–33, 1901–1933//.   2
Juvenile Gleanings. Medina, Ohio; A. I. Root, v.1–2, 1882–1883//.   2
Kansas Beekeeper. Columbus, Kans.; v.1–5, 1881–1885//   2
Modern Beekeeping. Clarkson, Ky.; v.1–40, 1916–1956//.   1
Modern Farmer and Busy Bee. St. Joseph, Mo.; v.1–21, 1890–1910//.   2
Moon's Bee World. Rome, Ga.; v.1–4, 1873–1877//.   2
National Bee Gazette. St. Louis, Mo.; v.1 nos. 1–3, 1892//.   2
National Bee Journal. Indianapolis, Ind.; Homestead and Western Farm   2
    Journal Print, v.1–6, 1870–1874//.
National Beekeeper. Dinero, Tex.; v.1, 1902//?   2

Nebraska Bee Tidings. Minden, Nebr.; v.1, nos.1–6, 1927//.   2
New England Apiarium. Mechanic Falls, Me.; v.1, nos.1–7, 1883//.   2
New Jersey Bee Culture. Pennington, N.J.; v.1–12, 1922–1933//.   2
New Zealand Beekeeper. Pungareu, Taranaki; National Beekeepers' As-   1
soc. of New Zealand, v.1– 1939–.
New Zealand Beekeepers' Journal. Dunedin; National Beekeepers Assoc.   2
of New Zealand, v.1–6, 1916–1922//.
New Zealand Honey Producer. Christchurch; v.1–2, 1929–1930//?   2
New Zealand Honeybee. Auckland; v.1–2, 1937–1939.   2
North American Bee Journal. Indianapolis, Ind.; v.1, nos.1–10, 1872–   2
1873//?
Pacific Bee Journal. Los Angeles; v.1–5, 1896–1902//.   2
Pacific States Bee Journal. Tulare, Calif.; v.1, nos.1–8, 1903–1904//.   2
Pennsylvania Beekeeper. State College, Pa.; v.4–36, 1929–1961.   2
Practical Beekeeper. Tillbury Center, Ont., Canada; v.1–2, 1893–1895//?   2
Progressive Bee-Keeper. Higginsville, Mo.; v.1–16, 1891–1906//.   2
Queen Breeders' Journal. Marlboro, Mass.; v.1, nos.1–6, 1889//.   2
Rocky Mountain Bee Journal. Boulder, Colo.; v.1–4, 1901–1904//.   2
Rural Beekeeper. River Falls, Wis.; v.1–3, 1904–1906//.   2
Scottish Beekeeper. Glasgow; Scottish Beekeepers' Assoc., v.1– 1924–.   1
South African Bee Journal. Johannesburg; South African Assoc. of Bee-   1
keepers, v.1– 1921–.
Southland Queen. Beeville, Tex.; v.1–9, 1895–1904//.   2
Success in Bee Culture. Highwood, Conn.; v.1, nos.1–8, 1893–1894//?   2
Thebesto Bee. Denver, Colo.; Colorado Honey Producers' Assoc., v.1–3,   2
1922–1925//.
Western Bee Journal. Hanford and Kingsbury, Calif.; v.1–2, 1904–   2
1905//.
Western Beekeeper. Denver and Boulder, Colo.; v.1–2, 1898–1900//?   2
Western Beekeeper. Des Moines, Iowa; v.1–6, 1889–1893//?   2
Western Honey Bee. Los Angeles; California State Beekeepers' Assoc.,   2
v.1–18, 1913–1930//.
White Mountain Apiarist. Berlin Falls, N.H.; v.1–2, 1891–1892//?   2
Wisconsin Beekeeping. Madison; Wisconsin State Beekeepers' Assoc.,   2
v.1–13, 1927–1937//.
Wyoming Bee Line. Cheyenne; Wyoming State Beekeepers' Assoc., v.1–   2
5, 1925–1929//.

C. Scholarly Journals

Using the citation analysis method previously described in this volume, we have generated the following list of journals with the titles arranged by frequency of citation, i.e., *Poultry Science* was most frequently cited in the references in the thirty-eight source publications, and the *Journal of Hered-*

ity ranked second, *Journal of Dairy Science* third, etc. In future studies of the historic agricultural scholarly publications, it would be advisable to extend the citation analysis to incorporate more journal articles as source documents in order to obtain more detailed information on important but less frequently cited journals.

In reviewing this list of the seventy-two most frequently cited titles in the particular group of source documents used for analysis, we find a strong correlation between those titles most frequently cited and their availability on microfilm. All of the twelve most frequently cited journals are available on microfilm. Microfilm copies of 87.5% of the top third of the titles on the list are available, 75% of the middle third, and 58% of the bottom third. For the complete list of seventy-two titles, fifty-three (or 73.6%) are available in some measure on film. It appears that a substantial portion of the scholarly literature used by animal scientists has already been preserved on microfilm.

A number of those titles not already available on film are journals related to specific breeds such as the *Jersey Bulletin*, the *Ayrshire Digest*, and the *Milking Shorthorn Journal*. Another group not already filmed are those which were not published on a fixed, periodic schedule such as the *Publications of the Carnegie Institution of Washington*, the *Proceedings of the World's Poultry Congress*, and the *Proceedings of the International Congress of Genetics*. In addition a number of foreign language journals, such as *Archiv für Geflügelkunde* and *Zeitschrift für Tierzüchtung und Züchtungbiologie,* are not currently available on film. These probably should be the preservation responsibility of the issuing country.

Thus it is evident that a substantial start has been made in ensuring that the scholarly journals related to this subject field will be accessible to future researchers.

Table 8.1 lists the most frequently cited journals derived from citation analysis arranged in order of number of times cited in the source documents. These titles represent those on which statistically valid data were accrued among the 600 titles cited. The availability on microfilm from one of three sources is indicated.

With the role of both agricultural books and periodicals in the development of successful farming in the United States from the mid-1800s to the mid-1900s being clearly evident, the need to preserve the most important of these publications for a complete understanding of the lives and times of our agricultural predecessors becomes significant. The identification of these publications has been one of the major objectives of the Core Agricultural Literature Project. Through the use of citation analysis and in-depth review by scholarly experts in the various fields related to animal science

Table 8.1. Most frequently cited scholarly journals

Journal	Microfilmed
Poultry Science	UMI
Journal of Heredity	UMI
Journal of Dairy Science	UMI
American Naturalist	UMI
Journal of Animal Science	UMI
Journal of Agricultural Science	UMI
Journal of Experimental Zoology	MI
Science	UMI
Journal of Agricultural Research	UMI
Genetics	UMI
Journal of Genetics	MI
Anatomical Record	UMI
U.S. Egg and Poultry Magazine	—
Scientific Agriculture	UMI
Biological Bulletin	UMI
American Society of Animal Production, Record of Proceedings	—
Society for Experimental Biology and Medicine, Proceedings	MI
Journal of Biological Chemistry	UMI
Journal of Nutrition	UMI
Zeitschrift für Induktive Abstammungs und Vererbungslehre	UMI
Endocrinology	UMI
Royal Society of London, Proceedings	UMI
Royal Agricultural Society of England, Journal	MI
World's Poultry Congress, Proceedings	—
Societé de Biologie, Paris; Comptes-Rendus	MI
American Journal of Anatomy	MI
Agriculture; Journal of the Ministry of Agriculture; London	UMI
Journal of Morphology	MI
Jersey Bulletin	—
Royal Society of London, Evolution Committee, Report	—
Archiv für Geflügelkunde	—
American Journal of Physiology	UMI
American Veterinary Medical Association, Journal	UMI
Biometrika	UMI
Nature	UMI
Académie des Sciences, Paris; Comptes-Rendus	PR
Carnegie Institution of Washington, Publications	—
Wilhelm Roux' Archiv für Entwicklungsmechanik der Organismen	UMI
Ayrshire Digest	—
U.S. Dept. of Agriculture, Yearbook	PR
Guernsey Breeders Journal	UMI
Holstein-Friesian World	UMI, 1980+ only
Hoard's Dairyman	UMI, 1950+ only
National Academy of Sciences, Proceedings	UMI
Royal Society of Edinburgh, Proceedings	PR
Biochemical Journal	UMI
Food Research	UMI

Journal	Microfilmed
Physiological Zoology	UMI
American Journal of Veterinary Research	UMI
Cornell Veterinarian	—
Empire Journal of Experimental Agriculture	UMI
International Congress of Genetics, Proceedings	—
Quarterly Review of Biology	UMI
Zeitschrift für Tierzüchtung und Züchtungsbiologie	—
Milking Shorthorn Journal	—
Breeders Gazette	UMI, 1949–1964
Archives of Biochemistry	—
Quarterly Journal of Experimental Physiology	UMI
Royal Society of Edinburgh, Transactions	PR
Royal Society of London, Philosophical Transactions	PR
Biologisches Zentralblatt	UMI
Scottish Journal of Agriculture	—
Zoologischer Jahresbericht	—
Heriditas	UMI
Deutsche Landwirtschaftliche Tierzucht	—
Bibliographia Genetica	—
Genetica	UMI
Cambridge Philosophical Society, Biological Reviews	UMI
Farmer and Stockbreeder	—
Veterinary Journal	PR, 1956+
Zoologischer Anzeiger	MI
Zoological Society of London, Proceedings	UMI

UMI = University Microfilms, Inc.; MI = Microforms International; PR = Princeton Microfilm.

and beekeeping, lists of books and journals have been produced that are authoritative, but also of manageable length. While not all reviewers have agreed on the value of all titles, a meaningful consensus has been produced which will enable the conservators assigned the responsibility of preserving these publications to establish priorities as they proceed with their important work of ensuring that the writings of past generations are available for those who come later.

D. Holdings at Kansas State University

The monographs and popular periodicals in this chapter were examined at the Farrell Library, Kansas State University, which has a substantial historical animal science literature collection. The staff at the Farrell Library carefully checked each item in the lists to ascertain which they owned. The resulting data should be helpful in cooperative planning for the systematic preservation of this literature on a national or regional basis.

Of the 612 titles in the animal science monograph list, the Farrell Library had 80% in one edition or another, but only 62% of the earliest editions. Of the 122 items it did not own, ninety-one were from commercial publishers, fifteen from associations or independent organizations, and the remainder from university, government and private printings. Of these 122 items, seventy were published in the United States and forty-four in the United Kingdom.

The Farrell Library staff also checked the beekeeping monograph core list of ninety-seven titles, of which it owned 45% in one edition or another. Of the forty-five titles not at Kansas State, twenty-three were published in the United States and twenty elsewhere.

Of the core popular periodicals in animal science, the Farrell Library had only forty-six of the 307 titles and most of these were broken sets.

EDITOR'S NOTE: The Mann Library, Cornell University checked its holdings for two of the historical lists. Of the Popular and Trade Journals (p. 372), 51.3% of the 341 titles were held in fairly complete sets. The Beekeeping periodicls (p. 387) were 79.5% complete at Mann or other libraries at Cornell.

Bibliography

Agricultural and Horticultural Periodicals, U.S. Dept. of Agriculture Report, 1867, pp. 404–409; 1868, pp. 608–611; 1870, pp. 544–548. Washington, D.C.; U.S. Dept. of Agriculture, 1868–1871.

Bailey, Liberty H. *Cyclopedia of American Agriculture*. 4th ed. New York; Macmillan, 1912. Vol. 4, "Current Agricultural Journals," pp. 78–87.

Barnett, Claribel R. "The Agricultural Museum: An Early American Agricultural Periodical," *Agricultural History* 2 (1928): 99–102.

Batten's Agricultural Directory. New York; George Batten Co., 1908. 271p.

Bee Research Association. "World List of Beekeeping Journals and Other Serial Publications Received by the Library," *Bee World* 49 (1968): 121–140.

Beekeeping in the United States. Rev. ed. Washington, D.C.; U.S. Dept. of Agriculture, 1980. 193p. (*USDA Agriculture Handbook* no. 335)

Bidwell, Percy W., and John I. Falconer. *History of Agriculture in the Northern United States, 1620–1860*. Washington, D.C.; Carnegie Institution of Washington, 1925. 512p.

Books for Bee-Keepers, Farmers, Market-Gardeners, Florists, etc. 5th ed. Medina, Ohio; A. I. Root Co., 1905. 21p.

Cobb, C. A. "The Contribution of the Press to Agriculture," pp. 24–30 in: *Silver Anniversary Cooperative Demonstration Work, 1903–1928; Proceedings of the Anniversary Meeting, Houston, Tex., Feb. 1929*. College Station, Tex.; Extension Service Agricultural and Mechanical College, 1929. 164p.

Crane, Eva, ed. *World List of Current Beekeeping Journals*. London; Bee Research Association, 1955. 12p.

Danhof, Clarence H. *Change in Agriculture: The Northern United States, 1820–1870*. Cambridge, Mass.; Harvard University Press, 1969. 322p.

Demaree, Albert L. "Agricultural Periodicals," pp. 393–398 in: *The American Agricultural Press, 1819–1860*. New York; Columbia University Press, 1941. 430p.

Dictionary Catalog of the National Agricultural Library 1862–1965. New York; Rowman & Littlefield, 1967. Under heading, "Agriculture. Periodicals," pp. 4–100 in vol. 3.

Edwards, Everett E. *A Bibliography of the History of Agriculture in the United States*. Washington, D.C.; U.S. Dept. of Agriculture, 1930. 307p. (*USDA Misc. Publication* no. 84)

Evans, James F., and Rodolfo N. Salcedo. *Communications in Agriculture: The American Farm Press*. Ames; Iowa State University Press, 1974. 264p.

Fusonie, Alan M., compiler. *Heritage of American Agriculture: A Bibliography of Pre-1860 Imprints*. Beltsville, Md.; U.S. Dept. of Agriculture, National Agricultural Library, 1975. Periodicals, pp. 58–71. (*Library List* no. 98)

Fusonie, Alan M., and Donna Jean Mason Fusonie. "Heritage of Apicultural Literature. A Bibliography of Pre- 1870 Monographic Imprints," *Associates NAL Today* 1 (1976): 26–48.

Goldberg, David H., and Stanislaw J. Kosecki, compilers. *World List of Poultry Serials*. Beltsville, Md.; U.S. Dept. of Agriculture, National Agricultural Library, 1989. 182p.

Great Britain. Ministry of Agriculture, Fisheries and Food. *Animal Health: A Centenary, 1865–1965*. London; H.M.S.O., 1965. 396p.

Hanke, Oscar A. *A History of American Poultry Journalism, 1870–1926*. B.S. Thesis, University of Wisconsin, 1926. 99p.

Hanke, Oscar A., et al. *American Poultry History, 1823–1973*. Madison, Wis.; American Poultry Historical Society, 1974. 775p.

Jeffers, Fred H. *A Selection of Old Poultry Books, English and Amerian with a Chronology of Significant Dates in Poultry History*. Windsor, N.Y.; Windsor Standard, 1954. 26p.

Johansson, T. S. K., and M. P. Johansson. *Apicultural Literature Published in Canada and the United States*. Bayside, N.Y.; The author, 1972. 103p.

Leavitt, Charles T. "Attempts to Improve Cattle Breeds in the United States, 1790–1860," *Agricultural History* 7 (1933): 51–67.

List of Agricultural Journals; U.S. Patent Office Report, 1845. Washington, D.C.; 1846. p. 1165.

List of Periodicals Currently Received in the Library of the U.S. Department of Agriculture. Washington, D.C.; U.S. Dept. of Agriculture, 1909. 72p. (*USDA Library Bulletin* no. 75)

Marquis, J. Clyde. "Social Significance of the Agricultural Press," *Annals of the American Academy of Political and Social Science* 40 (1912): 158–162.

Marti, Donald B. *To Improve the Soil and the Mind. Agricultural Societies, Journals, and Schools in the Northeastern States, 1791–1865*. Ann Arbor, Mich.; University Microfilms International, 1979. 309p.

McMunn, Earl W. "Great Men and Enduring Farm Magazines: A Commentary," pp. 193–211 in: *Agricultural Literature: Proud Heritage—Future Promise, A Bicentennial Symposium, September 24–26, 1975* . . . edited by Alan Fusonie and Leila Moran. Washington, D.C.; Associates of the National Agricultural Library, 1977.

Milum, V. G. *Information on Beekeeping Journals*. Urbana; University of Illinois, 1954. 12p.

Mott, Frank L. *A History of American Magazines, 1885–1905*. Cambridge, Mass.; Belnap Press, 1957. Chapter 19, "Agriculture, Horticulture, Livestock," pp. 336–345.

Pellett, Frank C. *History of American Beekeeping*. Ames, Iowa; Collegiate Press, 1938. 213p.

Periodicals and Society Publications Currently Received by the Department Library. Washington, D.C.; U.S. Dept. of Agriculture, 1894. 8 p. (*USDA Library Bulletin* no. 2)

Pickens, William. *A List of References for the History of Apiculture and Sericulture in America*. Davis, Calif.; Agricultural History Center, University of California, 1975. 18p.

Plumb, Charles S. *A Partial Index to Animal Husbandry Literature*. Columbus, Ohio; The author, 1911. 94p.

Punnett, R. C. *Notes on Old Poultry Books with a Bibliography up to 1880 by E. Comyns Lewer and R. C. Punnett*. London; The Feathered World, 1930. 40p.

Sanford, Albert H. *The Story of Agriculture in the United States*. Boston; D. C. Heath & Co., 1916. 394p.

Schlebecker, John T., and Andrew W. Hopkins. *A History of Dairy Journalism in the United States 1810–1950*. Madison; University of Wisconsin Press, 1957. 423p.

Stuntz, Stephen C., compiler. *List of the Agricultural Periodicals of the United States and Canada Published During the Century July 1810 to July 1910*. Washington, D.C.; U.S. Dept. of Agriculture, 1941. 190p. (*Misc. Publication* no. 398)

True, Alfred C. *A History of Agricultural Education in the United States 1785–1925*. Washington, D.C.; U.S. Dept. of Agriculture, 1929. 436p. (*Misc. Publication* no. 36)

Tucker, Gilbert M. *American Agricultural Periodicals: An Historical Sketch*. Albany, N.Y.; Privately printed, 1909. 9 leaves.

U.S. Dept. of Agriculture. *Index to Literature Relating to Animal Industry in the Publications of the Department of Agriculture, 1837 to 1898 . . .* by George Fayette Thompson. Washington, D.C.; U.S. Govt. Print. Off., 1900. 676p. (*USDA Bulletin* no. 5)

Wilson, Allen D. *Agricultural Periodicals in the United States*. M.A. Thesis, Library Science, University of Illinois, 1930. 76p.

Wiser, Vivian, Larry Mark, and H. Graham Purchase, eds. *100 Years of Animal Health, 1884–1984 . . .* Donald V. Robertson, technical editor. Beltsville, Md.; Associates of the National Agricultural Library, Inc., 1986. 230p. *Journal of the NAL Associates* 11 (1/4) (Jan.–Dec. 1986).

Wright, Muriel F. *Periodicals Related to Dairying Received in the U.S. Department of Agriculture*. Washington, D.C.; U.S. Dept. of Agriculture, 1926. 22p. (*USDA, Bureau of Agricultural Economics, Agricultural Economics Bibliography* no. 16)

Index

Authors and titles in the core list of monographs (pp. 86–185), the core list of journals (pp. 202–206), and the historically significant monographs (pp. 321–341) are *not* included in this index.

Library of Congress Cataloging-in-Publication Data

The Literature of animal science and health / edited by Wallace C. Olsen.
     p.   cm. — (The Literature of the agricultural sciences)
    Includes bibliographical references and index.
    ISBN 0-8014-2886-6
    1. Animal culture literature. 2. Veterinary literature. I. Olsen, Wallace C. II. Series.
SF22.5.L58 1993
636—dc20   93-7801